PHARMAPHOBIA

PHARMAPHOBIA

*How the Conflict of Interest Myth
Undermines American Medical
Innovation*

Thomas P. Stossel

ROWMAN & LITTLEFIELD
Lanham • Boulder • New York • London

Published by Rowman & Littlefield
A wholly owned subsidiary of The Rowman & Littlefield Publishing Group, Inc.
4501 Forbes Boulevard, Suite 200, Lanham, Maryland 20706
www.rowman.com

Unit A, Whitacre Mews, 26-34 Stannary Street, London SE11 4AB

British Library Cataloguing in Publication Information Available

Library of Congress Cataloging-in-Publication Data

Stossel, Thomas P., author.
Pharmaphobia : how the conflict of interest myth undermines American medical innovation / Thomas P. Stossel.
p. ; cm.
Includes bibliographical references and index.
ISBN 978-1-4422-4462-7 (cloth : alk. paper)—ISBN 978-1-4422-4463-4 (electronic)
I. Title.
[DNLM: 1. Delivery of Health Care--United States. 2. Inventions—United States. 3. Conflict of Interest—United States. 4. Consumer Product Safety—United States. 5. Health Care Costs—United States. 6. Marketing of Health Services—United States. W 84 AA1]
RA418.3.U6
362.10973—dc23
2014042834

∞™ The paper used in this publication meets the minimum requirements of American National Standard for Information Sciences Permanence of Paper for Printed Library Materials, ANSI/NISO Z39.48-1992.

Printed in the United States of America

There are, again, two methods of removing the causes of faction: the one, by destroying the liberty, which is essential to its existence; the other, by giving to every citizen the same opinions, the same passions, and the same interests. It could never be more truly said than of the first remedy that it is worse than the disease. Liberty is to faction what air is to fire, an aliment without which it instantly expires. But it could not be a less folly to abolish liberty, which is essential to political life, because it nourishes faction than it would be to wish the annihilation of air, which is essential to animal life, because it imparts to a fire its destructive agency.

—James Madison, *Federalist Papers*, Number 10, 1787

Thus the rule of law could clearly not be preserved in a democracy that undertook to decide every conflict of interests not according to rules previously laid down but "on its merits."

—Friedrich A. Hayek, *The Road to Serfdom*, 1944

Conflict is the essential core of a free and open society. If one were to project the democratic way of life in the form of a musical score, its major theme would be the harmony of dissonance.

—Saul Alinsky, *Rules for Radicals*, 1972

CONTENTS

IV: THE DAMAGE THEY DO, AND HOW TO STOP IT

ACKNOWLEDGMENTS

Many individuals have provided me with information, insights, and valuable criticisms. I also tried as much as possible to obtain fact and interpretation checking concerning the many diverse incidents and problems covered in the book from people who had direct involvement with them or who have specific expertise. Those contributing include, in no particular order, the following people:

Tom Sullivan, President, Rockpointe Company; Paul Rubin, PhD, Dobbs Professor of Economics, Emory University; George Chressanthis, MBA, PhD, Professor of Health Care Management, Temple University; Michael S. Brown, MD, University of Texas Southwestern; Michael Weber, MD, SUNY Downstate Medical Center; Joseph DiMasi, PhD, and Joshua Cohen, PhD, Tufts Center for the Study of Drug Development; Fred Southwick, MD, University of Florida; Brigham and Women's Hospital colleagues—Christopher Bono, MD; Barry Brenner, MD; Frank Bunn, MD; Julie Glowacki, PhD; Robert Handin, MD; David Mount, MD; Marc Pfeffer, MD; Paul Ridker, MD; and Michael Weinblatt, MD—David Steensma, Dana Farber Cancer Center; Raphael Dolin, MD, and Ananth Karumanchi, MD, Beth Israel Deaconess Hospital, Boston; Andrew Nierenberg, MD, Massachusetts General Hospital; Barbara Alving, MD, Director Emerita, National Center for Research Resources; Roque El-Hayek, Esq, MD, JD, Wolf Greenfield Company; Stephen M. Stahl, MD, University of California, San Diego; Tom Brownlie, Alliance Development Manager for U.S. Public Affairs and Policy, Pfizer, Inc; Glenn Treisman, MD, and Roger Blumenthal, MD, Johns Hopkins Medical

School; Daniel Sulmasy, MD, University of Chicago; Paul Offit, MD, Childrens Hospital of the University of Pennsylvania; Kevin Bozic, MD, MBA, University of California, San Francisco; Benny Dahl, MD, PhD, University of Copenhagen; Brian Caplan, PhD, George Mason University; Zachary Bloomgarten, MD, Mount Sinai Medical School; Patty Eisenaur, EVC Group, San Francisco; Brian Druker, MD, Director, Knight Cancer Center, Oregon Health and Science University; Will Hiatt, MD, University of Colorado Medical Center; Matthew Movsesian, MD, University of Utah Medical Center; Harry Sweeney, Director Emeritus, South Penn Square Associates; Rafael Fonseca, MD, Chief of Medicine, Mayo Clinic; Larry Hirsch, MD, Vice President for Diabetes Care, Becton Dickinson Corporation; George Lundberg, MD, The Cancer Collaborative; Professor Alan Silman, Medical Director, Arthritis UK; Peter Pitts, Center for Medicine in the Public Interest; Tom Huddle, MD, PhD, University of Alabama Medical Center; David Shaywitz, Chief Medical Officer, DNAexus and co-author with me of articles in The Wall Street Journal and other venues; George Rainbolt, PhD, Georgia State University; Martha Liggett, Esq, Executive Director, American Society of Hematology; Sally Satel, MD, and the late John Calfee, PhD, The American Enterprise Institute; Stephen Cull, PhD, Roche Products Ltd.; John Kamp, Esq, National Association of Medical Educators; and Gerald Williams, MD, Jefferson Medical College.

In addition to those mentioned above, I am especially grateful to the following individuals who contributed with detailed editing: the late Bill Glazer, MD; Lance Stell, PhD, Thatcher Professor of Philosophy Emeritus, Davidson College, and Ethics Director, Carolinas Medical Center; Bruce Gingles, Vice President, Cook Medical Company; and Herb Schaffner of Schaffner Media Productions, who served extraordinarily as editor and agent. I have liberally incorporated many cogent insights and trenchant comments these individuals provided.

Thanks to financial support since 2011 from the Searle Freedom Trust, I was able to take advantage of the talents an able research assistant, David Barton who made major editing contributions, including assiduous fact checking and bibliography management. My brother-in-law Patrick Maguire gave me permission to tell his story and helped me get it straight. My daughter Sage, a published author, conveyed candid criticisms—although not as candid as my brother John of Fox Business Television ("Holy shit, nobody talks like you write!"). Despite frequent admonitions for "Let's have a conflict-of-interest-free zone today, Hon," my wife, Kerry Maguire, DDS, MSPH, who epitomizes how private industry and public health can seamlessly work together, has been a constant inspiration and constructive critic.

INTRODUCTION

Why I Wrote This Book

Then too, if a man gives the best possible advice but is under the slightest suspicion of being influenced by his own private profit, we are so embittered by the idea (a wholly unproved one) of this profit of his, that we do not allow the state to receive the certain benefit of his good advice. So a state of affairs has been reached where a good proposal honestly put forward is just as suspect as something thoroughly bad.

—Thucydides, *History of the Peloponnesian War*

I am what is called a physician-researcher. I have been affiliated with Harvard Medical School for nearly 50 years. When I graduated from Harvard Med in 1967, young physicians were strongly encouraged to participate in medical research, and following two years of internal medicine residency, I obtained research training at the National Institutes of Health (NIH) campus in Bethesda, Maryland. I then returned to Boston's Harvard-affiliated Children's Hospital for further clinical experience in hematology. I joined the Harvard faculty in 1972 and have worked at its affiliate teaching hospitals ever since.

The length of my career allows me to reflect on how much more effective medical care is today than when I started it. But during medical school, postgraduate training, and my first 15 years of academic experience, I was only vaguely aware that the basis of this improvement was the culture, focus, financial wherewithal, and distributional skills of the medical products industry that provided the medicines—pharmaceuticals[1] and biotherapeutics[2]—and medical devices[3] that have enabled physicians to add such remarkable value to patient care. I was equally clueless as to how cooperation between physicians, universities, and industry and regulatory oversight of medical products by the government's Food and Drug Administration (FDA) has been essential for that progress.

And I knew little or nothing about the nuts and bolts or the economics of medical product development. The only consistent message I had absorbed from my immersion in academe was that great research being done in medical schools and nonprofit research institutes would accommodate health care innovation by bringing their discoveries "from the laboratory bench to the bedside."

In 1987 I was recruited to the Scientific Advisory Board of the biotechnology company Biogen. Founded in 1978, the company resided in Cambridge, Massachusetts. My selection to the Board was a result of my having achieved some notoriety as a cell biology researcher while maintaining a leadership role in clinical and administrative activities. The Board consisted of a dozen world-class scientists including Biogen's Nobelist founder and Harvard chemistry professor Walter Gilbert. The Scientific Advisory Board chair, MIT Professor Philip Sharp, also subsequently won the Nobel Prize. Having my opinion valued as the sole physician in such a company was humbling and exhilarating, and the experience was transforming.

The Biogen exposure woke me up to how ignorant I had previously been about economics in general and medical product development in particular and introduced me to the work ethic, fundamental honesty, and passion of most people in business. It also taught me the rudiments of what it takes to translate research discoveries into potential products. As a result, I have acquired patents based on my research, have licensed research projects to three companies for clinical development, and have participated in the founding of two. Most importantly, I began to understand how difficult medical product development is and how important freedom of action is to overcome those difficulties.

These epiphanies coincided with the abrupt emergence of a relentless ideological movement dedicated to attacking the partnerships that drive medical progress. Over the past 25 years, this crusade has downplayed private industry's contributions to medical innovation, discounted the immense costs and difficulties of achieving those contributions, accused the

FDA of lax oversight, denied the importance of university and physician partnerships with industry for medical innovation and education, and exaggerated problems related to such partnership. I refer to the anti-industry crusade as the *conflict-of-interest movement*, because it has adopted that term as its watchword.

"Conflict of interest" is an inexact term with diverse but unsatisfactory definitions. The anti-industry movement, however, confidently stamps it on relationships of which it disapproves and applies it as described in the quote above from Thucydides's *History of the Peloponnesian War*: it is an insinuation that the medical products industry and those who partner with it are corrupt, placing personal profit above providing medical value. Because of its for-profit basis no "proposal honestly put forward" by private industry is above suspicion. According to the conflict-of-interest movement, the performance and dissemination of research done by industry or by industry-sponsored academic researchers is untrustworthy, as are efforts by medical product companies or physicians paid by them to make practitioners aware of such products and how to use them. According to the conflict-of-interest movement, financial and social amenities that lubricate relationships between innovators, manufacturers, and customers in our general economy are nothing less than bribery in the context of medical innovation, education, and care where the medical products industry is concerned. The conflict-of-interest movement preaches that the only remedies for this corruption are total disclosure of corporate payments to physicians and researchers and management or elimination of the activities these payments support. The general term for these remedies is *conflict-of-interest regulation*.

The case underlying the conflict-of-interest movement is a mixture of moralistic bullying, opinion unsupported by empiric evidence, speculation, simplistic and distorted interpretations of complicated and nuanced information, superficially and incompletely framed anecdotes, inappropriately extrapolated or irrelevant psychological research results, and emotionally laden human-interest stories. I refer to this rhetorical weave as the *conflict-of-interest narrative*; the promoters of that narrative as *conflict-of-interest instigators*; and the authorities in academic institutions, medical professional organizations, medical practice management groups, and state and federal government that have responded to it by enthusiastically enacting the recommended remedies as *conflict-of-interest movement enablers and enforcers*. The conflict-of-interest movement qualifies as a *mania* because of its lack of substantive grounding. For example, the conflict-of-interest policy enacted by my health care system employer forthrightly cloaks its specific regulations with instigator rhetoric such as:[4]

> [c]onflicts of interest, and the appearance of conflict of interest, may arise from these [industry] interactions. These conflicts create a risk that integrity, independence, leadership, exercise of professional judgment, or the reputation of [the health care system] may be compromised.

This very litany lacks "integrity": because almost no evidence over decades supports that "integrity, independence, leadership, [or] exercise of professional judgment" has been compromised. Other than muckraking media reports concerning the "appearance" of conflict of interest, industry relationships have had no effect on the institution's reputation. By failing to make the effort to understand that the evidence underlying the conflict-of-interest narrative fails reasonably to support the instigators' claims or their demands for regulation, the enablers have inflicted rampant mandated disclosure, and management and elimination of collaborative relationships between physicians, universities, and industry.

Since its founding, the biotechnology industry has produced valuable biopharmaceuticals and made important contributions to the national economy. Thanks to this enablement of conflict-of-interest regulation, many of the financial incentives that led academic medical researchers to establish the biotechnology industry in the 1970s have been abolished. Industry support for research partnerships with physicians and for medical education and physician training have all declined. Widely banned are activities that benefit physicians' ability to care for patients. These activities include interactions with company marketing personnel, access to medical product samples, trivial reminder items, and payments to physicians for educating other physicians in convenient and pleasant circumstances about ever increasing numbers of products. Vast resources have been diverted from medical innovation, medical education, and medical care to comply with conflict-of-interest regulations and to violate physician privacy by mandating disclosure of their payments from industry. The conflict-of-interest narrative has contributed to a prosecutorial extortion racket that has extracted enormous sums away from industry's ability to develop new products by forcing it to pay fines for marketing behavior that has caused no damages and arguably provides mainly benefit.

The contrast between the corruption claims of the conflict-of-interest movement and my actual experiences as a Biogen consultant and in attempting to make my research findings clinically useful was striking. Also puzzling to me was the facility with which the conflict-of-interest narrative flooded the airwaves unencumbered by demands for critical accountability. This rhetorical free ride contrasted markedly with my personal experience doing research. I could never publish research results or interpretations without rigorous and nearly airtight evidence, and obtaining resources to translate my research into medically and commercially viable products required even more demanding evidence.

For the next 15 years I closely followed the relentless progress of the conflict-of-interest movement but limited my reactions to tedious complaints to friends and family. Then when in 2004 a *Los Angeles Times* reporter attacked colleagues who were researchers at the National Institutes of Health (NIH) because of their business consulting activities, I began to write and speak out. My first op ed article, "Free the Scientists," appeared in *Forbes* in early 2005.[5] Later that year, I published an article titled "Regulating Academic-Industrial Research Relationships—Solving Problems or Stifling Progress?" in the *New England Journal of Medicine.*[6] At that year's end, in an op ed in the *Wall Street Journal*, "Mere Magazines," I explained how academic institutions and medical journals falsely demonize the medical products industry.[7] Since then, I have published over 40 articles and op eds and participated in more than 150 lectures, panels, debates, or interviews on this topic. My experience with attempting to get the message out increasingly convinced me that doing so more effectively required a comprehensive documentation of medical innovation and how the conflict-of-interest movement damages it. That effort is what this book is about.

RESPONDING TO THE CONFLICT-OF-INTEREST MOVEMENT: THE STRATEGY OF THIS BOOK

The book consists of four sections. The first section contains two chapters, the first of which introduces my personal experience with some of the incredible advances that have come from partnerships between physicians, academics, and the medical products industry. The second section initially briefly reviews the history and working features of this partnership and the regulations under which it operates. It then recounts the emergence of the conflict-of-interest movement, the regulations it has introduced, the individuals and institutions responsible for the movement, and why I believe they promote it. The third section explains why the movement is ill founded and enumerates its specific scientific, policy making, and economic errors. The final section discusses the movement's costs to medical innovation and education and what I believe it will take to stop the movement and remove its costs.

This book concerns "health care," writ large. So, although for parsimony I refer mainly to "medicine" and "physicians," the subject matter pertains to all types of health care activities and the professionals and paraprofessionals who engage in them.

In putting this book together I have had several distinct advantages. One is that I am old. A long sojourn in medicine during which I have engaged in diverse activities means I have observed a lot of history and gotten to know a lot of people. Being able to draw on this experience and consult with many contacts has been very helpful. Another is that the quarter century of flourishing of the conflict-of-interest movement has deposited a very large paper trail that can be analyzed for soundness of facts and interpretation.

I have tried to execute this project with the seriousness that I have applied to my medical practice and research activities. I gathered as many facts as I could, thought about them in depth, and sought advice from many stakeholders and experts close to specific topics. Because the conflict-of-interest narrative is rife with unattributed assertions and misattribution, I have included extensive references to primary sources that sedulous readers can check for accuracy.

A strategic challenge is that medicine involves very technical knowledge that is unfamiliar to even highly educated laypersons. And, in addition, most physicians share the ignorance I possessed prior to my Biogen experience concerning the exceedingly complicated and difficult procedures used by the medical products industry to accomplish innovation, and the development of useful technologies and how they actually end up helping patients. In addition, the history of the appearance and evolution of the conflict-of-interest movement is long and convoluted. I have tried to convey the information about these topics as simply and concisely as possible, but the sheer volume of material requires perseverance. Therefore, to accommodate readers only interested in the "big picture," I have deposited some of the more detailed information in notes.

Undoubtedly, an effort of this complexity and scope will contain errors and omissions. I invite readers to call them to my attention. I will make corrections in future editions, should interest accommodate them.

I

Some Benefits and the Mechanics of Medical Innovation

I

THE STAKES

FOUR PERSONAL MEDICAL STORIES

Grace

Every year I serve as attending physician on the hematology service of my hospital to treat patients' blood diseases. Two years ago, I participated in the care of a 35-year-old woman whom I'll call Grace. Grace is a married management consultant who was 18 weeks into her first pregnancy. The week before her admission to my hospital she developed abdominal cramps and diarrhea. These symptoms persisted for several days, and when she noted that the diarrhea contained bright red blood, she called her primary care physician who told her to go immediately to the emergency room of a nearby community hospital. There, blood tests revealed alarming results. Grace's oxygen-carrying red blood cells were markedly deficient in number as were her platelets, the blood cells that participate in blood clotting. Most disturbing, however, was the fact that chemicals normally removed by the kidneys were accumulating in her blood, indicating kidney malfunction. Based on these findings, arrangements took place to transfer Grace to my hospital, a major referral center better positioned to manage complicated and unusual cases.

On arrival, Grace was admitted to the medical intensive care unit. The diarrhea had subsided, and her main symptom was drowsiness. But her blood abnormalities had worsened, and her kidneys had stopped producing urine altogether. In addition, whereas normal red blood cells viewed with a microscope are round and smooth, Grace's were jagged and misshapen. Grace's symptoms and laboratory results added up to a class of disorders known as a "thrombotic microangiopathy" (the literal English translation of this Greek terminology is "sick small blood vessels clotting up"). The specific constellation of Grace's history and laboratory findings assigned her to a particular variety of thrombotic microangiopathy, named "the hemolytic-uremic syndrome (HUS)."

The major cause of HUS is an ingestion of food contaminated with bacteria, usually a strain of the common intestinal *E. coli* that rarely produces a particular toxic factor named Shiga. White blood cells carry the Shiga toxin to cells lining small blood vessels, especially in the kidney, causing them to swell and partly or completely block blood flow. This obstruction leads to the destruction of red blood cells, trapping of platelets, and kidney failure. HUS is rare and more common in children than adults, although a recent outbreak of *E. coli* gastroenteritis in Europe generated many cases. [1]

Testing for Shiga toxin revealed its presence in Grace, confirming the HUS diagnosis. From the first description of HUS in 1955 and through most of my medical career, the condition was either a death sentence or else condemned patients to permanent kidney failure.

Thanks to medical innovation, however, Grace's outcome was far different. During a month-long hospitalization, she received treatments that allowed her to return home in a normal state of health and with her pregnancy preserved. Four and a half months later she delivered a normal baby girl.

In addition to general supportive care, several technologically sophisticated interventions minimized Grace's disease. One was the procedure called hemodialysis that takes over for nonworking kidneys by cleansing the blood of the chemicals normal kidneys remove. The patient's blood flows from a catheter inserted into an artery into a device that filters out the chemicals and then returns the cleansed blood through another catheter into a vein. Although dialysis can sustain life when kidneys fail, the ideal goal is to restore kidney function, a task that required interrupting the destructive underlying process that characterizes HUS. To this end, Grace's caretaker team applied two additional technological treatments.

The first was to remove on a daily basis several pints of Grace's plasma, the protein-rich blood fluid in which blood cells circulate, and replace it with plasma taken from normal blood donors. This procedure developed by trial and error and yielded some of the first survivors of HUS, although we do not really know how it works. The second treatment was to administer a drug named eculizumab (brand name Soliris) developed by a Connecticut-based company named Alexion for a different rare blood disease but recently documented to improve recovery in HUS.[2]

Standing at Grace's intensive care unit bedside I could reflect on the importance of technology contributed by the medical products industry to Grace's management and clinical improvement. Single technicians operated the compact dialysis device and the sophisticated machine that automatically performed the plasma exchange procedures. Because of sensors that monitored blood pressures and flows and intricate circuitry, the instruments practically ran themselves with ease and relative safety. Other devices enabled physicians to obtain precise images of Grace's organs or monitor her cardiovascular and metabolic status on a minute-to-minute basis without her having to leave her medical intensive care unit bed.

Dental Prevention in Zambia

A few weeks after my encounter with Grace, I made the long journey to Zambia in Sub-Saharan Africa, where I am a fully licensed medical practitioner and where my wife, who is a public health dentist, some colleagues, and I have established a nonprofit organization named Options for Children in Zambia.[3] Since 2004, Options has provided dental care and other services in a large urban orphanage, The Kasisi Children's Home, and in a remote rural village named Muchila. A visit to see medical colleagues at Zambia's principal academic health center, University Teaching Hospital, in the capital city of Lusaka reminded me that Grace wouldn't have had a chance of survival if she had been Zambian rather than American. But even in a poverty-ridden country like Zambia, the medical products industry is making a difference.

When we first came to Zambia in 2004, 20% of the population was infected with HIV-AIDS, and The Kasisi Children's Home had a hospice for dying infants and children. Over half of the Kasisi orphans and Muchila villagers were in pain due to advanced tooth decay. Thanks to the American President's Emergency Plan for AIDS Relief (PEPFAR) that provides HIV test kits, anti-HIV drugs (developed by the American pharmaceutical industry) and a countrywide program screening and treatment program for HIV-positive mothers about to deliver babies, the national prevalence of HIV infection has fallen to 14%. HIV-infected individuals in Muchila village previously had to walk for days to obtain anti-HIV drugs at a regional hospital. Now health workers have supplies of the drugs at the local village health center. The Kasisi hospice closed down in 2010. After a few years of applying fluoride varnish treatments to the children's teeth and placing plastic sealants in the grooves of molars—both accomplished with simple devices provided gratis by dental product companies—the prevalence of advanced tooth decay has declined by over 90% at Kasisi and is falling in Muchila.

Patrick

Patrick, my brother-in-law, lives in the Denver area. Strapping and handsome in 1997 when he was 35 years old, he worked as a quality control manager in a methanol factory. On weekends, he and his buddies climbed mountains in the Colorado Rockies higher than 14,000 feet, hoping to "bag all the fourteeners" in the state. But feeling progressively lightheaded and ill, he consulted a physician, who obtained some blood tests. The results revealed that his red blood cell count was down to one fifth of normal, a value that would have put less robust individuals into shock or heart failure. Further testing showed that the reason for the low blood count was that he was losing blood in his stools. This finding led to imaging studies that detected a mass attached to his small intestine. A surgeon removed the mass along with a segment of Patrick's intestine, attached the severed ends of the bowel, and sent the specimen to the pathologist for analysis. The pathologist diagnosed an uncommon cancerous tumor, known at that time as a leiomyosarcoma, the English translation for which a cancer of the muscular lining of the intestine that propels its contents from the stomach to the rectum.

At that time, the standard of treatment for this condition was surgery, and the definition of success was "clear margins," meaning that the pathologist examining the resected specimen provided by the surgeon under the microscope saw no cancer cells near the edge of where the surgeon had removed the specimen. Patrick's margins were clear, and thanks to his youthful vigor, he quickly returned to his normal life. His doctors considered him cured.

But in the spring of 2001, Patrick began to have lower abdominal pain. Imaging studies of his abdomen alarmingly detected a mass the size of a soccer ball in his pelvis and two ping-pong ball–size lesions in his liver. Either on their own or during the surgical removal of the intestinal mass, cancer cells had dropped into Patrick's pelvic cavity and seeded a new tumor. Offshoots of that tumor had produced the liver metastases.

In the past, such widespread tumors resisted all available chemotherapy or radiation treatments, and surgery only served to provide transient relief of obstructions and distensions inflicted by the relentless cancer progression. The patients suffered awful deaths.

Fortunately, just as Patrick's tumor relapsed, information was emerging that a drug named imatinib, originally developed for a form of leukemia might be effective against his cancer, the name of which by that time had changed from leiomyosarcoma to gastrointestinal stromal tumor (GIST). I helped arrange for Patrick to become a subject in a clinical trial at my hospital to formally determine whether the anecdotal preliminary evidence of the drug's efficacy could be confirmed. By the time Patrick was enrolled in the trial in September of 2001, the GIST had grown sufficiently to collapse his ureters, the conduits draining urine from the kidneys to the bladder, causing acute flank pain due to pressure within the kidneys, and Patrick had to have plastic tubes inserted to prevent his kidneys from being destroyed by the compression.

Patrick started treatment with the experimental drug in September. By December, his pelvic tumor had shrunk to the size of a softball, his pain was gone, and the ureteric tubes were removed. Over the ensuing months the size of the residual tumor remained unchanged, as did the two liver metastases despite continued drug treatment. The experts who pioneered the treatment of patients like Patrick concluded that it made sense to remove these residual cancer deposits. In the summer of 2003, a surgeon performed an extensive operation and excised the remnants of the pelvic tumor and the two liver lesions. Today, 15 years since the original appearance of his cancer, annual imaging scans have happily shown he remains free of disease progression. Nevertheless, based on the experience of other patients who relapsed if imatinib was discontinued, Patrick continues to take it at an annual cost of $123,000. Fortunately, his insurance pays for the drug.

My Bad Back

The previous three stories described medical interventions that due to industry contributions, resulted in unequivocally and durably favorable outcomes. The following example, a very personal one, deals with a situation that involves medical activities with far more ambiguous end points.

The extremely common affliction, variously labeled "acute back syndrome," or more quaintly, "lumbago," is excruciatingly painful, often set off by seemingly inconsequential movements and only partially relieved by pain medications, rest, and local applications of heat or cold. Minute movements of the torso cause large lower back muscles to go into excruciating spasms. Between spasms, the same muscles continuously hunch one over to one side or the other. Initially, walking and sitting are nearly impossible, and pain persists even when lying down. Simple essential tasks—like moving one's bowels—are torture. It is a major cause of time lost from work and, once experienced, creates anxiety that a wrong move will cause it to return. Back pain afflicts relatively young people who, if athletic, find the problem very frustrating. Believe me, I know, because I had my first attack when I was in medical training in my mid-twenties and was laid up for a week at a time annually for the next 15 years. Between attacks, I had no symptoms until, in my early 40s, I developed what is also common—chronic back pain associated with evidence of inflammation of the nerves that emerge from the spinal cord to mediate sensation and motor control to the legs. This inflammation causes severe lower extremity pain, pins and needles feelings, numbness, and weakness, a constellation known as "sciatica."

In medical school in the 1960s I was taught that bulging of "intervertebral discs," spongy material cushioning the spaces between the vertebral bones comprising the spine compressed surrounding tissues causing the symptoms of acute and chronic back pain. What I had learned was the basis of treatments recommended by orthopedic or neurological surgeons who dealt with these conditions. They documented disc bulges with a procedure that involved injecting dye into the spinal canal and taking X-rays. Having identified bulges, they would recommend prolonged bed rest, sometimes with traction, that supposedly would allow the bulges to recede; if improvement was not forthcoming, they performed surgery to remove the bulging disc material.

But by the time I was in the throes of this affliction, more rigorous monitoring of many back sufferers had concluded that most cases of acute back pain resolve spontaneously and that the benefits of all treatments were unclear. Improved and less invasive imaging procedures had also revealed that disc bulges are common yet may cause no symptoms.[4] Surgical specialists had backed off rushing into procedural interventions for back pain and could reassure patients that if they could manage their pain conservatively, the condition would most likely resolve and in most cases not progress to worse complications. They tended to resort to surgery only when neurologic complications were severe or when patients' frustration led them to demand that something more be done. One procedure, to inject inflammation-reducing substances into painful areas of the spine, has become very common. Patients believe that the temporary relief of pain it seems to afford is beneficial, although it does sometimes cause complications and does not influence long-term outcomes.

Confounding better understanding of how to manage this condition is the subjectivity of pain and the influence of psychological factors on its perception and the lack of anatomical evidence of what is going on, based in part on the fact that nobody dies of it.[5]

Depending on whether the patient has an acute attack, chronic pain, or neurological complications, or sees an orthopedist, a neurosurgeon, a neurologist, a physical therapist, or a chiropractor, the approaches to treatment differ, but the outcomes do not.[6] For patients who have severe chronic pain or neurologic complications or simply are desperate, surgeons intervene with more invasive procedures involving fusing vertebrae together. To stabilize the bony structures, some surgeons invented metal implant devices and later packed them with hormone-like substances that promote bone growth. Thanks to the uncertainties surrounding back pain, these interventions are controversial.

I avoided surgery and managed by taking relatively mild painkillers and engaging in daily walking and swimming rituals. Fortunately, the pain gradually abated, and by my late forties, I was back on the tennis court, although I have a numb patch on my left thigh and muscles in my lower legs twitch as if there were worms under the skin, a symptom known as "fasciculations," which attests to the presence of spinal nerve compression. I can also confirm what people told me back then—that everyone would remember me forever for having been a back sufferer because of the ritualistic antics for dealing with it (like lying on the floor of my office).

THE MEDICAL STORIES IN CONTEXT

Good health is not necessarily a result of medical interventions. Indeed, those who through no efforts of their own enjoy a genetic heritage that renders them relatively resistant to disease, who live where conditions minimize exposure to infectious diseases, and who avoid risky behaviors detrimental to health may have few encounters with the health care system. Sooner or later, however, everyone sickens and dies. And in contrast to the aforementioned outcomes, many of these instances involve diseases that do not respond or respond minimally to available therapies. Human nature drives people to accept treatments, even if they are expensive, poorly effective, and sometimes ridden with unpleasant side effects. The way Patrick's GIST would have been addressed prior to the availability of imatinib is one example of such desperation. The management of chronic back pain for those less fortunate than I was remains controversial and marginally satisfactory. Mental health conditions, such as anxiety and depression, when not severe, are similar to back pain in being of uncertain cause and unpredictably responsive to treatment. [7]

Nevertheless, the overall trend, based on metrics of longevity and life quality has been steady health betterment. This statistical abstraction is palpably obvious to physicians who have practiced medicine for a long time, and formal analyses by economic scholars credit a synergy between the medical profession, researchers advancing knowledge potentially relevant to medicine, and private industry—the synergy I define as "the medicine-industry interface"—with immense advances responsible for the good health outcomes. Far less appreciated is the fact that the scientific advances and commercial contributions that mediate the positive accomplishments require overcoming immense scientific and economic obstacles. Emerging scientific knowledge is far less readily translatable into clinical progress than popularly believed, and we must rely on a frustratingly high level of serendipity, trial and error to achieve it, and adaptation to frequent and unpredictable failure.

Most discussions about health care emphasize its global costs. Since science and medicine merged in the late nineteenth century, they have risen exponentially. Grace's HUS management and dental prevention and care in Zambia represent opposite ends of the spending spectrum. Dental prevention, like vaccination against infectious diseases, is a highly cost-effective way to improve health. Indeed many preventive measures such as wearing seat belts, not smoking, keeping body weight and blood pressure under control, and avoiding substance abuse all save health system costs. But most of these relatively inexpensive measures also require industry contributions: someone has to manufacture seat belts, blood pressure measuring machines, blood pressure medication, and smoking cessation aids. On the other hand, HUS "prevention" was not practically possible for Grace, and the large expenses associated with her treatment saved her and her baby's life, and returned her to economic productivity. The expense of Patrick's imatinib pales before the benefits it has afforded him. The story of my back pain, while far less satisfactory than the others in terms of pointing to benefits of medical intervention, does have some positive attributes. Compared to when I was a medical student, we can be more confident that conservative management can work. Today's pain medications, developed by industry, are better and allow for more treatment options. Operative procedures, when necessary, are far safer thanks to improved technical tools available to surgeons.

The examples presented in this chapter are representative of thousands that illustrate the benefits of medical innovation based on physician- and academic-industry partnerships. The next chapter explains some fundamentals of this innovation and partnership.

Subsequent chapters describe the rise of the conflict-of-interest movement and how it obfuscates the benefits we have received from the efforts of the medical products' industry and threatens to compromise future partnership-based medical innovation.

2

A PRACTITIONER'S HISTORY OF MEDICAL INNOVATION

Health, defined as absence of disease and physical and mental well-being, has improved immensely since the beginning of the last century, especially in the developed world. Early on, improvements in housing, nutrition, and sanitation accounted for much of this progress.[1] Subsequently, reduction in infant mortality due to antisepsis and of infection-mediated early childhood deaths by vaccination and antibiotics were important contributors to this advance.[2]

The population's aging afforded by these successes, however, created new health problems: failing vital organs, bones, and joints. But the incidence of heart attacks and strokes, which became the leading cause of mortality in the United States, has steadily fallen, and today is half of its 1950s peak.[3] Improved detection and treatment have brought cancer mortality to an all-time low.[4] New treatments have prevented the crippling effects of rheumatoid arthritis[5] and slowed the bone softening of osteoporosis with its scourge of fractures.[6] A seven-year annual increase in hospitalizations and death due to the 1980s HIV/AIDS epidemic elicited dire predictions it would overwhelm our health care system. But in 1996 HIV/AIDS mortality in the United States fell precipitously and was negligible a year later.[7] As exemplified by former basketball star Magic Johnson, HIV-infected people can now live relatively normal lives.[8]

Replacement of degenerated hips with prostheses now rapidly returns previously disabled pain sufferers to their athletic activities. The hips came first, but now knee, elbow, and other prostheses became available and are constantly improving.[9] A frequent complication of heart diseases is compromise of the electrical circuitry that governs our hearts' normal "lub-dub" pumping that keeps our blood circulating. Cumbersome boxes with attached paddles to be applied to patients' chests to deliver electrical currents and restore the circuitry had just appeared when I was in medical training, and users had to be careful not to electrocute themselves. Now, far simpler and safer "AED" devices, which anyone can use, are ubiquitous in public places. Also, cardiologists implant tiny current sensors and emitters that automatically allow patients with heart disease to survive without seeking—possibly too late—hospital intervention for heartbeat deviations. When I was in training, we had no way to restore circulation to a heart compromised by having its arteries blocked, thereby preventing delivery of oxygen-carrying blood. Today, we have coronary artery by-pass surgery and drugs and devices, specifically artery-opening "stents" that not only restore but preserve—by releasing artery-protective drugs—the lifesaving blood circulation.

The accumulation over time of knowledge concerning biology in general and human physiology in particular contributed materially to these accomplishments. But absent private industry most of them would not have occurred. No amount of scholarly knowledge about diseases helps patients without practical tools to diagnose and treat them.

Throughout history, individuals created medically useful inventions, but making them widely available demanded businesses capable of mass-production. To this end, apothecaries formulated medicines, and companies formed to assemble medical devices invented by surgeons. In the 19th century, industry began discovering drugs and devices on its own. It identified drug candidates by screening chemicals' or biological extracts' effects on chemical reactions known to mediate diseases, the growth of disease-causing microorganisms or the shrinking of cancers in experimental animals. It modified chemicals to optimize their effects and make them amenable to introduction to the body as pills, injections, or other means (achieving this accessibility is known as "formulation"), scaled up their manufacture, and established elaborate systems for control of their quality. Toxicology and veterinary experts in the industry determined whether products' benefits compared to side effects justified their evaluation in human subjects.

CHANGING MEDICAL HISTORY
THROUGH PARTNERSHIP

Physicians and university researchers have worked with companies making medical products since such entities existed. For example, Paul Ehrlich, a German physician who was one of the founders of modern immunology and received the Nobel Prize for these contributions, interacted at his Frankfurt-based academic institute with several chemical companies to develop the first drug effective against any infectious disease, the arsenic-containing compound Salvarsan, for the treatment of syphilis. [10] But the late arrival of knowledge applicable to medical innovation kept such interactions relatively uncommon in contrast to business administration, chemistry, and engineering fields concerning which universities had developed policies that encouraged faculty to work with companies. [11] Typically, universities permitted faculty to devote one day a week to consulting activities, and these interactions resulted in the founding of many successful technology companies. Some purists argued that academic research commercialization would discourage public dissemination of research results, but after the Second World War the ideas that universities should contribute to technological progress and that commercialization was the optimal way to achieve this end largely overcame such reservations. [12]

In the 1970s, academic inventors of recently developed genetic engineering technology joined venture capitalists to found the first biotechnology companies. These companies succeeded in producing natural human hormones such as insulin that resulted in replacement products that were less likely to induce side effects than the previous variants purified from animal organs. They also introduced other natural agents such as blood cell and immunologic stimulants that were very potent but present in such small amounts that extracting them from animals or humans was impractical. In addition, they made designer antibodies that inactivated toxins or body cells causing diseases. The eculizumab product that helped my patient Grace survive her HUS is an example of such a substance. It is a modified form of a natural blocker of reactions designed to help fight infections but that can get out of control and damage normal body parts— like Grace's kidneys. At the same time, entrepreneurial surgeons worked with industry to invent or improve medical devices such as the implantable catheters that allowed Grace's caregivers to infuse fluids and drugs and do the dialysis and plasma exchange procedures without having to resort to repeated invasions of blood vessels. In these interactions, the relative freedom of academic physicians and researchers compared to usually more regimented and project-focused company scientists contributed a constructive synergy. Company financial support enabled academic researchers to undertake projects that would not have been possible to fund by government or other agency grants.

In 1971, the U.S. Congress raised concerns that much government-funded biomedical academic research was not resulting in inventions with patent protection. Such protection that grants inventors a temporary monopoly to market their inventions is necessary for inventions to become useful products because of the high risk of failure and because success requires long and arduous effort. If a pioneer developer lacked patent protection, competitors would step in after the innovator had made enough progress to reduce the risk. In response to these concerns, Congress passed the Bayh-Dole Act. The act encouraged universities to obtain patents and license them to companies for product development. Bayh-Dole often receives credit for a marked uptick in industry partnerships between universities and physicians, but mechanisms to encourage such "technology transfer" preceded Bayh-Dole by many years,[13] and the technological advances that produced translatable projects were arguably more important factors.[14]

Universities acquired intellectual property rights based on faculty research and licensed them to companies for development. In doing so, they shared with faculty inventors licensing fees, other payments for achievements of milestones such as a green light from the FDA to run a clinical trial, and—in the event the FDA approved a technology for marketing—royalties from product sales. Because most academic research involves early steps in innovation and requires much additional validation of its potential, academics were more likely to license inventions to venture capital-backed start-up companies than to established or publicly traded ones, which concentrated on projects further in development and closer to market. The cash-strapped start-ups compensated academic inventors with stock and stock options. If success enabled these new companies to obtain public investment or acquisition by larger corporations, appreciated equity afforded profits, sometimes large, to faculty members and their employer institutions. In the unusual cases when these projects resulted in clinical products in the marketplace, inventors and institutions received royalty payments.[15] More commonly, prominent faculty members served as advisers to start-ups, and their cachet helped unlock investment. In return the advisers received fees, stock, and stock options.[16]

As companies developed more products, they increasingly recruited physicians to test them in clinical trials required for FDA approval. The largest interface between physicians and industry, however, emerged from marketing strategies to make companies' wares known to practicing physicians. Companies bought advertising in medical journals and purchased reprints of medical journal articles reporting favorable results. The number of industry exhibits at medical professional society meetings grew, and these organizations turned to companies to sponsor their educational programs. Corporate support of such societies enabled them to grow and diversify their activities without raising members' dues. Some medical professional conventions became very large, because companies subsidized physicians and researchers worldwide to attend them. The professional groups holding the meetings recognized company support by affixing their logos on signage and meeting paraphernalia, such as tote bags given to registrants.

Industry also supported physicians' education outside of professional organizations. One strategy was to hire specialist physicians to present lectures about newly introduced products to small physician audiences. Typically, such talks, officially designated "promotional speaking" by the FDA, took place after working hours in restaurants, sometimes upscale ones, and in the past, physicians could bring spouses to the events. In many instances, the speakers were specialists in the field concerning the product or had participated in clinical trials of it. They traveled to venues with other speakers for training where they heard experts present properties of the products and presentation scripts. The companies often provided didactic materials for speakers to use in the presentations. The emergence of brokers to identify potential presenters led to the creation of "speakers' bureaus," a term previously applied for finding celebrity speakers for business and professional meetings.

Another approach was for companies to subsidize education programs in academic centers, at professional meetings, or at resorts concerning diseases for which they have products (a company manufacturing insulin might sponsor programs concerning diabetes) without exerting direct control over the choice of speaker or what the speaker says. Physicians attend such programs to comply with state licensure requirements for continuing medical education (CME), and accreditation agencies emerged to vet the educational material for quality and balance. By the end of the past decade, the medical products industry funded about half of the over $3 billion of U.S. CME activities. An education planning industry also evolved to raise funds for and organize such events.

A major mechanism for conveying product information has been sales representatives paying calls on practicing physicians' offices, an activity known as "detailing."[17] These detailers routinely employed strategies to gain access to busy physicians, such as bringing lunch for the physician and staff. They also left product samples for physicians to gain familiarity with them as well as small reminder items (pens, mugs, sticky pads, calendars) bearing company and product logos. Company representatives sometimes established more intimate relationships with physicians, treating them to sports events or other entertainment. As the subsequent text will reveal, these accoutrements of the medicine-industry interface, pejoratively labeled as "gifts," evolved into a major polemical battleground.

REGULATIONS AFFECTING THE HEALTH CARE PRODUCTS INDUSTRY

Far more regulation affects companies that make most health care products than the physicians who use or prescribe them.[18] One set of rules, intellectual property (patent) law, grants companies temporary monopolies over sales of products for which patents are in force. The trinity of patentability is that an idea must be "novel, non-obvious and 'enabled' [reducible to practice]." Currently if a patent issues, the inventor has 20 years of monopoly protection starting from the time of filing. Because the average time from product discovery to market for drugs is 16 years, and the follow-on time of competing products has shortened, the patent monopoly time is relatively short.

Patents fall broadly under two categories. "Composition of matter" patents cover a chemical entity or a specific device for whatever purpose it is used. A "use" patent covers the novel, nonobvious, and reducible to practice application of a chemical or device not patentable for its own sake (because they were never patented or have lost patent protection). Composition-of-matter patents are considered superior to use patents, but broad-use patents can be quite defensible.

Inventors frequently file initial patent applications with the U.S. Patent Office as "provisional" applications that afford protection of an invention for a year during which the inventor obtains additional information to solidify the basis of the application. The filing fee for such applications is relatively low, but inventors usually outsource the filing effort to attorneys who specialize in the arcana of patent prosecution, and the resulting legal fees can be high. The usual follow-up to a provisional application is a "Patent Cooperation Treaty (PCT)/International application." This filing stipulates intellectual property protection in jurisdictions that have large medical markets (Canada, Europe, Japan, China, Korea, and potentially more countries). PCT applications enable an additional 18 months of delay before "national phase applications" are required, with filings in many additional countries. The costs incurred for these procedures include filing fees in the various jurisdictions and the expert legal work required to prosecute a lengthy adversarial process. Patent filers want to obtain the broadest possible claims for their invention, whereas the patent examiners' goal is to narrow claims to be commensurate with specific technical information included in the patent application. Negotiations to define allowable claims can go on for years. Adding to expense is the adaptive mandate to follow initial patent applications with new ones as refinements to technology evolve or new information suggests topics for use patents. A broad portfolio of patents is a bulwark against infringement. Because most successful projects end up in patent litigation, having such a barrier is very important.[19]

Since the beginning of the 20th century, the U.S. government has ruled whether companies can market their products.[20] Passage of the Food and Drugs Act in 1906 was a reaction during Theodore Roosevelt's administration to instances of adulterated or contaminated drugs and vaccines. The initial role of the agency was to assure that manufacturers conform to quality standards. In 1938, after a Tennessee company used an antifreeze chemical to make a liquid form of an antibiotic, and the additive killed a number of children, the agency, renamed the Food, Drug and Cosmetic Agency (FDA), imposed the obligation that product developers provide evidence for product safety testing prior to approval for sales.

Starting in 1959, Tennessee Senator Estes Kefauver held hearings that questioned the utility of many drugs on the market, the pharmaceutical industry's promotional and pricing practices, and the quality of product safety testing. The pharmaceutical industry and its supporters in Congress mounted resistance to Kefauver's efforts to increase government regulation of drug development and might have succeeded were it not for the thalidomide tragedy.

A German company developed thalidomide as a tranquilizer and a treatment for pregnancy-associated nausea. In 1957, it was approved for sale—without a prescription—in Europe. Two established American pharmaceutical companies declined to license the product for introduction to the United States based on their assessment that it was not safe. A third company, relatively inexperienced in drug development, distributed thalidomide tablets to over a thousand physicians who in turn gave them to tens of thousands of patients. But the company did not intend this widespread distribution to serve as an evaluation of safety and effectiveness. In 1960, they submitted a request for FDA approval without any formal testing. Dr. Frances Kelsey, a Canadian-born physician employed by the FDA handled the request and delayed thalidomide's approval. In the following year horrendous birth defects of offspring of women who took thalidomide during pregnancy became public knowledge. The riveting images of babies with hands and feet attached directly to their torsos dissolved political resistance to most of Kefauver's proposed regulations. President John F. Kennedy signed the Kefauver-Harris amendments to FDA legislation in June of 1962 and awarded Frances Kelsey the Presidential Medal for Distinguished Federal Civilian Service.

The 1962 Kefauver-Harris Amendments stipulated that companies must now demonstrate that their products are effective as well as safe. The definition of effectiveness is that the products' results need to be shown—in "adequate and well-controlled" studies—to be better than no treatment, although they do not have to surpass the efficacy of existing products. Randomized controlled trials, introduced around that time, in which subjects were randomly assigned to receive either a test or a sham (placebo) product, and neither the physician participating in the trial or the subject were aware of which it was, superseded earlier haphazard testing procedures epitomized by the thalidomide story.[21] Other stipulations of the Kefauver-Harris Law were that companies could not promote their products prior to FDA approval (as they had in the past) and that the FDA, not the Federal Trade Commission, was to regulate drug advertising. The 1951 Durham-Humphrey Amendment to the 1938 FDA law had previously legislated that most drugs were purchasable only from pharmacies when prescribed by physicians. However, some products with longstanding safety profiles were directly obtainable by consumers (known as "over-the-counter (OTC)" products).

The operational process that evolved from the 1962 FDA legislation is for a product manufacturer to submit an "Investigational New Drug (IND)" application to the FDA, based on evidence from laboratory tests and safety assessments in animals that a drug can feasibly be administered to humans and exert a therapeutic effect with acceptable risks. The next step is a "Phase I" trial in which one administers the drug to volunteers or very ill patients with otherwise untreatable diseases such as cancer to establish doses that the subjects can tolerate and measure the persistence and elimination of the drug in and from the subjects, an exercise known as "pharmacokinetics (PK)." If the outcome of the Phase I study is acceptable, a small "Phase II" trial in patients with the disease to be targeted can establish whether the efficacy and safety profiles inferred from the preliminary laboratory and animal work hold up in humans. Should this "proof of concept" analysis hold up, additional "Phase III" trials determine whether the drug is sufficiently effective and safe to warrant approval. Specific circumstances determine the size of such trials. The value of an antibiotic that effectively eliminates a particular infection, for example, is discernible in a small number of patients. By contrast, to show that blood cholesterol lowering statins, discussed in Chapter 10, protect heart attack or stroke victims from further attacks, requires large numbers of subjects, because the incidence of these complications is relatively low. The FDA usually requires two Phase III trials for product approval.

Throughout the product development process, companies work with the FDA to define the various studies' analytical requirements. Upon completion of the Phase III trials, if successful, companies submit a "New Drug Application (NDA)" to the FDA laying out the specific information incorporated into the drug's "label," the information the company will be permitted to inform physicians about concerning the drug. The Agency reviews the entire voluminous documentation package and negotiates with the company regarding the label's content. In some circumstances, the FDA requires additional evaluation after approval: if questions regarding safety arose in the Phase III trials, the Agency may ask for further ("Post-marketing" or "Phase IV") studies.[22] Companies often avoid testing drugs in children because of liability concerns, and the FDA counters this reticence by providing extended marketing exclusivity if companies evaluate approved drugs in pediatric populations.

Since 1976, the FDA has also regulated medical devices. Devices associated with absent or minimal risk, such as throat swabs or bandages, need not undergo any review. The FDA defines such devices as "Class I." However, the Agency requires extensive premarket analysis of "Class III" devices deemed potentially high risk, such as implantable heart pacemakers, and only demonstration to FDA's satisfaction that the objects are safe and effective eventuates in their approval for clinical use. In between reside "Class II" devices that the manufacturer must convince FDA are "substantially equivalent" to a "predicate" preexisting device. Based on the statutory definition for the review process of such devices, they carry the designation "501(k)."

As an incentive to innovate, the FDA grants drug manufacturers a temporary monopoly interval on product sales (five years in the United States) from the time of regulatory approval, irrespective of whether the product has ongoing patent protection.[23] An unintended consequence of the Kefauver-Harris FDA amendments was that the product development cost increases incurred by the requirement to demonstrate product efficacy discouraged product development for disorders affecting relatively few patients that therefore would be insufficiently profitable to justify the increased development costs. To address this problem, Congress in 1983 passed the Orphan Drug Act, which conferred extended marketing exclusivity, tax incentives, development cost sharing provisions for, and expedited approval of products related to diseases affecting less than 200,000 patients in the United States.[24] Since the Act's passage, the number of drugs available for uncommon diseases has grown enormously,[25] and economic analysis shows a correlation between orphan drug approvals and a decline in mortality due to orphan diseases.[26]

Another important amendment to FDA law, the Drug Price Competition and Patent Term Restoration Act passed in 1984, commonly known as the Hatch-Waxman Act, encourages the entry of "generic" versions of approved brand products when their patents expire. The FDA allows companies developing generics to obtain product approval based on much less stringent information than required for new drugs. A company introducing a generic drug need only demonstrate that the generic product is chemically identical to the brand compound (known as "bioequivalence") and has a similar duration of action in patients receiving the product. The companies developing such generics also receive short-term exclusive selling rights at the brand price. When this exclusivity runs out, the generic products sell at steep discounts that usually force the company that developed the original brand product out of price competition.[27]

Above and beyond its product approval decisions, the FDA stipulates what marketing claims companies can make about approved products (known as what is "on-label") and closely monitors what companies advertise. Although no product can be prescribed that is not FDA approved,[28] once approval of a product for some indication has occurred, physicians can prescribe it for unapproved uses. This "off-label" prescribing is common,[29] but FDA law mandates that companies cannot generally *promote* products for other than approved uses. This odd anomaly is the compromise hammered out between Congress' wish to have the government regulate medical *products* and the medical profession's insistence that the government not regulate medical *practice*. Chapter 14 addresses the consequences of this contradiction in detail.

The FDA also has the ability to require companies to inform physicians of product shortcomings or untoward effects. The most extreme sanction, short of demanding removal of a product from the market, is to attach a "black box warning" to the product label. Encased in a black border, the warning appears prominently at the top of the package insert label and describes the reasons for caution. In addition to displaying the warning prominently in the written material describing the product, company representatives have the obligation to inform physicians prescribing the product of that warning. The FDA also inspects manufacturing facilities and quality control procedures of product-producing companies as well as of the suppliers of product ingredients.

Over the century of its existence, the FDA has had to deal with the tension between protecting the public from unsafe and ineffective products, and preventing patients from obtaining timely access to others that improve longevity and life quality. Although its purview encompasses over a fifth of the U.S. economy (in addition to drugs and medical devices, the Agency regulates vaccines, blood products, food, cosmetics, radiation-emitting substances, and most recently, tobacco products), its size and budget are relatively small compared to other government agencies, such as agriculture and defense. When in 1992 lengthening times for drug approvals raised concerns, Congress authorized companies to increase the FDA's financial assets by paying fees upon submission of

NDA applications. The industry funds authorized by this "Prescription Drug User Fee Act (PDUFA)" transiently enabled the Agency to clear out a backlog of unapproved drugs, and the Act has been reauthorized repeatedly since that time.[30]

The majority of products the FDA has approved are beneficial and cause few problems, but the few that do, attract public attention. Delayed approvals of potentially useful products, however, do not. FDA officials who approve a problematic product have a lot more to lose than they gain when they approve perfectly safe and effective ones. Another inherent problem is that medical illnesses, medical science, and the health care workforce evolve far faster than statutory bureaucracies assigned to regulate them can adapt. Nevertheless, in my view FDA has performed as well as can be expected in the face of the fact that it is a complex bureaucracy; its resource constraints; and most importantly, medical uncertainty, a concept I repeatedly emphasize in this book. At times it has succumbed to political pressure—possibly instigated by the legal profession that benefits from more stringent regulation and its promotion of compliance—and such pressure has been particularly prevalent in the domain of off-label prescribing. On the other hand, the Agency has adapted to advances in technology and public demands to handle products deemed important for medical needs on a prioritized basis. Approximately half of drugs under review receive priority reviews (mainly anticancer and anti-HIV drugs). Moreover, the FDA approved the first blood cholesterol lowering "statin" drug to prevent heart attack or stroke recurrences based on the indirect outcome of reductions in blood cholesterol years before direct effects on clinical results were demonstrated. Such indirect consequences are known as "surrogate" or "biomarker" outcomes. It also flexibly streamlined the process for approving the drugs that became available to treat HIV/AIDS, again based on surrogate markers, before their effects on mortality were proven. These fast-tracked medications rapidly rendered this formerly uniformly lethal disease manageable. The FDA worked cooperatively with the company that developed the drug Grace received for her HUS and approved it rapidly in 2008 because of the seriousness of the medical condition it affects.

However, I also sympathize with the frustration medical product developers, investors, and patients with serious illnesses for which inadequate treatments are available express when the FDA refuses to approve products or requires more layers of expensive and time-consuming evaluation before doing so. But I disagree with the idea that desperation arbitrarily justifies unleashing unproven products. History has revealed that confidence in scientific theories in fashion believed to predict the effectiveness and safety of medical products is often unwarranted. A current conviction is that the now increasingly accessible knowledge of patients' genetic makeup can reliably permit bypassing the brute force testing of whether something works in patients.[31] This information may sometimes be useful, but on balance I think it is not.

In addition to the aforementioned regulatory controls, the medical products enterprise is subject to the same product liability and fraud and kickback laws that affect all commercial endeavors. The Office of the Inspector General and state and federal prosecutors monitor the industry for such violations. Furthermore, approval of a drug by the FDA does not exempt pharmaceutical companies from litigation in multiple legal jurisdictions resulting from claims that the product caused injury to patients, and the adequacy of information supplied by the company to warn physicians and patients about the potential for such injury becomes the substance for deciding such cases.[32]

To summarize this chapter, the ability of physicians and researchers to partner with a large and diverse family of corporate entities, ranging from struggling start-ups concentrating on early inventions to global giant companies marketing multiple products, has contributed enormous value to human health. As later chapters will explain in detail, this value accrues with great difficulty and requires huge financial investments.

The regulatory apparatus described above is a major reason for the difficulty and expense. Another is the fact that medicine abounds with great uncertainty and controversy that resolve slowly and more by trial and error than by intelligent design. Any such enterprise, especially one as large and varied as medicine, will inevitably suffer not only from bad luck, poor judgment, and inadvertent errors but also from outright criminal activity. The conflict-of-interest movement, introduced in the next chapter, distorts the reality that the former adverse influences far outweigh the latter. Rather, it lays disproportionate blame for medicine's mistakes on the profit motivation of the medical products' industry and on those who work with it. It promotes the fantasy that the mistakes are avoidable if we create total transparency that enables omniscient overseers to police the behavior of the industry and of those who work with it.

II

Why We Have A Medical Innovation Crisis

3

ENTER THE CONFLICT-OF-INTEREST MANIA

PHASE ONE: THE DECLARED "CONFLICT-OF-INTEREST CRISIS" IN MEDICAL RESEARCH

Although an undercurrent of criticism of the medical products industry by a few academics has long existed,[1] "conflict of interest," a term traditionally used to connote self-dealing by public officials, rarely was articulated in the context of medicine prior to the late 1980s. Then following what has been termed "canonical incidents" involving medical academics conducting research sponsored by the medical products' industry,[2] its mention in medical journals and the public media as a serious problem rose explosively. The National Library of Medicine listed 9,500 references to the term as of December 2012.[3] The first part of this chapter briefly describes some of the aforementioned canonical cases in the order they occurred and how academic institutions, medical journals, and the government responded to them by mounting legislation. The second part of the chapter recounts the expansion of conflict-of-interest criticism and regulation from research relationships with industry into every aspect of medical practice and medical education. Chapter 5 discusses how the canonical cases do not quantitatively or qualitatively merit the influence they had in imposing policies. Chapters 6 and 7 describe the process and substance flaws of the evolved conflict-of-interest policies.

SOME CANONICAL CASES

The Spectra Case

In October of 1988, a *Boston Globe* article titled "Flawed Study Helps Doctors Profit on Drug" claimed that Scheffer Tseng, a physician in training at Harvard Medical School's affiliated hospital, the Massachusetts Eye and Ear Infirmary, had unethically manipulated a clinical trial and then engaged in insider trading to profit from his findings.[4] Tseng was reportedly participating in a study evaluating the ability of a vitamin concoction made by a company called Spectra to treat a condition called "dry eye syndrome." The Eye and Ear Infirmary's management fired Tseng and his immediate supervisors in response to these allegations.

The Dong Case

A pharmaceutical company named Boots contracted Betty Dong, a clinical pharmacist at the University of California in San Francisco (UCSF), to compare the effectiveness of its chemical version of a thyroid hormone with crude animal thyroid gland extracts to treat patients with defective thyroid hormone production. Dong concluded from her results that the two treatments had equivalent safety and efficacy. Dong had signed a contract giving the sponsoring company control over the right to publish results, and when she proposed to publish these results in a medical journal in 1994, the company attempted to suppress publication. UCSF academics complained, the company relented, and Dong published the study findings in the *Journal of the American Medical Association* (*JAMA*). A *JAMA* editor wrote a scathing accompanying editorial titled "Thyroid Storm" (thyroid storm is a severe form of an overactive thyroid) that became an early *J'accuse* of the conflict-of-interest movement.[5]

The Deferiprone Case

The oxygen-carrying protein hemoglobin in red blood cells contains iron, and over time the red blood cell transfusions used to treat anemia can cause accumulation of iron in toxic amounts, damaging the heart, liver, and other organs. A blood specialist and researcher at the University of

Toronto who was participating in a clinical trial of a drug called deferi-prone that was being evaluated by a Canadian company named Apotex for its ability to remove iron deposits from the bodies of patients with chronic anemia (low red blood cell counts) publicly alleged in 1996 that the medication being tested was unsafe and ineffective, thereby violating a confidentiality contract with Apotex. When university officials subse-quently restricted the researcher's activities, including removal from par-ticipation in the deferiprone study, academics inside and outside of Cana-da accused the university of impinging on academic freedom. They claimed that the university's motive was to curry favor with Apotex, because rumor held that Apotex had promised to make a major donation to the university.[6]

The Gelsinger Fatality

The most notorious and most frequently invoked adverse incident as-cribed to financial conflict of interest in research concerned the untimely death of a teenager named Jesse Gelsinger in 1999. Gelsinger suffered from a rare genetic disorder that caused deficiency of a key liver enzyme. James Wilson, a researcher at the University of Pennsylvania, attempted to replace Gelsinger's defective gene by injecting a normal one into his liver. Following injection of the gene preparation, Gelsinger suffered a fatal allergic reaction.[7] Investigations of the incident revealed numerous procedural lapses, but the most sensational reporting focused on the fact that Wilson had equity interests in the company sponsoring the gene therapy research and reportedly had not disclosed them to the Gelsingers. The Gelsinger family sued the University of Pennsylvania, and the suit rapidly eventuated in an undisclosed financial settlement.[8]

The Calcium Channel Blocker Controversy

One class of drugs introduced to medical practice during the 1980s and 1990s and credited with contributing to a steadily declining risk of death due to the number one killer, cardiovascular disease, were "calcium chan-nel blockers."[9] These medications were initially used to prevent recur-rences of heart attacks but later became widely applied to treat high blood pressure, also a risk factor for heart attacks and strokes. Around 1990 a few heart specialists raised concerns that calcium channel blockers might be responsible for patient deaths, but their concerns did not attract much notice until epidemiologists published an analysis in 1995, based on 16 clinical trials involving a particular calcium channel blocker, suggesting that calcium channel blockers increase mortality.[10] Many prominent cardiologists disputed these claims, but in early 1996 an investigative report by the Canadian Broadcasting Company's television program *The Fifth Estate*, titled "The Heart of the Matter," blamed the skepticism concerning the dangers of calcium channel blockers of some of these physicians, one of whom advised the Canadian health regulatory agency, on their having financial relationships with calcium channel blocker manufacturers.

Following up on this theme, Canadian physicians published an article in the *New England Journal of Medicine* in 1998 titled "Conflict of Interest in the Debate over Calcium-Channel antagonists."[11] The paper reported on a survey of physicians who had published views concerning the safety of calcium channel blockers and correlated the published opinions with authors' financial relationships with pharmaceutical companies. The survey revealed that physicians with any industry relationships discounted the risks of these drugs compared to physicians lacking such relationships. The article concluded: "Our results demonstrate a strong association between authors' published positions on the safety of calcium-channel antagonists and their financial relationships with pharmaceutical manufacturers. The medical profession needs to develop a more effective policy on conflict of interest."

The National Institutes of Health Consulting Violations

Being government employees, researchers at the National Institutes of Health (NIH) research facility in Bethesda, Maryland, known as the intramural program, had historically not been permitted to serve as consultants to private industry. In this respect, intramural researchers differed from their university counterparts who received research grants from the NIH but were allowed to do such consulting work. In 1995, noting that the consulting ban together with low salaries compared to academic institutions was having an adverse effect on NIH's ability to recruit and retain the best researchers, the then NIH director lifted the consulting restrictions. NIH intramural researchers could now consult for industry but were required to report their industry relationships in advance to the relevant NIH authorities.

In 2003, a *Los Angeles Times* reporter alleged that hundreds of intramural NIH researchers were serving as paid consultants without having obtained the required permission from the agency.[12] As a result of these allegations, the Commerce Committees of the Senate and House of Representatives held hearings in 2004 at which the legislators berated the NIH leadership for its failure to enforce "integrity." An NIH researcher accused her supervisor, an Alzheimer's disease researcher, of having been paid by a pharmaceutical company to provide it with samples of body fluids from Alzheimer patients. When called to testify in Congress, the researcher pleaded the Fifth Amendment.

CONFLICT-OF-INTEREST POLICIES AT ACADEMIC HEALTH CENTERS

In 1990, the Harvard Medical School administration reacted to the Spectra scandal by creating the first policy in any university for oversight and management of the faculty's research relationships with private industry.

The rules established by Harvard Medical School mandated that faculty members disclose all relationships with industry to the university administration and that the disclosures trigger oversight or outright prohibition of some activities. Because of the equity issues in the case, stock ownership weighed heavily in the Harvard policy. The policy precluded, without exception, consulting fees or equity above an arbitrary ($30,000) value from a company to which a faculty member had licensed intellectual property if that company sponsored the faculty member's research; whether the research involved patients, animals, or simply chemical compounds in a laboratory was immaterial. In addition, only equity from a "publicly widely traded" company was acceptable, and the allowable stock value was the shares' current sale price.

As a result of the uproar associated with the Dong incident, university policies now stipulate that faculty must be allowed to publish outcomes of industry-sponsored research, although universities permit companies specified times to review drafts of publications and they recognize that premature publication or presentation of research can compromise a company's legitimate competitive edge or invalidate intellectual property rights. [13]

The Gelsinger case led the Association of American Medical Colleges (AAMC), an umbrella organization for medical schools, to convene a commission to make policy recommendations concerning academic-industry relationships related to human subjects research. The principal recommendation was a "rebuttable presumption" that individuals with financial relationships with the company sponsoring a human subjects research study should not participate in that study ("rebuttable" referring to exceptional cases in which such participation might be allowed). [14] Most medical schools adopted this recommendation as part of their policies.

The Gelsinger incident also reversed a rumored loosening of the Harvard conflict-of-interest regulations to address faculty recruitment concerns. Instead, the rules became stricter. The minimal equity or consulting fee amounts permitted for academic researchers undertaking corporate-sponsored research dropped to $20,000 (and fell again to $10,000 in 2010). Faculty members were now required to disclose their industry relationships to their students. The remuneration of faculty with patented projects under development by companies, such as from licensing fees and milestone payments, was severely limited until the technologies achieved FDA approval, and faculty members were prohibited from having their names on publications describing research concerning those technologies while under development.

THE GOVERNMENT

The NIH stipulated in 1996 that universities receiving grants from that agency must put conflict-of-interest policies in place but left considerable discretion to the grantee institutions, based on the premise that NIH did not have the resources to monitor behavior of researchers at numerous external sites. The NIH required grantees receiving more than $10,000 annually from private industry to report that fact to their employers. Justifying this relatively hands-off policy was the fact that by that time, many medical schools had established conflict-of-interest policies affecting research relationships between their faculty and industry.

This leniency ended, however, under pressure from Senator Charles Grassley, Republican senator from Iowa, and the Office of the Inspector General. In 2011, the NIH administration increased the reporting requirements for institutions with NIH-funded researchers.[15] NIH grant applicants and recipients were now required to report not only payments exceeding $5,000 received from industry but also other outside payments such as travel and meal reimbursement *requests* from private foundations "related to institutional responsibilities"—*within thirty days*—to their grantee institutional authorities. Institutional officials must then determine whether the payments represent "a significant financial conflict of interest" and, if so, report them to the NIH with an explanation as to how the conflict will be managed or eliminated. Grantee institutions and the NIH must make these disclosures available to anyone who asks for them within five days of a request. In addition, if NIH grantees fail to make timely disclosures, NIH can mandate a "bias" investigation concerning the investigators' research.

The most severe restriction of industry partnerships related to the government took place at the NIH intramural program. In response to the commotion launched by the *Los Angeles Times* and the ensuing congressional investigations, the NIH director convened a committee of senior academic officials to review the NIH's industry consulting policy. The committee recommended that NIH researchers be allowed to consult with industry but with stricter institutional oversight.[16] Nevertheless, in response to relentless media attention and congressional pressure, in 2005 the director banned all paid consulting at the NIH.[17]

MEDICAL JOURNALS

Four years prior to the Spectra case, increasingly industry-phobic editors of the *New England Journal of Medicine* began to ask authors of papers it published to disclose whether their research was industry sponsored. Because article authors had long acknowledged funders of their research, mainly charitable foundations or the NIH, to give them due credit, this requirement was not objectionable—nor was it rigorously enforced. But in response to the Spectra allegations, the same editors banned individuals with industry relationships from writing editorials or review articles concerning products related to those relationships.

Medical journals successively imitated the *New England Journal of Medicine* in imposing industry payment disclosure requirements on authors of published papers, and by 2008 almost all such journals had disclosure policies.[18] In many cases, the listed financial relationships of multi-authored papers were so lengthy that they nearly exceeded the space given to the science (more recently, journals took to moving these lists to searchable web links). Basic science journals initially engaged in some foot dragging, questioning the value of financial relationship disclosure,[19] but later caved in and followed the example of the medical periodicals.[20] Some medical journal editors have recommended authors disclose *all* affiliations, religious, political, or ideological.[21]

In 2005, the editors of *JAMA* introduced a requirement that papers reporting industry-sponsored studies include statistical analyses of the study data performed by academic statisticians independent of the sponsoring company.[22] This discriminatory move led to some objections[23], but the policy persisted for eight years, and the *JAMA* editor in chief publicly stated that if an industry refused to submit papers to the journal, it was because it had something to hide.[24]

IMPLEMENTATION OF THE RESEARCH REGULATIONS

The regulations that appeared in the early 1990s requiring institutional oversight of academic research relationships with industry and limiting faculty remuneration became progressively stricter at medical journals and in academic health centers and the government. In contrast to other industry-related activities discussed below, however, little information exists concerning the enforcement of these rules and their effects on research or innovation. For example, almost no data exist as to how many research projects have been subjected to management procedures or prohibited outright because of conflict-of-interest concerns. Management varies with the zeal of the managers. One "case study" at the University of California, San Francisco, where the management was particularly zealous, reported imposing management strategies on 26% of faculty relationships including giving up company stock, reduced payments for promotional speaking, and giving up management positions and leadership roles in clinical trials.[25] Absent feedback from faculty members about how these interventions affected their productivity, the effects are difficult to determine. Chapter 15 describes some consequences of the research rules on university and NIH intramural program efforts to partner with industry.

PHASE TWO: BANNING EVERYTHING

The Brennan Article and Its Effect

In early 2006, Troyen Brennan, a physician administrator at Harvard's Brigham and Women's Hospital, and 10 additional authors, three of whom previously held high-ranking administrative positions in academic medicine, published a "special article" in *JAMA* titled "Health Industry Practices That Create Conflicts of Interest: A Proposal for Academic Medical Centers."[26] The Brennan article called for an end to prevalent practices related to physician–industry interactions in academic health centers, and it explicitly stated that the recommendations should percolate throughout the entire medical profession. The article took as established that corporate medical marketing is fundamentally deceptive and that it inveigles physicians to prescribe unnecessary, unnecessarily expensive, and even dangerous products. It exhorted academic centers to limit or eliminate company marketing by banning all "gifts" including trivial reminder items such as mugs, calendars, and sticky pads as well as meals and product samples provided by sales representatives. Speakers' bureaus should disappear. Industry payments for research or education should go to institutions rather than individuals. Nearly every institutional conflict-of-interest policy cites this paper, which I subsequently refer to as the "Brennan *JAMA* article."

The Brennan *JAMA* article crystallized a set of ideas contemporaneously promoted in articles and full-length books by journalists and academics, including some prominent figures such as a former Harvard University president and editors of prestigious medical journals.[27] In addition to the criticisms of industry-marketing practices raised by Brennan, these books condemned the very value and probity of the medical products industry. The critics also claimed that the user fees industry provides to the FDA under the Prescription Drug User Fee Act rendered the relationship between the two entities "too cozy" and that as a result, the FDA was approving ineffective and unsafe products.

Two contemporaneous incidents contributed plausibility to this depiction of industry. In 2004, Merck withdrew from the market a pain-killer medication brand named Vioxx, which had been FDA approved in 2001 and was subsequently suspected of having lethal cardiovascular side effects. In the same year, the pharmaceutical giant Pfizer pleaded guilty to criminal charges and agreed to settle civil penalties of $450 million for alleged illegal off-label marketing of a drug named gabapentin (brand name Neurontin) manufactured by Parke-Davis, a company it had recently acquired. This case was the first of an ongoing string of guilty pleas and settlements adding up to billions of dollars. As reported in the media, the cases were open-and-shut examples of illegal behavior, but in reality the government extorts these settlements by threatening companies with a corporate death penalty known as debarment, as discussed in Chapter 14.

Several foundations and medical journals, the AAMC, the Institute of Medicine (IOM) of the National Academies of Science, and the American Medical Association endorsed some or all of the Brennan article's recommendations. Responding to growing pressure, academic health centers, states, and the federal government enacted regulations based on these recommendations.

WHAT GOT BANNED OR RESTRICTED

The rest of this chapter briefly reviews the activities that have been regulated. Chapter 7 returns to this list and explains the incidents at length and why the bans and restrictions are not factually or logically warranted. Because of its complexity and importance, Chapter 12 separately covers bans and restrictions on industry marketing.

Gifts

In 1993, long before the Brennan article, the Minnesota State Pharmacy Board enacted a ban on gifts (reminder items, meals, entertainment, educational subsidies) from medical products companies other than payment for specific services, such as consultation or research. It also required pharmaceutical companies to report all payments to physicians residing in the state, beginning in 1997. This reporting was ignored until a front-page *New York Times* article in 2007 highlighted large payments to a few physicians, notably a kidney specialist.[28] Although the story acknowledged that he was a leading authority on kidney disease, it insinuated that the payments were unsavory. The article proved popular, revealing that reporting industry payments sells copy and embarrasses recipients, providing a template for many such articles to come.

Academic health centers rapidly imposed bans on gifts. In 2008, the Massachusetts State legislature passed a law requiring a publicly searchable registry of industry payments to health care professionals and eliminating product samples, gifts, and industry-sponsored meals outside of physicians' offices. The regulations became known as the "Gift Ban Law."[29] Vermont passed similar legislation in 2009.[30] California, Maine, Nevada, West Virginia, and the District of Columbia have implemented less comprehensive statutes regarding industry payments. Between 2009 and 2010, lawmakers in Colorado, Connecticut, Illinois, Maryland, New Jersey, New York, Oregon, and Texas contemplated or enacted similar laws regarding payments to state employees.[31]

Chapter 13 describes how the disapproval of gifts dominates the logic of the conflict-of-interest movement narrative. This demonization has persisted despite the fact that the pharmaceutical, biotechnology, and medical device industry trade associations revised their voluntary codes concerning industry interactions with health care professionals to recommend eliminating all gifts to physicians except "modest" "educational materials." They also recommended restricting detailing-related meals to physicians' offices, banning subsidies for entertainment at professional meetings, declaring consulting activities in resorts off-limits and stipulating arbitrary caps on payments for physicians' speaking to other physicians about products.[32]

Professional Writing (Ghostwriting)

The conflict-of-interest movement uses the term "ghostwriting" to denote the use of undisclosed or inadequately disclosed professional writers to draft manuscripts and the inclusion of individuals as authors who it alleges may have made minimal or no contributions to the work. Such ghostwriting is now routinely banned by university conflict of interest policies, yet most policies do not define the term and those that do, define it vaguely and disparately. As discussed in Chapter 7, medical writers have a legitimate role in medical science, and authorship decisions can be contentious.

Commercial Support of Continuing Medical Education

Beginning in the 1970s, states imposed requirements on physicians to participate in ongoing education concerning their specialties as a condition of continuing licensure, and a large industry emerged catering to those demands. Academic health centers initially dominated this activity, but professional societies and private medical education companies competed for this increasingly large continuing medical education (CME) business. To try to assure the quality of CME offerings, the American Medical Association, the American Hospital Association, the American Board of Medical Specialties, and the AAMC established the Accreditation Council for Continuing Medical Education (ACCME) in 1980 to regulate the content of educational programs.

As industry funding of CME increased, through provision of grants to academic institutions, professional societies, and scientific meetings, it collided with the conflict-of-interest movement as it emerged in the 1990s. The movement's promoters wanted to reduce or eliminate company support of CME, which now exceeded half of CME funding. They averred that even if sponsoring companies did not control the specific content of educational presentations or who gave them—although they insisted that companies had such control and that presentations promoted the use of the sponsor's products[33]—the sponsorship skewed education toward conditions susceptible to treatment with the sponsor's medications and devices, because companies would support only topics relevant to their products.

As a result of these accusations, several medical institutions, such as the University of Michigan Medical School and Sloan Kettering Cancer Center, announced that they would no longer accommodate corporate support of their CME offerings unless such support went to an institutional fund with no restrictions as to educational topics. Not surprising, companies have expressed little interest in such giveaways, although in 2010 Pfizer awarded Stanford Medical School a $3 million unrestricted educational grant.[34]

The ACCME attempted to resist attacks from the conflict-of-interest movement by imposing what it termed "firewalls" between corporate sponsors and specific educational events. Sponsoring companies cannot select specific topics or speakers (although they may choose what general topics to fund). Presenters must disclose all their corporate relationships, declare whether they will discuss off-label product uses, and submit presentations for content review. Course managers must determine whether the presenters need to change or remove content that promotes or appears to promote specific products. The ACCME requires voluminous documentation verifying that these requirements have been met. ACCME has therefore become a large bureaucracy, and institutions must pay significant sums for its vetting work, which has become more complex in response to criticism of inadequate regulation of corporate influence.

Commercial Support of Professional Organizations

Subsequent articles modeled on the Brennan *JAMA* article recommended curtailing or eliminating commercial subsidy of professional societies and health advocacy organizations.[35] The Council of Medical Subspecialty Societies (CMSS), the umbrella organization for 40 professional societies, formalized a code in 2010 "for interactions with companies." Encased in rhetoric concerning "professionalism," the voluntary code emphasized appearances, as epitomized by the recommendation to exclude company logos from tote bags and other paraphernalia given to participants at society meetings. It encouraged reducing and diversifying corporate support. In a more severe measure, it recommended excluding professional society members with industry relationships from leadership positions in the organization, peer-reviewing corporate-sponsored presentations, prohibiting presenters with "unmanageable" conflicts of interest, and monitoring presentations by reviewers "trained to recognize bias."[36] Many major professional societies have dutifully complied.

Product Samples

The conflict-of-interest movement considers samples, usually small amounts of drugs or disposable devices, a specific "gift" species needing prohibition. Unlike most gifts, samples are intended for patients. The conflict-of-interest movement denounces samples because obtaining samples increases physician contact with sales representatives. The only concession conflict-of-interest movement promoters pay to samples having value is that they might benefit indigent patients, but they counter that such patients do not obtain most of the samples provided by physicians.[37]

Promotional Speaking (Speakers' Bureaus)

The 2006 Brennan article singled out promotional speaking as an unsavory activity for academic physicians. In 2007, a psychiatrist in private practice in Massachusetts published a *New York Times Magazine* article titled "Dr. Drug Rep" condemning this speaking practice. He expressed remorse for accepting what he deemed excessive hospitality from a drug company during training for speaking. He also alleged company marketing personnel pressured him to be more enthusiastic about a drug's benefits.[38] Academic institutions framing conflict-of-interest policies limited or banned such speaking by faculty, declaring it "unprofessional," because of the use of presentation graphics prepared by companies. As mentioned above, Massachusetts and Vermont passed laws in 2009 banning promotional speaking at restaurants.

Key Opinion Leaders

Marketing analysts coined the term "key opinion leader" (KOL) in the 1940s when they observed that consumers adopt products based on recommendations from persons known to them; if these individuals occupy positions of high respect, the adoption effect becomes stronger.[39] With passage of the Durham-Humphrey Amendment to FDA law in 1951, companies could not sell most of their products directly to patients. They therefore sought out physicians to fulfill the role of influential promoters of their wares, and such physicians came to be called KOLs.

The conflict-of-interest movement has denigrated such physicians, characterizing them baldly as industry shills. A prime example is an article that appeared in the *British Medical Journal* in 2008 titled "Key Opinion Leaders: Independent Experts or Drug Representatives in Disguise?" An accompanying illustration depicting a hideously deformed physician puppet being manipulated with strings obviated any doubt as to the answer to the question posed by the article's title.[40] Focusing mainly on promotional speakers, the article's emphasis was on the size of payments physicians earn in collaborating with industry, and it featured a testimonial by a former drug rep claiming that speakers' employment by industry depends solely on their prescribing volume of the sponsoring company's products. Another theory holds that physicians become KOLs purely for the perks and a sense of self-importance. Neither theory allows that promotional speaking might provide valuable information.

IMPLEMENTATION OF THE BANS AND RESTRICTIONS

In the 1970s, medical students unhappy with what they considered the American Medical Association student organization's too tepid opposition to the Vietnam War founded the American Medical Student Association (AMSA). AMSA's platform now supports alternative medical therapies and calls for industry to redirect its efforts toward making products for diseases affecting emerging nations. Recently, its main focus has been to encourage apartheid between medicine and industry. Since 2007, it has awarded "grades" to medical schools based on the stringency of their conflict-of-interest policies: a university gets an "A" for banning nearly all relationships considered inimical by the 2006 Brennan *JAMA* article and an "F" if lenient or lacking a policy, with grades in between for intermediate degrees of severity.

AMSA's grading of medical schools according to their conflict-of-interest policies is one benchmark for evaluating the march of conflict-of-interest regulation at academic health centers. The first scorecard, in 2007, a year after the Brennan *JAMA* manifesto started the regulatory thrust, reported that 115 of America's 152 medical schools had conflict-of-interest policies (and responded to AMSA's requests to obtain them). Of those, 9% received grades of A or B. Five years later, in 2012, 92% of schools received As or Bs. With the caveat that AMSA has a vested interest in demonstrating that its grading system has promoted policy direction, the Brennan article recommendations appear to have become widespread policy.

Even nonacademic practices have adopted the recommended policies.[41] Although figures vary according to specialty, between 19% and 55% of medical practices have imposed moderate limits on the access of company marketing representatives, and between 1% and 14% impose severe limits.[42]

One prominent manifestation of the "ban-everything" juggernaut was the passage of The Physician Payments Sunshine Act as part of the Affordable Care Act in 2010. Its title came from a famous quotation in a 1913 *Harper's Weekly* article by Supreme Court Justice Louis Brandeis: "Sunshine is said to be the best of disinfectants." Amplifying its insinuation that something is "infected" is the substance of the law: medical product manufacturers must publicly report, through the Centers for Medicare and Medicaid Services, all "transfers of value" (money or "gifts") to physicians in excess of *$10*. This law, implemented in 2013, fully embodies the spirit of the conflict-of-interest mania. It is clearly intended to limit, if not abolish, all payments from industry to physicians. This pressure to ban everything has the potential to dampen innovation and impair the exchange of information about new medical products, as discussed in Chapter 15.

4

THE MANIA MONGERS

Two sets of protagonists drive the conflict-of-interest movement. One set I designate the "instigators," those who initiated and propagate the conflict-of-interest movement. Another major population of conflict-of-interest movement protagonists I call the "enablers and enforcers" is the administrators who manage universities, professional organizations, medical journals, and even the medical products' industry itself. They have been the main conflict-of-interest policy framers. This chapter catalogs the instigator and enabler roster, exposes the organizations that provide them with financial support, and explains why universities and medical journals so strongly promote the conflict-of-interest narrative.

THE MANIA'S INSTIGATORS

One instigator subset, the Utopians, embraces idealized concepts of medicine and higher learning. The Hippocratic tradition, they claim, since ancient times differentiated profit-seeking charlatans from altruistic physicians, who although deserving of "modest" remuneration for services, always put patients' interests before their own, justifying quasi-priestly elevation to an exceptional position above "mere business." This special status earns them the trust of vulnerable patients. *Altruism* is, to these Utopians, the heart of "professionalism," which enables physicians to self-regulate. Commercialism, they aver, has tarnished medical professionalism, causing it to descend from a former state of exaltation.

The conflict-of-interest movement instigators' research equivalent of medical professionalism is scientific integrity, the selfless disinterested, objective, and bias-free search for truth for truth's sake. This quasi-robotic disinterest is what they allege justifies public support of higher learning and subsidy for research. They call for an absolute divide between medicine (and academe) and commerce: physicians' fiduciary responsibility is to patients, academics' to truth seeking, and industry's to profits. Attempts to straddle the demands of medical professionalism or academic purity with the nether world of business profits compromise the moral high ground of scientific integrity and professionalism and cause neglect of duty (disloyalty) to patients. The Utopians impose their ideals as *obligations* rather than as difficult if not nearly unattainable *aspirations*. This absolutism renders inevitable deviations from perfection serious transgressions rather than inevitable errors. It also enables these instigators to deride articulated claims of industry to having an interest in promoting patient welfare, because its fiduciary responsibility to make profits renders these claims hypocritical.

While some conflict-of-interest movement instigators may be sincerely committed to these lofty ideals, later chapters explain why they are false. They are artifacts of medicine's pre-scientific past and misrepresentations of scientific inquiry. Principles aside, legitimate or not, however, many instigators have exploited industry relationship criticism and its regulation as a vocation: they garner academic advancement by publishing articles in accommodating medical journals and in books and further the agendas of their sponsors. These activities have elevated their status to becoming declared experts on conflicts of interest, and this status gains them access to and often dominance of policy deliberations concerning industry relationships. Some serve as plaintiffs' or prosecutors' witnesses in lawsuits against medical products companies. In the mental health field, Scientology adherents who oppose psychiatry and non-physician therapists who lack drug-prescribing privileges can promote their agendas by attacking the use of psychiatric medications. Purveyors of food additives, "natural" medications, and "supplements," ("nutraceuticals") are also conflict-of-interest movement instigators. They claim that the pharmaceutical industry is behind a conspiracy, condoned by the FDA, to overmedicate the population that would be far better off if allowed freely to purchase the nutraceutical promoters' wares.[1]

A handful of former medical products industry sales representatives or physicians who once served as promotional speakers have, in turncoat fashion, flipped to become conflict-of-interest movement instigators and reveal what they claim are unsavory industry practices of which they allege to possess insider knowledge.

Politician conflict-of-interest movement instigators gain attention by prosecuting the corruption allegations served up by the conflict-of-interest narrative. The most active conflict-of-interest movement's political agitator has been Iowa Senator Charles Grassley. In 2004, when he was the ranking member of the Senate Commerce Committee, he held hearings concerning the Vioxx withdrawal and the NIH consulting fracas. Chapter 15 discusses in detail how, beginning in 2008, Grassley demanded that medical schools provide him with information regarding consulting payments from companies disclosed by selected faculty physicians as required by the schools' conflict-of-interest policies and compared the reported sums with amounts the companies paid the consultants. This exercise revealed large discrepancies in over a dozen instances.

Joining the politicians in stepping on the conflict-of-interest movement bandwagon have been populist advocacy organizations such as the AARP, *Consumer Reports*, and Public Citizen.

Another conflict-of-interest movement instigator set with a commercial agenda is the news media that sell copy based on sensationalized corruption claims. The reported material abets the conflict-of-interest instigators who profit most from the conflict-of-interest movement, the lawyers who prosecute medical products companies, or the physicians who work with such companies.

THE MANIA'S ENABLERS AND ENFORCERS

Many of these individuals forthrightly *articulate* the importance of industry's contributions to medical innovation and the value of relationships for medical advances. Moreover, they claim to disavow the sanctimony of the extreme Utopians.

But these enablers embellish their rhetoric with the instigators' demands for "trust," "integrity," and "avoidance of bias." These disclaimers, especially when they routinely wander into concerns about *appear-*

ances of conflict of interest, tacitly affirm that the medicine-industry interface has or is likely to compromise "trust" and "integrity" and promote "bias." They therefore open the door for the instigators to spin almost any behavior as untrustworthy.

Enablement also permeates the health care products industry itself. With rare exceptions, top industry leaders have failed to rebut the corruption allegations. Most importantly, the industry has neglected to defend the economic realities and profitability requirements on which it depends to stay in business. Accomplished physicians and academic researchers that companies routinely appoint and handsomely remunerate for service on corporate and scientific advisory boards have also been resoundingly silent. The reticence, presumably intended to avoid gratuitous attacks from conflict-of-interest movement instigators, is very unfortunate, as these advisors, many of whom have substantive track records of scholarly accomplishment and include Nobel and other prestigious prizewinners, have far greater credibility than the conflict-of-interest instigators and enablers.

THE MANIA'S PAYMASTERS

Individuals and institutions with ideological or other personal agendas have allowed the conflict-of-interest movement to thrive and freely publicize its messages. Proceeds from settlements related to prosecutions of medical products companies have been one source of financial support for the conflict-of-interest movement instigators. The billionaire George Soros's Open Society Foundation donated $7.3 million to a Columbia University sociologist and co-author of the 2006 Brennan *JAMA* manifesto to found an "Institute of Medicine as a Profession (IMAP)."[2] Other university-based conflict-of-interest movement policy operations include the Safra Center at Harvard's Kennedy School of Government, dedicated to exposing and eliminating "institutional corruption," and the Mongan Institute for Health Policy, based at Boston's Harvard-affiliated Massachusetts General Hospital.

The Josiah Macy Foundation has spearheaded efforts to eliminate industry support of medical education. It has funded IMAP and the Mongan Institute as well as underwritten an Institute of Medicine (of the National Academy of Sciences) commission that recommended restrictive industry relationship policies.[3] The Pew Charitable Trusts, funded by the past profits of Pennsylvania oil companies, has liberally subsidized a number of conflict-of-interest movement organizations including "Community Catalyst" and a "Prescription Project." The 2013 version of the Prescription Project website explicitly states that it advocates for the principles articulated by the 2006 Brennan *JAMA* article.[4] The Pew Trust has also underwritten the American Medical Student Association (AMSA), which as discussed in chapter 3, "grades" medical schools on the stringency of their conflict-of-interest policies.

WHY DOES THE ACADEMIC MEDICAL ESTABLISHMENT PROMOTE THE CONFLICT-OF-INTEREST MOVEMENT?

The history of modern American medicine reveals the answer to this question. The medicine presently practiced by most practitioners, based on current understanding of human biology and knowledge regarding the effects of drugs, vaccines, and surgical procedures, is defined as "allopathic." Allopathic medicine won out by the 1950s over competing practices such as homeopathy. University-affiliated medical schools sat at allopathic medicine's pinnacle,[5] because 40 years earlier, the Carnegie Foundation's Flexner Report had catalyzed the European-styled control of universities over medical pedagogy that previously took place in apprenticeships or in commercial diploma mills.[6] Organized medicine used the report to promote legislation that limited medical licensure only to graduates of accredited university-associated medical schools. Although these developments provided medical graduates with a firmer grounding in medical science, this foundation did not accomplish much to improve their clinical performance. Physicians of any type in the early 1900s still had little at their disposal to help patients. For example, at that time, most serious diseases encountered by physicians were of microbial origin, and lacking antibiotics, physicians could diagnose infections but do little else to treat them.

What the Flexner effort did accomplish, however, was to increase markedly the control universities came to wield over American medicine. The elimination of competing pathways to a medical career meant that a relatively small number of medical schools were available for a larger pool of potential students than they could accommodate. This monopoly limited the number—and raised the incomes—of medical graduates and elevated the prestige of now far more selective educational institutions.

A benign economic climate for medicine up through the 1960s muted concerns about the top-down hierarchical management of medical schools. Reliable and generous Medicare reimbursements at its 1964 enactment for services that indigent patients could not previously provide allayed physicians' suspicions of the government capitalizing medicine. Medical schools expanded in number and size thanks to liberal government subsidies for construction, faculty recruitment, and stipends for physicians in training (interns, residents, and fellows receiving specialty training).

Prior to the 1950s, most American medical research took place in a handful of universities or at a few freestanding charitably endowed research institutes. A marked expansion of the NIH changed this landscape.[7] Most research that the NIH funds is done by university-based investigators who submit grant applications that reviewers drawn from the academic research community prioritize for funding on the basis of their assessments of proposal quality. The NIH's enlarged granting program enabled medical schools to expand their faculties and build an extensive research enterprise. Academic health center leaders competed with one another to recruit star researchers and prided themselves on how many papers their departments published in journals and presented at professional society meetings.[8] At that time, scholarly accomplishment was an absolute requirement for leadership positions in medicine. Most chairs of medical specialty departments in universities, editors of medical journals, and heads of professional societies had made medical research contributions. On the other hand, the management of academic health centers' business affairs was a relatively small and casual enterprise, and the individuals responsible for it were anonymous and few.

The era of economic benignity and the academic bubble it accommodated, however, was short lived. Relentlessly rising medical costs and competition for federal spending in the 1970s and 1980s forced the academic ecosystem to increase its engagement in reimbursable clinical activities, irrespective of their educational or research value. Obtaining NIH funding became more difficult and highly unpredictable. Dependent on fluctuating federal budgets, NIH funding has, adjusted for inflation, declined, and presently only a minority of grant applications submitted to the agency achieve funding. Moreover, grant payments have been reduced in amount and duration. A downside of the years of generous NIH funding was that academic institutions became dependent on it, and many lacked financial reserves to replace federal dollars when they declined. Reductions in Medicare and other reimbursements for clinical services also eliminated the cross subsidy these payments had provided earlier for time spent in research. A prediction that these forces would diminish the number of physicians participating in medical research has been born out.[9]

One response of academic health centers to address rising medical costs and reduced reimbursements for clinical services was to absorb community physician practices. Many practitioners, facing reduced public and private insurance reimbursements and increasing bureaucratic impediments to obtain them, willingly exchanged the independence of private practice for what they perceived as the relative security of institutional employment. The earlier sharp distinctions between academics focused on research and education and physicians in the business of clinical practice progressively blurred. The "local medical doctors," at whom academics had sneered for supposedly mismanaging patients that ended up in their university hospitals, became coveted allies to recruit patients and even to join hospital primary care practices.

Today academic health centers, while predominantly being nonprofits, are large businesses headed by highly paid executives, and they advertise their services aggressively and hyperbolically and generate most of their operating revenues from clinical services.[10] The administrations of academic and nonacademic health centers are large bureaucracies focused predominantly on cash flow. Not only are their top leaders no longer anonymous, they are often local celebrities. The enfranchisement of a dominant manager class increasingly separated culturally from practitioners, researchers, and educators in medical centers is not a conspiracy. It is, rather, a consequence of the growth in size and complexity of medicine. Charisma plus business and political savvy are adaptive characteristics of successful medical managers.

As the few employees of academic health centers with large hardwired salaries, top administrators have a compelling reason to prevent disruptions that could threaten their power and profits by accommodating restrictive conflict-of-interest regulations. This plausible assertion reliably evokes indignant protest from those in authority. But to accuse them of self-protectionism by attempting to prevent theoretical criticism is no more offensive than conflict-of-interest movement instigators and enablers declaring perfectly justifiable activities of individuals remunerated for industry-related activities to be perceived as corrupt—and legislate against them. Furthermore, as discussed in Chapter 6, the regulations imposed by conflict-of-interest movement enablers conveniently spare them from most personal consequences.

The rank and file professional employees of these institutions who *do* suffer the consequences are predominantly passive. They submit to cumbersome anachronistic academic promotion practices that confer largely financially irrelevant titles on them. In many, especially private medical schools, only success at garnering external salary support guarantees "academic freedom." Promotion to senior faculty ranks can confer what universities may define as "tenure," but increasingly the position has no set remuneration; a faculty member who fails to obtain external support is expected to leave the institution. Struggling to maintain clinical practices, research programs, and educational activities, faculty members lack the time to study the regulations' justification and fear administrative reprisals. Potential consequences include withdrawal of academic promotion prospects or financial support and public opprobrium. Most medical professionals, selected on the basis of having obediently jumped through a long series of academic hoops, are not constitutionally inclined to resist authority. The more top-heavy hierarchical structure of today's medical centers and the intrusion of more and more bureaucratic compliance requirements as well as the greater difficulty in obtaining external funding have eroded faculty independence. Because the NIH funding constraints affect all American medical research institutions, the ability of employees in most businesses to address employer abuse by moving to another firm for better treatment is not an option for most medical academics. In addition, hindrances to mobility include the facts that researchers require expensive equipment and highly trained assistants, and many clinicians have loyal patients.

In the past, when the number of medical products was relatively small and most medical research took place in academic institutions, medical product companies predominantly looked to medical schools to test their products and depended heavily on academic medical authorities for promoting the credibility of those products. This deferential attitude on the part of industry toward academe persists, presumably contributing to industry's tolerance of the abuse academe inflicts on it, even though industry contributes more to practical medical innovation than universities do (discussed in Chapter 8). But as clinical trials have increased in number, size, and sophistication, companies began fleeing what they experienced as an increasingly bureaucratic, entitled, and expensive culture with which American academe approached clinical trials and looked to private clinical trial organizations (CROs) that managed research performed by community physicians or to academic centers outside of the United States. American academic centers faced with a loss of revenues from their clinical trial business have complained about the "ethics" of using such venues for clinical research.[11] In doing so, they pounced on a few incidents in which volunteer research subjects were harmed by trials in these nonacademic CROs.[12] But harm also befalls research subjects in clinical trials with no commercial sponsorship.[13]

Industry's investment in medical research surpassed NIH's in 1987, is currently twice that of the NIH, and is a logical source from which to supplant disappearing federal monies for academic activities. But although a few companies and medical schools have formed research partnerships over the years, this potential sustenance for university research remains largely untapped. If the leadership of academic medical centers was truly passionate about innovation, it might be more cautious about the adversarial attitude toward industry it has accommodated in welcoming the principles of the conflict-of-interest narrative and in enacting the regulations it calls for.

HOW AND WHY MEDICAL JOURNALS FOSTER THE CONFLICT-OF-INTEREST MANIA

Medical Journals Promote the Conflict-of-Interest Narrative

In addition to books and media reports, medical journals have been the backbone of the conflict-of-interest narrative. The relevant content in medical journal articles has consisted of some original research, primarily surveys of physicians describing their self-reporting of the nature, extent, and perceived effects of their interactions with the medical products industry (described in detail in Chapter 12) or of patients' attitudes toward physicians' industry relationships and summaries of institutional conflict-of-interest policies. Most of the material, however, has been commentaries conveying writers' opinions regarding such relationships.

Having closely followed the march of the conflict-of-interest movement, I was intuitively aware that its coverage by medical journals was extremely one sided. Over a decade lapsed between publication of a lone paper in the *JAMA* in 1993, titled "Conflict of Interest: The New McCarthyism in Science,[14] and one I managed to get accepted for publication by *The New England Journal of Medicine* (*NEJM*) defending academic and physician-industry relationships in 2005.[15] In 2010, I initiated a formal analysis of over a hundred such articles published in four prominent medical journals, *NEJM*, *JAMA*, *The Lancet*, and *Lancet Neurology*. The exercise led to the striking finding that almost 90% of the published articles emphasized the downside risks of such interactions.[16] The emphasis was not subtle, as many of the articles had tendentious titles such as "dancing with the porcupine," "in the grip of the python," "the impugning of medical science," "uneasy alliance," and "is academic medicine for sale?"

More remarkably, less than half of these risk-emphasizing articles provided any evidence whatsoever to support their conclusions regarding risk, and to the extent they presented evidence, it was at best anecdotal and at worst speculative or even false. Less than a fifth of them even mentioned that relationships might be beneficial, and only a few attempted to explain why the risks offset benefits. Of the handful of articles emphasizing benefits of industry interactions, all of them presented evidence and discussed the risk elements.

Medical journals have clearly been extremely influential in spreading the gospel of the conflict-of-interest movement. Ideological predilections of their managers are one explanation for this behavior, but more important, it is a reflection of a conceit that medical journal managers sell: namely that the most important repository of truthful and valuable medical information resides in what these journals publish. By inference, information provided by the medical products' industry—denigrated as "marketing"—is inferior. The journal managers' success in promoting that message is a reflection of the journals' dominance in the academic medical establishment and the great public adulation they enjoy. The remainder of this chapter describes the errors of much of that journal manager sales pitch.

Who Medical Journal Managers Say Medical Journals Are for and Who They Are Really For

Is this statement true?: "Physicians and patients rely on medical journals as trusted sources of medical information."[17] No. The founding of the first scientific journal in the 17th century has been appropriately hailed as one of the great steps in modern intellectual history.[18] People engage in scientific pursuits for diverse reasons, but contrary to the Utopian dream that they seek truth for truth's sake, most scientists want recognition for their accomplishments. Prior to the existence of journals, they had no reliable way to stake claims for the priority of their discoveries.[19] As a result, they resorted to hoarding information about their findings, occasionally publishing large tomes describing years or decades of effort, or like Leonardo da Vinci, recorded encrypted messages describing his scientific insights. In the 17th century, the first scientific journal, The Philosophical Transactions of the Royal Society of London, solved this identity problem by publishing, within a few months, relatively brief "letters" in the order of their receipt containing descriptions of diverse scientific contributions. This system accelerated the dissemination of scientific information and enabled affording credit to discoverers of that information.

As science evolved from an activity of independently wealthy or patronized amateurs to one of professionals working in universities, articles submitted to journals for publication predominantly originated from such institutions. The number and quality of faculty members' publications determined academic promotion and the awarding of research funding by granting agencies. Academics communicate with one another in many ways: through correspondence, seminars, and informal conversation at scientific meetings, but the journal publication is the currency that affords academic status. The adage "publish or perish" is a venerable truism.

Over the centuries, as science grew in scope and magnitude, the number of journals increased, as did their differentiation to focus on different scientific disciplines. Medical journals were latecomers to the mix, but their primary purpose—communication between professionals—and their service as mechanisms for affording credit to academic scholars were no different than those of the nonmedical periodicals.

Given this history, medical journals existed for medical academics and researchers, not for physicians and patients. Indeed how could journals help patients? Can patients learn important and useful health information from them, as they gather other information from newspapers, magazines, radio, television, or the Internet? Hardly. The language of medical journal articles is highly technical and impenetrable to nearly all but trained experts. In addition, as discussed below, most medical journals are not immediately accessible to the public.

Perhaps if medical journal articles were like technical manuals enabling physicians to find specific instructions for how to minister to patients, the citation at the head of this section might make more sense. But for many reasons medical journal articles are rarely precise how-to descriptions. Journal articles have a contrived stereotypical style that only aficionados can decipher. The design of research articles describing clinical trials of drugs, diagnostics, or devices, for example, is supposed to instruct experts on how the study was done in sufficient detail to permit their replication. To save space, however, journals relegate study methods and many study results to fine print and to supplemental repositories that readers must track down. Based on these features of medical journals, the inescapable conclusion is that they do not inform practicing physicians' management of patients.[20] Common sense supports this conclusion, and Chapter 12 explains further the limitations of journal articles as sources of information to instruct physicians.

Journals as Brands

The oversold importance of medical journals as conveyances of practical clinical information is the result of highly successful marketing that has brought status, power—and wealth—to a few medical journal managers. For the first three centuries of their existence, journals appeared and disappeared, and they were shabby genteel enterprises that struggled economically.[21] Some journals survived financially because of sponsorship by scientific and medical professional societies that required their members to be paid subscribers. But recent developments turned a few journals into highly successful businesses.

One reason was the sheer growth of the scientific enterprise. At face value, expanding the size and number of journals could have accommodated the increase in material to communicate. But nothing attests more eloquently to the role of vanity in journal publishing than the fact that on balance the journals' market evolved just like any other—by successful branding.

If scientific publication were truly logical, researchers would submit papers only to journals covering their specialty, and other specialists would subscribe to those journals. Such a system would be efficient in that scholars could keep abreast of their field by reading a limited number of journal sources. But the perception that publishing per se does not get a researcher's signal above a cacophony of science output noise played into the hands of a few "general" journals. They branded themselves as "interdisciplinary," claimed to select articles of general interest to all scientists and thereby managed to get themselves at the top of a prestige pecking order. Such one-stop shopping may make sense for groceries and hardware purchasers, but the notion that geneticists or cell biologists really benefit intellectually from having their papers next to articles by quantum physicists, astronomers, or geologists does not. Similarly, as medicine has become increasingly specialized, the chance that cardiologists, ophthalmologists, or spine surgeons will find the same papers of interest is small. The perceived benefit of publishing one's research in general journals is not intellectual but rather is predominantly social.

The documentation of journal prestige has become an industry. The principal statistic defining a journal's prominence is its "impact factor," the number of times papers it publishes are cited by others over a fixed time period. Journals therefore court certain types of articles such as large clinical trials that raise their impact factors. Medical school administrators may rely on journal impact factors as benchmarks to decide faculty promotions. Rather than examine the content of publications, they simply compile the number of articles faculty members have published in the highest impact factor periodicals.[22]

A key ingredient mediating a journal's ascent to the top of the prestige hierarchy is to capture articles authored by the leading figures of a research field. Others reliably flock to compete for having their work associated with that of these stars. Journals exploit this herd behavior by making no effort to accommodate the rising rate of accumulating scientific information. Rather, they simply become more selective by rejecting the majority, in some cases over 90%, of submitted papers. The desperate yearning of researchers for high-profile space in such journals and the arbitrary limitation of that space, further constrained by the "interdisciplinary" imperative, make the probability of success extremely low. Economists refer to this behavior as the creation of a "false scarcity."[23]

Within a short reign of nine years (1967–1976), a charismatic editor named Franz Ingelfinger turned the NEJM into the world's most prestigious medical periodical. He astutely recognized a growing public interest in medicine in the 1960s, courted the lay media, and encouraged the crafting of readable editorials with catchy titles. Most importantly, Ingelfinger put a stop to researchers' holding of press conferences to announce discoveries that had been slated for publication in the NEJM. He established an embargo system in which the NEJM releases papers to the press a week prior to publication to allow reporters to write their stories, but the stories cannot appear until the embargo date. This prohibition became eponymous as "the Ingelfinger rule." Most journals have since adopted it, claiming the rule protects physicians and the public from premature exposure to incomplete medical information. But it is really about increasing the journals' notoriety by nudging the press to give them credit for medical findings of public interest.[24] This tactic has the effect of making the public associate such information with specific journals that are far more visible than the researchers who actually do the research work; were the researchers to call a press conference after the embargo, the novelty is past, and the press no longer has any interest.

Ingelfinger also welcomed publication of emerging clinical trials, shortsightedly considered too lowbrow—viewed as comparing commodities, like beer brands—by the editors of the then most prestigious medical science journals. He also embraced epidemiologic studies, such as correlations between diet and disease, to which the public could relate. He promoted false scarcity. Despite a marked increase in the number of submitted papers, he kept the number of published papers per issue constant. This rationing enhanced the NEJM's exclusivity, and the rapid growth in clinical trials benefited other general medical journals, notably JAMA and The Lancet, because they were able to pick up the spillover from arbitrarily rejected NEJM papers.

Peer Review

Selectivity in journal publication based on opinions of referees lagged years behind their founding. The first journals exercised no discrimination whatsoever, and they explicitly denied responsibility for the quality of the published content. Only when the volume of submitted papers exceeded these journals' capacity to accommodate them did editors begin to pick and chose what they published.[25]

In its idealized depiction, peer review is a voluntary public service altruistically provided by scholars to uphold community standards of excellence. To the rank-and-file scientists, the reality is far less sanguine. Operationally, peer review consists of journal editors selecting reviewers deemed knowledgeable with the field, represented by submitted papers, to read the papers critically and make recommendations to the editors based on their assessment of the paper's importance to the field, interest to potential readers, clarity and readability, and most important, soundness of conclusions based on presented evidence.

Having served as author of many research papers, a reviewer for journals, and a journal editor, I can attest to and have documented flaws of this system.[26] An editor familiar with a field can usually determine the critical outcome simply by selecting reviewers. The age, experience, personalities, and competitive relationship to authors of reviewers all determine the character of reviews. Young referees are more likely to provide in-depth critiques but tend to be hypercritical, whereas senior scientists frequently deliver offhand imperial opinions. Reviewers most competent to review papers are frequently paper writers' competitors—or else cronies. When researchers are vying for priority or embroiled in disputes, the temptation to hide behind the anonymity afforded reviewers to prevent or delay publication by adversaries is strong. Experienced advocates can cleverly disguise obstructionist reviewing with rhetorical artistry. The principal value of peer review is that it imposes some accountability. To the extent that researchers and commentators know that what they claim must convince reviewers and collect the best possible evidence to accomplish that goal, the accountability is useful. But when researchers must pander to reviewers' prejudices and personal agendas—as frequently occurs—utility dissipates.

Journal Content Quality

Despite the vaunted gatekeeper functions of peer reviewers and editors, analysts have documented that a large number of journal publications do not report findings that withstand subsequent scrutiny. One reason for this poor reproducibility is a convention of deeming experimental results publishable when statistical analysis implies that the outcome of the experiments is not simply due to random chance. Experience reveals that when, as is often the case, the effect is relatively small or the experiments are performed a limited number of times, the significance does not hold up to further study. Another factor may be that once research results appear in high-profile journals, they achieve a status that discourages other researchers from challenging them.[27] Recently industry researchers have documented an inability to reproduce seemingly promising research results potentially relevant to clinical drug targets published by academics in prestigious scientific journals.[28]

For all its flaws and the frustrations it inflicts on researchers as recounted, the medical (and research) journal remains as the most if not entirely reliable repository for documenting the steady, inefficient advance of medical science. In the fullness of time, most research gets published.[29] But the lasting effect of research revolves far more on the persistence of researchers and the ultimate reproducibility and utility of their findings.

Journal Economics

Prior to the Internet and electronic publishing, journal financing required covering fixed costs of correspondence with authors and reviewers, printing and binding of papers, and periodically distributing the volumes to subscribers who paid for these expenses through subscription charges. The professionalization of science resulted in academic libraries becoming dominant subscribers, initially accumulating print versions of the journals and, more recently, licenses to enable faculty to download electronic versions of papers. In recent years, the increased number of journals has severely strained university library budgets.

A large disparity now divides the economics of the elite journals from others. Most journals nowadays have been taken over by large publishing houses that make marginal profits off of specialty journals with relatively few subscribers and little or no advertising. An intermediate class of journals that represent large professional societies is more profitable because association members are compelled to pay subscription fees as a membership condition. Most of the low- and intermediate-subscription journals extract fees from authors, charging for paper handling and article reprints. Although electronic access has largely eliminated reprint purchases by academics, industry buys them for marketing purposes. Advertising also generates revenue for clinical journals covering medical specialties that involve brand products. The top-tier general journals, however, have been extremely profitable. Large subscription bases attract advertising by the medical products industry and by medical service providers seeking to hire physicians and who pay for want ads. The top journals do not publicly reveal their profits, but 2009 tax records of the Massachusetts Medical Society, owner of the NEJM, reported "publication" revenues of $90 million with $20 million in "advertising."[30] Hence, these journals have a lucrative market, and it behooves their managers to sustain the illusion that they are, contrary to much evidence presented here, the most reliable and effective modalities for physician education.

Where does all the money go? It depends on who owns the information factory. The nonprofit Association for the Advancement of Science controls Science, the JAMA belongs to the American Medical Association, the Massachusetts Medical Society is the parent of the NEJM, and a subsidiary of the private British publishing company Macmillan, the Nature Publishing Group, manages Nature and a stable of specialty spin-off journals. Commentators have decried the emergence of "predatory publishers" who have created new open-access electronic journals promising easy and rapid dissemination of research, mainly motivated by acquisitioning submission fees from authors.[31] Because authors submitting papers pay for almost all journal publication, it is unclear that these opportunists are any more "predatory" than the mainstream journals.

The profits from the various journals benefit the purposes of these diverse entities. None of them revert to the researchers who create the value of these journals. Nor do they go to right the education topic distortions conflict-of-interest movement critics allege result from commercial subsidy of medical education.

III

Why They Are Wrong

5

ABUSING EVIDENCE

Until relatively recently, a fanciful theory hatched in antiquity guided medical therapy: imbalances in the four humors—blood, black and yellow bile, and phlegm—caused diseases, and the useless and harmful practices of bleeding and purging were supposed to restore balance and effect cures.[1] Only in the past two centuries has scientific evidence based on direct observation informed medical diagnosis and treatment, and presently, "evidence-based medicine" is in vogue.

This chapter reviews a paradox: the conflict-of-interest narrative, on the one hand, is reminiscent of ancient medicine in that it prescribes on the basis of authoritatively presented, subjective *beliefs* for which little or no evidence exists. The narrative also freely extrapolates from a handful of isolated and misrepresented anecdotes to draw sweeping conclusions. This chapter exposes the specific misrepresentations of some of these anecdotes. On the other hand, the conflict-of-interest narrative presumes that evidence exists or is easily attainable to accommodate a Utopian standard of comprehensive scientific knowledge to justify the introduction of new products into our medical repertory. It promotes the conceit that only after vast amounts of information have been published in medical journals and analyzed by academic statisticians who may comprehend little or nothing about the data content or how it was obtained will we know the benefits and risks of medical therapies. It also advances the idea that industry deliberately suppresses data "transparency" and all evidence that bears adversely on its products. The conflict-of-interest movement's case for such suppression rests on an elaborate smokescreen that obscures the fact that the most relevant evidence for medical product efficacy and safety is the data that companies submit for evaluation to the FDA. This evidence is far more complete and rigorously analyzed than what academics publish in medical journals. With that obfuscation in place, the conflict-of-interest narrative trumpets what it alleges are the devious tactics industry allegedly uses to misrepresent the far less relevant evidence disseminated by medical journals.

AUTHORITY AND SPECULATION MASQUERADING AS EVIDENCE

The relentless march of conflict-of-interest regulation is a tribute to the confidence and authority with which the conflict-of-interest narrative presents its case. For example the 2006 Brennan *JAMA* article begins with this ringing indictment:[2]

> The current influence of market incentives in the United States is posing extraordinary challenges to the principles of medical professionalism. Physicians' commitment to altruism, putting the interests of patients first, scientific integrity, and an absence of bias in medical decision making now regularly come up against financial conflicts of interest. Arguably, the most challenging and extensive of these conflicts emanate from relationships between physicians and pharmaceutical companies and medical device manufacturers.

This statement exemplifies how the conflict-of-interest narrative abounds with confident imperial and *quantitative* assertions: "*extraordinary* challenges," "physicians' commitments…*regularly* come up" "*the most challenging and extensive* of these conflicts emanate from [industry] relationships."

The conflict-of-interest narrative plays fast and loose with evidence. The Brennan *JAMA* manifesto's opening paragraph, cited above, contains a reference to a 2004 article written by Arthur Schafer, a philosophy professor at the University of Manitoba, that was published in *The Journal of Medical Ethics*.[3]

Although Shafer took a dim view of industry's intrusion into the academy and concluded it should withdraw from it, *nothing* in his article supports the forthright assertions of the Brennan *JAMA* article's opening salvo quoted above. Schafer's piece concerns *research* relationships, not the corporate *marketing* activities targeted by Brennan and his co-authors. The conflict-of-interest narrative abounds with such false attribution, selective citation, and as explained in the previous chapter, lack of balance.

Another signature of the conflict-of-interest narrative literature is speculation. For example, an editorial commentary buttresses its forthright assertion that physician-industry relationships "can . . . have serious negative effects" with an impressive array of hypotheticals:[4]

> But physician–industry relationships can also have serious negative effects. For example, doctors with ties to industry *may* be more inclined than their colleagues to prescribe a brand-name drug despite the availability of a cheaper generic version. The provision of free samples *may* reinforce this behavior and *perhaps* stimulate off-label use of medications, which *can* pose risks for some patients. Industry relationships *may* stimulate the premature adoption of novel treatments, which *could* lead to serious health problems for patients. Industry inducements *may* reduce physician adherence to evidence-based practice guidelines in favor of company medications or interventions that are not recommended in independently developed guidelines. Finally, the financial rewards from industry relationships *may* reinforce a culture of entitlement among physicians, which *could* limit their ability to honestly acknowledge and manage the potential negative effects of these relationships [emphasis added].

Although such authors suggest that negative outcome *may* happen, they don't concede the possibility that they also *may not* happen.[5]

THE CANONICAL CASES DON'T MAKE THE CASE— QUANTITATIVELY OR QUALITATIVELY

The Cases' Numbers Don't Add Up

Chapter 3 summarized some of the most commonly mentioned incidents ascribed to financial conflicts of interest in medicine. In and of itself, the list of actual incidents of conflict of interest is small in comparison to the thousands of industry relationships that have been sufficiently neutral or positive over the two and a half decades that the conflict-of-interest movement has been in force.

Also conspicuously missing from the cases discussed in Chapter 3 are examples of research misconduct, formally defined as plagiarism; fabrication; or falsification of research results.[6] A review of 106 of such misconduct cases reported over an eight-year interval revealed that 105 took place in nonprofit institutions and had no commercial involvement.[7] Of 98 English language research papers retracted over a 40-year interval because of research misconduct, 96% had no declared industry support.[8] These findings invalidate the assumption underlying the rules limiting or eliminating industry payments or equity for research that financial gain or prospects of such gain from commercial sources cause serious problems in conducting or reporting research. The findings are not surprising in view of the far more stringent oversight of industry research compared to that in academe (discussed further below) and the fact that the consequences of research misconduct are much greater for companies than for universities. Fabricated or falsified research never leads to useful medical products, because their lack or reproducibility cannot withstand the rigors of FDA analysis. Companies, compared to universities, not only are more sensitive to the financial waste incurred by such flawed research but also to the potential for criminal prosecution.

The Cases' Facts Don't Add Up

As the following cases exemplify, additional information and interpretations about the incidents invalidate these stories as a serious justification for conflict-of-interest regulation. Although addressing all of the canonical incidents commonly cited by the conflict-of-interest narrative is beyond the scope of this book, the pattern of incomplete framing and misrepresentation exposed here is broadly applicable to the collection of canonical incidents commonly cited in the conflict-of-interest narrative.

The Spectra Case

According to the *Boston Globe*'s reporting of this incident, the involved researcher, Tseng, treated more patients than the institution's ethical review board had approved. In addition, the *Globe* alleged that Tseng had shares of stock in Spectra and sold them based on his impression that the treatment was not clinically effective, anticipating that the share value would fall when this negative information became publicly known.[9]

An internal review of this incident concluded that the management of Tseng's research activities at the Massachusetts Eye and Ear Infirmary was lax, and this conclusion resulted in the firing of his superiors. But Tseng's alleged human subjects violations potentially subjected him to reprimand or medical license revocation by the state medical board. His sale of company stock, if true, represented insider trading—a Securities and Exchange Commission felony. But investigations by the Massachusetts Board of Registration in Medicine and the Securities and Exchange Commission exonerated him. Following his termination by the Massachusetts Eye and Ear Infirmary, Tseng moved to the University of Miami, Florida, where he continues to practice ophthalmology and do eye research to this day.[10]

The Dong Case

The Boots company that sponsored Dong's research could well have allowed her to publish her paper; thyroid specialists today almost all prescribe the synthetic form of thyroid hormone Dong found equivalent to crude animal thyroid extracts. The reason is that in practice rather than in a clinical trial, maintaining desired blood levels of the hormone is far more reliable with the synthetic hormone.[11]

The Deferiprone Case

Marian Shuchman, a psychiatrist and medical writer, initially reported the canonical version of the deferiprone story at the University of Toronto. With passage of time and additional due diligence, she came to a very different set of conclusions summarized in an award-winning book, *The Drug Trial*.[12] According to Shuchman's revised version of the events, clashes with university authorities had more to do with the whistleblowing researcher's treatment by University of Toronto officials than with deferiprone. European Union regulators approved the drug in 1999, specialists in the United States prescribed it for iron-overloaded patients under the auspices of "compassionate use" waivers from the FDA,[13] and the American agency did finally approve it in 2011.[14] Iron toxicity is a serious and treatment-resistant condition. One of its complications is heart failure, and deferiprone is the only iron-removing agent shown thus far to reduce iron deposits in the heart with concomitant improvement in cardiac function.[15] Thanks to the conflict-of-interest movement, North American patients with iron overload only recently gained ready access to this potentially lifesaving drug.

The Calcium Channel Blocker Controversy

Although cited as a smoking gun for the risks of financial conflicts of interest,[16] the *New England Journal of Medicine* (*NEJM*) article correlating cardiologists' opinions concerning these drugs with their industry consulting activities was no such thing. A superficial reading leads one to conclude that authors with the fewest concerns about calcium channel antagonists felt that way because of their relationships with manufacturers of those drugs and that their "conflict of interest" was a tension between an objective assessment of scientific data and a self-interested desire to support the companies that paid them. But a more careful perusal reveals that authors consulting for companies producing other and *even competing products* were also less concerned about calcium channel blockers' safety than were nonconsultants. So what is their conflict of interest? The *NEJM* article did not even *mention* the intuitively obvious fact that company consultants are likely to be the most prominent and competent scholars, a conclusion supported by evidence based on consultants' publication productivity and noncommercial grant support[17] and an FDA review of advisory board members.[18]

Reflecting these facts, the test of time has vindicated these consultants' opinions. Despite the introduction of many new treatments for high blood pressure and heart disease, calcium channel blockers remain in wide use today. And in 2004, two Canadian courts awarded the highest punitive damage awards under that country's libel law to the physicians accused by the Fifth Estate "Heart of the Matter" reporters of endangering patients because of their conflicts of interest concerning calcium channel blockers.[19]

The Gelsinger Fatality

Jesse Gelsinger's death from the gene therapy experiment at the University of Pennsylvania, while tragic, had many origins, the least of which is directly ascribable to financial conflicts of interest. At the time, the obsession with disclosure of financial interests, while building, was not as prevalent as it came to be. A far more important influence was the fact that gene therapy, hyped for years, had no success to show for much effort. The gene therapy researcher, James Wilson, who treated Gelsinger had ample institutional and academic motivations to demonstrate progress that would have vindicated the University's investment and brought academic kudos to himself. The University of Pennsylvania's investigation of the Gelsinger incident revealed management lapses that, if avoided, might have prevented the sad outcome.[20] Moreover, nothing supports the idea that had Wilson either disclosed or lacked his corporate relationship Gelsinger would be alive today.

The NIH Consulting Violations

The ban against paid industry consulting by researchers working at the NIH remains in force. In surveys following the ban, a majority of intramural NIH researchers reported resentment of the regulations and believe that the ban has impeded recruitment and retention of scientists at the Institutes. Consultancies and board memberships have decreased by half,[21] and the transfer of knowledge, materials, and technologies from the NIH to industry was lower in the four years following the ban than it was in the previous five years.[22] The "hundreds" of undisclosed consulting relationships alleged in the press during the height of the scandal ended up totaling fewer than 50, and most were for researchers consulting for companies prior to receiving administrative approval to do so.[23]

The single legal prosecution arising from this scandal involved the NIH researcher who had allegedly sold clinical samples deposited at NIH to a company. In 2006, he pled guilty in a federal district court for having transferred the samples without permission and was sentenced to two years of probation, return of $300,000 in consulting fees he had failed to report to NIH authorities, and 400 hours of community service.[24]

THE EVIDENCE QUALITY SPECTRUM: FROM SELF-EVIDENT TO EDUCATED GUESSWORK

Evidence sufficient to inform practice is sometimes straightforward, but more often elusive. The conflict-of-interest narrative ignores this distinction: no medical practice should take place until declared certifiably "evidence based."

One example of straightforward evidence is the science that directs the treatment of pneumonia caused by a particular type of bacteria, the pneu-

mococcus. The organisms responsible for this disease are routinely iden-
tifiable in patients or animals with this type of pneumonia and, when
cultivated in the laboratory, are transferable to other animals, where they
produce the same disease in which more organisms are detectable. After
penicillin administration reliably cured a handful of patients, penicillin
therapy instantly became the standard of care for treating pneumococcal
pneumonia without performance of formal clinical trials. Similarly, early
imaging devices such as X-ray machines, capable of detecting anatomical
abnormalities that previously remained hidden or required invasive procedures to find, occurred with little or no formal testing beyond simple
observation.

In the mid-1980s, a German surgeon named Erich Mühe developed a
procedure addressing the common and painful problem of inflamed and
stone-infested gall bladders. The method involved insertion of a catheter
through which the operator could observe the patient's abdominal contents, cut the affected gall bladder, and remove it. Patients rapidly demanded this procedure for its cosmetic advantage and rapid convales-
cence compared to earlier operations requiring a large abdominal incision, considerable irritation of the abdominal contents, and a long conva-
lescence. Insurers also welcomed the lower hospitalization costs even
with higher equipment expenditures. All the data available were initially
anecdotal, but early adoption was explosive and subsequent analysis and
refinement have made such procedures universal.[25] Similarly, academics
bemoaned wide adoption without clinical trials of coronary bypass surgery, using leg veins to circumvent blocked heart arteries and provide
relief from the pain of angina pectoris.[26] Nevertheless, this procedure
remains a major mainstay of heart disease management, and subsequent
clinical trials have validated it and informed its best uses.

Following World War II, controlled experimentation, long a mainstay
of laboratory research, began to facilitate the evaluation of therapies for
medical conditions beset with greater uncertainties. The antibiotic
streptomycin, for example, was clearly effective against advanced tuberculosis, but its efficacy in milder infections was unclear. The first randomized controlled clinical trials revealed that the drug was indeed useful
in that condition.[27] Since that time, the randomized controlled trial has
appropriately been considered to represent the best standard for revealing
risks and benefits of many medical treatments.

A prevalent optimistic belief holds that "comparative effectiveness" or "patient-centered outcomes research" done by number-crunching of experimental results from published clinical trials or clinical trial registries will purge the health care system of interventions that are costly but no better than cheaper ones (or none at all). This belief's validity is debatable. What is "best" in theory is not always, indeed often, knowable, practical, or even possible.

Many diseases, especially chronic ones, are not nearly as straightforward as pneumonia caused by the pneumococcus, and many procedures do not yield clear cut results exemplified by X-ray imaging, Mühe's laparoscopic gall bladder procedure, or coronary bypass surgery. For example, some but not all patients with narrowed arteries due to fatty deposits, the condition called atherosclerosis, develop complications of impaired blood flow to the heart, brain, and other organs requiring bypass surgery or angioplasty. If and when they do, however, they occur unpredictably in time and with highly variable severity. The incidence of such complications depends on many other factors such as age, other illnesses, lifestyle, and genetics. As a result, the evaluation of preventive therapies such as cholesterol-lowering statin drugs (discussed in detail in Chapter 10) requires large randomized clinical trials. Sophisticated statistical analyses can be helpful in detecting valid conclusions within such trials that often have highly variable and even contradictory outcomes. But when treatment effects are small or influenced by atypical outlier responses, conclusions based on such studies may not be reliable. A technique known as meta-analysis, examining pooled data culled from many clinical trials regarding a particular treatment, has the advantage of augmenting the number of evaluated subjects, thereby increasing the power of the statistical analysis. A disadvantage of meta-analysis, however, is that poorly designed studies or studies with aberrant results can distort the analytical conclusions.

Many medical conditions are poorly amenable to randomized trials due to rarity, and even if they are common such as severe back pain and influence (discussed below), many lack uniform clinical properties amenable to measurement. Epidemiologists, statisticians, and other theorists who specialize in analyzing clinical trials often identify correlations between patient characteristics and treatment outcomes that may not be causal. These analysts often are not versed in the minute underlying details that lead to the numbers they analyze, nor do they necessarily have the specialized background to determine whether plausible mechanisms point to causality rather than coincidence. The worlds of data generation and data analysis can be frustratingly at odds, especially when the analysts have ideological predilections.[28]

For example, the University Diabetes Group Program, a large government-sponsored trial in the 1960s of the drug tolbutamide, taken by mouth to enable some diabetic patients to avoid using insulin shots or to make their insulin management easier, concluded on purely statistical grounds that the drug slightly increased patient mortality. Many physicians specializing in caring for diabetes patients who participated in the trial did not believe this statistical conclusion. The controversy was never resolved.[29] The principal problem is that complication rates being studied are often very low, and even if increased by a drug, the effect may be small. Attempting to get to an answer therefore requires studying huge numbers of subjects over very long time periods. The price tag for such research may be astronomical, and paying it diverts scarce resources from more straightforward mechanism-related research that involves close observation of individual cases, preferably by experienced specialists. My patient Grace's HUS case, for example, is a disorder studied by a very small number of blood disease experts. Their insights helped the company Alexion develop the eculizumab product that helped save her life. Randomized clinical trials documented the benefit of eculizumab for *atypical* HUS, but no such trial has yet shown it to work in *typical* HUS, the condition that afflicted Grace.[30] Should I therefore have withheld treatment? Often all we have to go on is our clinical judgment.

Nevertheless, treating patients without extensive outcomes data from randomized trials is anathema to conflict-of-interest movement Utopians. For example, some journalists decreed that medical journal articles and practice guidelines concerning treatments not validated by randomized trials are worthless, especially when compiled by individuals who are industry consultants. These allegedly conflicted recommendations have also supposedly blinkered government agencies such as the NIH and the Centers for Disease Control who endorse the guidelines and are remiss for not demanding more randomized trials to obtain what the Utopians confidently assume will be perfect and definitive evidence.[31]

THE EVIDENCE THAT MATTERS

The evidence that matters most to industry is that which leads to its product approvals by the FDA, and the FDA regulates how industry passes that evidence on to physicians and the public. The FDA, while far from perfect, is the best game in town for vetting such evidence. In the preapproval development phase of a product, the Agency's *paid full-time staff* has access to *all original data* possessed by product manufacturers determined in advance to be relevant to potential approval. In addition, the FDA can call on expert outside consultants for advice. Despite the uneven quality of randomized clinical trial results it analyzes, the FDA has rejected the cynical view that, on balance, this all-too common departure from the ideal is the result of deliberate attempts by industry to overrate product benefits and cover up risks. This clear-headed attitude exists despite the fact that FDA officials risk far more by approving products later revealed to be unsafe than failing to approve safe and effective therapies. Furthermore, the companies seeking product approvals cannot select data to reveal to the FDA, and the Agency makes random, unannounced visits to audit companies' data concerning a product under development. As explained earlier, this analytical process is far more rigorous than the unpaid and anonymous refereeing of processed data by cronies and competitors loosely overseen by editors of medical and scientific journals.

Medical journal managers and other conflict-of-interest movement critics often ignore the primacy of FDA analysis and fixate on industry-related research published in medical journals. According to the conflict-of-interest movement, for example, research *sponsorship* trumps research *quality*.

The editors of several medical journals recently declared they would not publish research articles describing studies sponsored by tobacco-industry funds.[32] A former *British Medical Journal* editor has recommended that this tobacco funding censorship policy extend to pharmaceutical company–sponsored research.[33] What transgressions of that industry place it in a circle of hell as low as Big Tobacco's? The former editor's answer is to point to publication of poorly designed or executed clinical trials sponsored by industry that oversell benefits and discount or deny risks.

Selective Publication?

The conflict-of-interest movement claims that its analyses have supposedly revealed that a majority of industry-sponsored clinical trial result publications report favorable ("positive") outcomes. Its interpretation of this supposed skew is that it results from the deliberate suppression of unfavorable ("negative") outcomes.[34] Although examples of such behavior exist, a tilt toward positive outcomes has long been a characteristic of medical journal articles in general, and several reasons account for it. The major one is that negative results are usually far less interesting to researchers than positive outcomes. As a result, journals have been disinclined to publish such studies.[35] Nevertheless, recent reviews of clinical trials involving drugs for rheumatoid arthritis, cancer, or cardiovascular disease found no difference in the prevalence of positive studies as a function of commercial or academic sponsorship.[36]

In addition, legitimate factors exist to account for a predominance of positive outcome reports of industry-sponsored trials in medical journals. Industry-sponsored trials are more likely to compare a new product they have developed with an old one in hopes of demonstrating better results, whereas academic trials may compare effects of existing products without expectations of superiority of one product over another. Companies want to maintain secrecy so as not to attract competition while they validate the possible utility of products under development. In this circumstance, they do not operate with the pressure academics endure to present and publish findings to support university promotion and research grant funding. Rather, companies developing products and their investors may consider proprietary information to be an asset. When such validation has been established, the delay means the chances that a publication will report *accurate* positive results are enhanced. Furthermore, the expense of product development forces companies to choose carefully what projects they will pursue. As a result, reported outcomes reflect more highly selected studies than are routine in academe.

Defective Research Quality?

Examples of poorly designed or performed industry-sponsored trial results published in medical journals have certainly been identified.[37] Some publications describing clinical trials in which a drug failed to improve outcomes downplayed the negative findings and touted favorable results not initially anticipated but identified by retrospective reviewing of the data (a strategy known as "post hoc analysis"). Publications have also reported clinical trial outcomes based on only the subjects who completed their allocated treatment (a form of reporting defined as "per protocol") rather than analyzing the results based on all originally enrolled subjects (known as "intention to treat" analysis). Other publications have described clinical trials in which the dosing of a company's drug made it look better or safer, whereas more appropriate comparisons would have negated such outcomes. Nevertheless, poorly planned, performed, and reported research occurs irrespective of who funds it. And on balance, corporate-supported clinical research, especially concerning clinical trials for evaluation by the FDA regarding approval, is of higher quality than similar research lacking such sponsorship, because industry has more resources to perform larger trials and assure their quality.[38]

Why Publishing or Not Publishing Industry-Sponsored Trial Results in Medical Journals Is Not the Right Question

Although the listing alleged deficiencies and deception of industry-sponsored research, one source the former *British Medical Journal* editor cites to justify banning medical journal publication of industry-sponsored research actually makes a recommendation that is the exact *opposite* of the former *British Medical Journal* editor's: *all* clinical trial results, whatever their sponsorship, must get published in medical journals so that academics can analyze them:[39]

> If I toss a coin a hundred times, for example, but only tell about the results when it lands heads-up, I can convince you that this is a two-headed coin. But that doesn't mean I really do have a two-headed coin: it means I'm misleading you, and you're a fool for letting me get away with it. This is exactly the situation we tolerate in medicine, and always have. Researchers are free to do as many trials as they wish, and then choose which ones to publish.

Two key fallacies invalidate these sentiments. One is the commentator's equating of clinical trials with coin flipping. The word "evidence" belies immense complexity when it comes to medicine. Many sophisticated skill sets and procedural and analytical elements, for example, must go into the proper conduct of a clinical trial. Once completed, proper interpretation of the trial results requires extensive biological insight, not just statistical expertise. Often the findings are ambiguous and subject to different interpretations. Only individuals with deep experience in the relevant research field are well positioned to navigate these shoals.

When companies undertake clinical trials prior to FDA approval, they work closely with the FDA to ascertain its regulatory requirements and thoroughly understand what evidence the FDA wants to see to countenance product approval. This vetting process occurs irrespective of whether academic collaborators participate in the performance of such trials. By contrast, no such review interaction takes place in the majority of trials undertaken by academic researchers without corporate sponsorship. Far more quality control characterizes industry's acquisition of evidence than academe's.

The second fallacy is the idea that the "truth" about clinical trial results must—or even can—reside in medical journal descriptions. As Chapter 4 discussed in detail, however, medical journals themselves bear responsibility for overrating the quality and utility of the evidence they publish. And, after all, *they* have published the allegedly biased and defective industry-sponsored studies highlighted by conflict-of-interest criticism.

Statistical analysis has powerfully abetted medical research, but its limitation is that its output is no better than the original data. Conclusions based on results derived from poorly designed or inadequately controlled studies or confounded by unappreciated variables will not be valid. And while the impetus for public research data dissemination arises from the assumption that industry hides unfavorable information, companies' competitors, stock short sellers, litigators, muckraking reporters, and data analysts themselves all have their own reasons for gaining access to data sets that may not advance innovation or medical care but rather promote their own agendas.

Furthermore, the incentives to publish differ for industry and nonindustry physicians and researchers, and the differences arguably account for some of the "failure" of industry to publish clinical trial results. Whereas academics, especially basic researchers, depend on journal article publication to communicate research results to colleagues and attain credit for research achievements, the importance of journal publication to industry for product introduction and sales is far less compelling. Regulatory agency approval, not journal publication, is the absolute requirement for product sales, and companies can and do use marketing to promote those sales (Chapter 12 defends the accuracy and clinical value of such marketing against conflict-of-interest movement criticism). The only clear benefit of journal publication for industry is that the FDA stipulates that the only way companies can inform physicians about off-label product uses is to provide them with published, peer-reviewed journal articles concerning such uses. Even in that case, however, the company selling the product cannot have done the research described in the article and therefore would have no control over publication. If the industry's academic collaborators who perform some of its trials didn't demand publications for academic advancement, industry might invest far less time and effort to publish. And, if they did, the ghostwriting witch hunt would go away!

The double standard of evidence analysis discussed above and the existence of predators bent on abuse of that evidence when they can access it goes a long way to explaining why companies might be reluctant to have academics with hostile agendas having license to reinterpret their clinical trial data and then publicize those reinterpretations through the less rigorous medium of medical journals. The following cases concerning a back pain procedure and influenza illustrate this point.

TWO EXAMPLES OF ABUSED EVIDENCE ENTREPRENEURSHIP AMID UNCERTAINTY

InFuse

As my own experience recounted earlier reveals, the management of back pain is controversial and often unsatisfactory. One approach to severe chronic back pain has been to weld vertebral bones together, a procedure called spinal fusion designed to reduce excess mobility between vertebral bones ("instability") believed to contribute to pain. A few clinical trials have reported better outcomes as a result of such surgery compared to conservative management.[40] Some fusion operations involve harvesting bone strips from the pelvis and depositing them as bridges between vertebrae (bone grafting) to stabilize them. Others use screws to connect vertebrae or apply various implants to stimulate bone growth to connect vertebrae. Surgeons pioneered the development of the screws and implants in conjunction with companies.

A more recent modification of the implant procedures has been to embed naturally occurring substances in the devices that stimulate bone formation between vertebrae selected for fusion to avoid additional surgery to obtain bone for grafting. Device companies developed particular stimulant and device combinations. One specific strategy taken by the Medtronic Corporation was to place a substance called bone morphogenetic protein 2 (BMP2) in a metal cage that surgeons implant at vertebral fusion sites, and the device-BMP2 combination goes by the brand name InFuse. The FDA approved this procedure for fusion of lower back vertebrae using a defined surgical technique in 2003. Subsequently, many such procedures took place as well as unapproved variations involving different surgical techniques and fusions of upper back and neck vertebrae.

In 2011, a series of articles concerning InFuse appeared in a periodical named *The Spine Journal*.[41] The publications called attention to papers published in the same journal during the initial development of the InFuse procedure. According to the 2011 publications, the earlier articles allegedly had touted the procedure's benefits and claimed that it was essentially risk free, supposedly reporting no complications following treatment of 780 patients. The 2011 *Spine Journal* article series also proffered that subsequent experience with a larger number of patients and reported in medical journal articles contradicted that rosy picture: the complication rate associated with InFuse was actually allegedly 10 to 50 times higher than that associated with bone grafting. Some of the authors of the earlier articles allegedly inappropriately favorable to InFuse were Medtronic consultants, and a few had received large payments from the company. Not surprising, therefore, a major insinuation of the 2011 *Spine Journal* articles was that these consultants downplayed InFuse's risks and promoted its benefits to curry favor with Medtronic for personal profit.

Possibly in response to these allegations, the InFuse treatments declined steadily over the next three years to nearly half of their 2011 peak.[42] Arguably spurred on by information provided by tort litigators, the Senate Finance Committee issued a report in October 2012 accusing Medtronic of the usual menu of conflict-of-interest narrative accusations such as bribing physicians, employing ghostwriters, and engaging in inappropriate off-label promotion.[43] Medtronic categorically denied all of the charges.[44]

All bone fusion procedures promote inflammation, because inflammation is part of the process that leads to repair reactions such as the annealing of broken bones. The reported side effects of InFuse, involving swelling and damage to spinal nerves, would not be surprising if the presence of the BMP2-containing device led to a greater than desired inflammatory response. Other complications of BMP2 reported in *The Spine Journal* publications, however, such as a small increase in cancers, are hardly compelling. The idea that a short-term localized exposure to BMP2 could result in diverse cancers at distant sites is simply not plausible. The alleged underreporting of toxicity due to InFuse in medical journals notwithstanding, the FDA had all the evidence of side effects and nevertheless approved the procedure. A follow-up analysis of the articles concerning InFuse criticized by the 2011 *Spine Journal* contradicted the accusation that no adverse events had been reported in those publications.[45]

The latest word in this saga emerged in six articles appearing in a June 2013 issue of the *Annals of Internal Medicine*. Two of the articles were detailed analyses of all clinical trial information provided by Medtronic comparing spinal fusion procedures using bone grafting or InFuse, published and unpublished. Commissioning the studies was a Yale University "Open Data Access" (YODA) program, a clinical trial result clearinghouse run by a prominent epidemiologist and dedicated to collecting large data sets for statistical analysis. Medtronic paid YODA $2.5 million to oversee this research. One of the two data reviews reported a small improvement in spinal fusion due to InFuse, but both reports concluded that the clinical benefits and risks of the two approaches were comparable.[46]

Three other articles were editorials. One, written by the *Annals* editors and subtitled "Closing In on the Truth," praised YODA, Medtronic, and themselves for having collated and carefully vetted so much information that provided physicians and patients with "reproducible research."[47] A second piece subtitled "A Historic Moment for Open Science" was authored by data-sharing enthusiasts, including the director of the YODA project, and called upon other companies to emulate Medtronic in providing clinical trial data for similar scrutiny.[48] The third article, written by a senior Medtronic official, also endorsed the analytical effort:[49]

> I see Medtronic's interest in pioneering open access of industry-sponsored research at the raw, individual-patient level as being centered on

a commitment to explore objective evaluation processes of Medtronic products.

Buried in the litany of self-congratulation expressed in these articles were some allusions to problems that can beset wholesale regurgitation of data. But, in this particular instance, the idea that the commissioned analyses were likely to lead to conclusions different from what Medtronic already knew seem highly unlikely. After all, Medtronic provided most of the raw data, and in light of the marked decline in use of InFuse and the negative publicity incurred by previous criticism of it, the company had little to lose by accommodating YODA's request for its data. Medtronic officials presumably believed that their magnanimity in funding all the participants in this exercise might have a public relations benefit, an unlikely outcome given the relentless march of conflict-of-interest rhetoric.

One could conclude from the analyses reported in the *Annals* that surgeons should never treat patients with InFuse because it is, according to the latest results, no better than bone grafting in terms of positive clinical outcome. The sixth article in the *Annals* series, however, written by prominent academic orthopedic surgeons—including a spine surgeon who actually performs the procedures analyzed in this series—belies that conclusion and raises the question as to whether after all this analytical effort at great expense, we are really that much closer to "the truth."[50] Although recommending against using InFuse for certain spine fusion procedures "without a compelling reason," the authors stated:

> Using either autograft or rhBMP-2 [InFuse] to enhance fusion rates in patients . . . seems clinically reasonable. Patients should be counseled on the relative benefits and harms of each option and should be allowed to actively participate in decision-making. In some procedures . . . , graft harvest is a separate procedure and avoiding a second incision and associated graft site pain may be well worth the exceedingly small risk for cancer.

If anything, the *Annals* reviews exonerated InFuse from the sensational allegations made by *The Spine Journal* that the procedure is 10 to 50 times more dangerous than bone grafting.

Tamiflu

Another example of "big data entrepreneurship" concerns a drug named Tamiflu for prevention and treatment of influenza. Influenza, or "the flu," is a dreary and all too familiar illness, typical in the winter. Caused by a family of contagious viruses, the flu involves the symptoms of the common cold but with more extreme symptoms of fever, achiness, and fatigue. Although unpleasant, most people get over the flu in the course of a week or so, but its respiratory effects can persist and it predisposes to bacterial infections causing bronchitis and pneumonia. However, the flu can be lethal for the elderly, the very young, or patients suffering from compromised lung function or immune systems. While the run of the mill flu is relatively benign to otherwise healthy people, more virulent strains sometimes arise, and epidemics of these strains disproportionately kill the young. The current explanations for this paradox are that older individuals may have partial immunity due to previous exposures to flu viruses and that younger people have more vigorous inflammatory responses to virus infections that are more likely to spiral out of control. The most flagrant example of such an infection was the pandemic of 1918 that killed between 50 and 100 million people, over 3% of the world's population at the time.[51] More recent pandemics, such as one occurring in 2009–2010, have been far less devastating, in part due to improved surveillance and medical management but also for reasons that are not entirely clear.

Treatment and prevention of the flu consists of three components.[52] One involves hygienic measures such as hand washing, wearing of masks, discouraging afflicted patients from frequenting public places, and occasionally, more aggressive quarantine procedures such as closing schools. The second is to vaccinate against the disease. The difficulty associated with vaccination is the fact that the flu virus changes over time, and this mutability confounds the ability of previous infection or vaccines from providing durable immunity. Vaccination programs therefore depend on ongoing surveillance that attempts to isolate prevalent virus strains to use for vaccine manufacture and subject the population to annual vaccination against the most recently defined virus strain. This approach is far from perfect; estimates of protection due to vaccine range from 50% to 70%.[53] The third approach, in addition to purely symptomatic therapies for fever and respiratory manifestations of the flu, is to treat infected patients Tamiflu (manufactured by Roche) that inhibits an enzyme that the virus uses to infect body cells (GSK produces a related drug brand named Relenza).

Randomized trials leading to regulatory approval of Tamiflu revealed that when inhaled by patients, it prevents symptoms in some individuals exposed to the flu virus and reduces by a day or so the duration of flu symptoms when they occur. The studies did not show a diminution of flu complications or mortality in elderly or debilitated patients. Nevertheless, the FDA approved its use and subsequently extended that approval to use in infants as young as two weeks of age.[54] Despite its modest clinical benefit in seasonal flu, Tamiflu has been profitable for Roche, principally because governments have purchased and stockpiled it as a precaution against the possibility of a particularly virulent flu pandemic.

Conflict-of-interest movement activists have attacked Roche for failing to publish the results of 60% of its Tamiflu clinical trials, although all but one of the omitted studies had been presented at a medical conference. These critics lament that despite incomplete publication in medical journals and the drug's modest efficacy it resides on the World Health Organization's list of essential drugs.[55] Nevertheless, an "[anti-]Tamiflu Campaign" that has recruited politicians and the media has failed to unearth evidence to implicate Roche in a medically important cover-up. Background information concerning the campaign reveals that Roche offered to supply its data to one of the activists requesting the proprietary information, but the investigator refused to sign a confidentiality agreement, a common procedure intended to assure the responsible use of proprietary information.[56]

Ultimately, Roche provided a UK-based health statistical analysis center, The Cochrane Collaboration, with patient-level data from all its 77 Tamiflu clinical studies. Of these, the Collaboration analyzed only the 20 randomized clinical trials, involving 9,623 subjects. GSK also provided an unspecified number of Relenza trial reports, and the Collaboration reviewed 26 of them (14,628 treated subjects). Compared to what the manufacturer had reported, the Collaborative concluded that the drugs showed less reduction in the risk of flu symptoms developing in exposed persons and had a higher incidence of side effects.[57] In response, a Roche investigator criticized the methodology underlying the Cochrane Collaboration conclusions as superficial and incomplete.[58]

What the Tamiflu activists hope to accomplish is unclear. We already know that the drug's benefits are marginal for treating seasonal flu. Flu victims have so many symptoms that blaming some of them on Tamiflu is hard to prove. The facts that seasonal flu is difficult to manage, the high frequency of the disease in diverse populations, and the high mutation rate of the virus all make it difficult to conduct informative research such as randomized trials. Conversely, the infrequency of the more severe flu epidemics and the—fortunately—small numbers of patients usually affected also preclude such studies. The assertion that more number crunching of aggregate outcomes will better inform clinicians, public health officials, and medical product regulators—not to mention miserable patients who want *something* for their symptoms—is highly debatable.

GETTING TO THE BEST EVIDENCE AMID UNCERTAINTY IS POSSIBLE—BUT REQUIRES HUMILITY

An appreciation of the uncertainties and controversies surrounding health is not intuitively obvious to most people in this technological age. We construct and operate complex machines such as jumbo jets. The engineers, technicians, and pilots who work with them can predict with great accuracy how they behave under different circumstances. Parts may wear out and need replacement, but the fundamental composition of the machines does not change. The difference between jumbo jets and humans, however, is that *we built* and completely understand the airplanes, whereas humans *evolved*. Living organisms survive as individuals and species by constant adaptation. Physical and chemical inputs may predictably affect specific body components in controlled laboratory circumstances, but in the intact organism they set in motion cascades of effects that are often impossible to predict. In fact, if our biological responses were totally predictable, pathogens and predators would have eliminated the human species long ago. The immense diversity of responses to influences, most importantly infectious organisms, ensures that the species survives, even if many individuals do not.

The aforementioned uncertainties and contradictions, however, are not inconsistent with practical efforts to move knowledge forward. The history of science is replete with cases of opposing passionate advocacies that seemed irreconcilable until new information broke the impasse, usually revealing that both adversaries were partially correct.

However, the fact that scientific progress and medical practice often require decision making based on tenuous evidence in no way vindicates the sloppy standards of the conflict-of-interest movement. Back pain and influenza, for example, are real afflictions and sufficiently disabling to demand action in the absence of definitive evidence. The damages alleged to flow from "conflicts of interest" are hardly real and do not warrant the action the movement has foisted on us.

6

BAD POLICY PROCESS

People who pronounce on matters about which they are ignorant are apt simply to absorb ideas propagated or taken up by other elite or establishment groups. Nature abhors a vacuum not only in the physical world but also in the world of politics and ideas. [1]

AVAILABILITY CASCADES, CONFORMITY CASCADES, AND GROUP POLARIZATION

Institutional administrative officials, senior academics, and conflict-of-interest movement promoters have dominated nearly all university, professional organization, and government conflict-of-interest policy deliberations with which I am familiar. The target of regulation, the medical products industry, has largely been marginalized in such discussions. Industry representatives and a few conflict-of-interest movement opponents, like myself, have been permitted to provide *testimony* to some of the forums, but in the absence of continuous opportunities to raise dissenting views, this participation was token. The Association of American Medical Colleges (AAMC) included the names of industry CEOs as participants in some of its policy activities, but in reality most industry representatives to the meetings were midlevel officials and compliance officers. As explained below, this composition of policy framers guaranteed that what economists define as "conformity and availability cascades," and "group polarization" contaminated the policy process.

When issues arise—especially technically complex ones unfamiliar to common experience—most people who encounter them do not have the time or interest to examine them carefully. As a result, addressing the perceived problems becomes a collective exercise in which those making policy tend to go along with opinions of others, especially those they consider like-minded, socially compatible, and in positions of authority. [2] Economists' description for this behavior is a *conformity cascade*. When such groups form opinions, reproducible habits surface. These tendencies include favoring stronger impressions, neglecting statistical data, focusing on the most easily available information, and failing to consider particular elements of an issue as parts of *systems* in which preventing something defined as bad can cause the unintended consequences of inhibiting good outcomes.

The conflict-of-interest movement, by dominating information content in the professional and popular literature (medical journals, mass media, and books)—as discussed in Chapter 4—has also created what economists dub an *availability cascade*: a relentless advertising of facts and interpretations of facts that favor its negative emphasis on industry relationship risks. [3] The media have a built-in motivation to promote nonrepresentative but titillating information and automatically play into the conflict-of-interest movement's agenda. Politicians making hay by corruption mongering have the same goals.

For example, the death of Jesse Gelsinger in the gene therapy research experiment described earlier leaves a strong impression. The thousands of unspectacular day-to-day events that occur at the medicine-industry interface, however, do not. Attention-riveting events galvanize policy makers into demanding restrictions. The effects of such restrictions on humdrum but overall important activities go unnoticed.

The progressive ratcheting up of conflict-of-interest policies is not, based on the factual record, a result of escalating adverse outcomes or even marginally coherent evidence that industry relationships are bad in terms of objective outcomes. Rather, it reflects *group polarization*. In deliberations dominated by conflict-of-interest narrative proponents, the promoters versed in the movement's narrative come across as most informed about the issues and convey the greatest enthusiasm for their views. Others, who are indifferent to the discussion or might even disagree, remain silent out of disinterest, deference, or fear. The antidote to these policy behaviors is vigorous rational dissent. Empiric evidence reveals that without the moderating influence of dissent, recommendations and policies migrate to extreme positions. [4]

DISMISSAL OF NUANCE

Conflict-of-interest policy deliberations have approached what is a highly granular and detailed set of practical interfaces between industry and medicine as if they were a broad "ethical" issue to be loftily managed from on high with general principles, speculation, and authority. As a result, the policies lack empiric evidence obtainable through experience, expertise, and effort. A health system analogy would be the establishment of guidelines for managing heart disease based not on clinical data and ongoing research collated by experienced experts but rather on abstract principles deduced by "disinterested" armchair analysts. Heart specialists who have day-to-day encounters managing heart disorders would be excluded from the deliberations because they might have strong management preferences—preferences in fact that might be good for patients.

SELF-DEALING

Economics thus concerns mainly the processes and outcomes produced by voluntary exchange, where of course, all participants benefit. Politics, on the other hand, mainly concerns processes and outcomes produced by group decisions which are practically binding on those who cannot resign from the group. Hence, in politics there are losers as well as winners—and it is politics, not economics, that is the dismal science. [5]

The playing field is not level. Chapter 4 discussed how conflict-of-interest movement promoters have self-serving agendas. The conflict-of-interest movement instigators' job is to agitate, and because their negative messages are attention riveting, it's an easy one. University-based instigators garner funding, notoriety, academic advancement, and even positions of authority by doing so. Muckraking journalists sell copy. Medical journal managers and others peddling medical information branded as sanitized from industry influence promote their businesses. Demagogue politicians receive attention. Whether they sue or defend physicians or medical product companies, the lawyers profit. The conflict-of-interest regulations are a gold mine for compliance bureaucrats and compliance trainers. Well-paid authorities managing medical schools, academic health centers, professional societies, and even patient advocacy organizations see far more job security in avoiding controversy than in promoting innovation or defending the truth.

BAD POLICY THEORY

Prophylactic Rather than Appropriate Therapeutic Regulation

Each year, tens of thousands of people die or suffer grievous permanent injuries in car accidents due to speeding. Nevertheless, no rules prevent drivers from owning cars capable of exceeding speed limits. Rather, speeders are subject to being pulled over by the police and fined. In the same fashion, we retrospectively manage rare but sometimes heinous cases of scientific misconduct in which an individual fabricates, falsifies, or plagiarizes research results and which can raise legitimate concerns about the use of public research funds. The motives underlying research fraud are often unfathomable but have rarely been financial. Chapter 3 reviewed how such behavior rarely occurs in industry or in industry-sponsored academic research.

Fraudulent scientific research has and always and presumably always will exist and often rises to public attention. When a spate of incidents involving scientific research fraud by investigators in universities surfaced in the 1970s and 1980s, they drew public attention including congressional investigations, because by that time the federal government was the major funder of academic research.[6] Most seasoned investigators believe that the prevalence of fraudulent research is vanishingly low, because the gold standard for a researcher's validation is duplication of results by others and fabricated findings are almost never replicable.

University managers have adapted to these fraud incidents by establishing procedures for investigating cases. The NIH instituted an Office of Research Integrity, to which universities report the results of their investigations of research misconduct allegations by faculty funded by NIH grants. When this office examines the evidence and determines misconduct, the NIH imposes penalties, which in come cases, may include criminal charges.

Aside from the "scientific integrity" education efforts, no academic institutions attempt *prophylactic* management of research conduct. Rather, universities investigate and, if necessary, prosecute misconduct *after* the fact. Conflict-of-interest regulation, however, *is* prophylactic: disclosed conflicts are subject to "management or elimination." Moreover, in contrast to conflict of interest, the definition of research misconduct has been very limited and precise: fabrication, falsification, or plagiarism of research results. A coalition of biomedical research societies resisted efforts in the early 1990s to extend the definition to "other practices that seriously deviate from those that are commonly accepted within the scientific community for proposing, conducting, and reporting research."[7] They rightly argued that research is competitive and controversy ridden and that disputes between researchers with diverse personalities and passions resolve over time in a manner that accommodates scientific progress.[8] The vagueness of the proposed extended definition would invite frivolous litigation and oppressive intrusion into research programs based on personal grievances rather than on legitimate suspicion of malfeasance. Unfortunately, appropriate corralling of excessive latitude in defining research misconduct has not taken place in the realm of medicine-industry relationships.

The Slippery Definitions of "Conflict of Interest"

Prior to its emergence at the medicine-industry interface, the term "conflict of interest" addressed concerns in law, financial management, and government about self-dealing, pandering to special interests, or lack of requisite impartiality in financial advising, legal advocacy, or judicial decisions. Even in those contexts, its application to policy and individual behavior has been problematic. Determining the level of "interest" that compromises behavior is subjective and speculative. Attesting to this fact, the treatment of conflict-of-interest violations in government as criminal offenses routinely failed to result in convictions due the inability to prove the required evidence for violations "beyond a reasonable doubt." When government addressed this impotence by taking civil legal actions that demand less stringent evidentiary standards, the same outcome resulted from the failure of prosecutors to prove damages caused by alleged violations. [9]

Medical conflict-of-interest movement promoters have routinely likened conflicts of interest issues in medicine to those in government and law. [10] But the analogy is inapt. Physicians and researchers do not reside in the same functional universe as judges, government officials, the military, or the clergy. [11] Physicians and researchers do not have arbitrary powers, and conversely, litigants or citizens do not have contractual relationships with judges and public officials. Other than limited and complex appeals, litigants and plaintiffs have no recourse to second opinions.

The definitions of conflict of interest framed by conflict-of-interest movement instigators, not to mention reference to the *appearance* of conflict of interest as applied to medicine, represent fuzzy logic and considerable subjectivity. Two examples illustrate this point:

> A conflict of interest is a set of conditions in which professional judgment concerning a primary interest (such as a patient's welfare or the validity of research) tends to be unduly influenced by a secondary interest (such as financial gain). [12]

> Conflicts of interest occur when physicians have motives or are in situations for which reasonable observers could conclude that the moral requirements of the physician's roles are or will be compromised. [13]

How does one possibly determine "undue influence" in advance of actual events? Who is a "reasonable observer?" The philosopher John Stuart Mill invoked a version of "reasonable observer" to establish or prioritize preferences concerning complex problems but stipulated that such an observer would have deep experience in the subjects being prioritized. [14] Regulators, however, demand *exclusion* of experts from such prioritizations because of their "conflicts of interest." The conflict-of-interest narrative's approach to defining conflict of interest represents a framing bias that for political advantage ascribes malignancy to hidden motives that must therefore be "disclosed, managed, minimized or eliminated." [15] If an individual's "character or actions" were not suspect, these measures would not be necessary.

Because the only conflict-free situation is the grave, the question often arises as to why the conflict-of-interest narrative singles out *financial* conflicts. The standard responses provided by the conflict-of-interest movement are that financial conflicts differ from other ubiquitous ones because they are "optional" and because they are easier to identify:[16]

> Financial conflicts of interest are discernible, measurable, volitional, manageable, and well understood by the public. However, in focusing on financial conflicts of interest, this policy does not intend to minimize the importance of nonfinancial conflicts, which can and do influence professionals' judgments, choices, and decisions.

Another case made for the singularity of financial conflicts is that they are supposedly uniquely durable:[17]

> We agree that financial conflict is not the only cause of bias. . . . [L]ong-standing scientific viewpoints, career considerations, and even political opinions might color the study design interpretation. However, these types of individual biases tend to cancel themselves out among large groups of scientists over the long term. While one investigator's career may rise on a cherished theory, another's may arise by debunking that theory. We contend that financial conflict of interest is qualitatively different, providing selective bias that acts consistently in one direction over time.

Neither of these arguments is defensible. Why are financial conflicts "optional" ("volitional")? The underlying assumption that activities unrelated to a faculty member's or physician's industry relationships are subject to a different reward system compared to those that are is false. The competition for academic promotion, acquisition of research grants, and professional esteem is not uncoupled from financial consequences. The financial ramifications of success or failure in these spheres are especially acute nowadays when physicians and academics face increasingly diminished resources for financial survival. If they spend time and effort on industry-related projects, they deserve compensation, especially because such effort may divert them from other revenue-generating activities. Worth noting is that such diversion may also reduce the income of private clinical practice groups or academic practice operations so that considerations other than ethics and reputation certainly must motivate the administrators of these businesses.

Empiric evidence reveals a powerful influence of nonfinancial motivations in the promotion of pet theories (the conflict-of-interest narrative is a prime example), whereas no such data support that such impulses are any less enduring than when researchers obtain financial rewards for their work. [18]

Conflicts of interest are ubiquitous: we have conflicts with ourselves when we engage in self-destructive behavior. Such conflicts cannot be easily eliminated. Yet, by definition, conflict-of-interest policies' emphasis on "managing or eliminating" financial—but not nonfinancial conflicts—"minimizes" "the importance of nonfinancial conflicts." The comment cited above, that nonfinancial conflicts—or financial remuneration unrelated to industry—"can and do influence professionals' judgments, choices, and decisions," is a colossal understatement. These conflicts are far more common, pervasive—and costly—than are financial relationships of academics and physicians involving industry. On average, less than 5% of the revenues of academic health centers arise from student tuition. Over half comes from clinical services and the rest from external grants. [19]

Medicine has become an enormous business operation faced with financial conflicts and addressed in ways that nearly always maximize profits: fee-for-service care promotes providing more services; paying set amounts for managing a panel of patients no matter how much treatment they receive (capitation) encourages providing less; fixed salaries unhinged from productivity promote slacking off and finding other income sources. The conflicts of interest related to these dominant activities in medical centers are no less "discernable and manageable" than those related to payments from industry. Universities know exactly who is up for promotion and who is submitting grant proposals, and clinics know who is treating what patients with what modalities. All that would be required to "disclose and manage" these activities is inquisitional bureaucracies modeled on those created for disclosure and management of industry relationships. Of course, to do so would be prohibitively time consuming and costly.

In summary, the conflict-of-interest movement's core concern is riddled with arbitrary and debatable ideas, contradictions, and inconsistencies. It speculates on invisible impulses set in motion by financial opportunities (that may encourage useful actions) when no way exists to understand the relationship between those opportunities and impulses. It purports to impart conscious analysis—through ad hoc management—of invisible motivations. It applies subjective judgments to the evaluation of what is supposed to be objective information.

Conflict-of-Interest Management Is Inconsistent with Rule of Law

At my academic institution, annual (or, as mandated by current NIH regulations, monthly) industry payment disclosures move on to several courts. One is my supervisor, a second is an Office of Industry Interactions, a third is an institutional conflict-of-interest committee, and a fourth is the conflict-of-interest oversight bureaucracy of its affiliated medical school. The most recent version of my health care system's conflict-of-interest policy calls for review, management, reduction, or elimination of industry payments. Other than references to "fair market value," the instructions explicitly license layers of supervision to make arbitrary and subjective decisions. This approach is inconsistent with American legal tradition. [20]

"Bias" Bashing and the Exiling of Expertise

The NIH's articulated reason for requiring grantee institutional policies to maintain oversight over researcher's relationships with industry has consistently been to avoid research "bias": [21]

> To ensure that the design, conduct, or reporting of research funded under Public Health Service grants will not be biased by any conflicting financial interest of those investigators responsible for the research.

> The NIH must ensure that the research it funds on behalf of US taxpayers is scientifically rigorous and free of bias.

A call to monitor commercial "bias" based on the assumption that such "bias" in biomedical research diminishes "scientific rigor" demands an empiric assessment as to whether researchers' relationships with industry have actually compromised NIH-funded research. No such evidence exists. A voluminous Institute of Medicine report published in 2009 and cited in the revised NIH regulations, while confidently declaring that industry relationships pose dire risks, acknowledged this lack. The emphasis on risk is therefore a manifestation of belief, not of evidence. It is *in itself* an example of profound subjective bias.

The key word is *evidence*. Despite its nuances and limitations discussed in the previous chapter, evidence is the bedrock of science in contrast to adherence to belief systems such as religion that can persist in the absence of evidence. Scientific evidence-based beliefs, however, are not free of bias. Indeed, evidence creates perfectly reasonable biases: evidence, for example, leads sensible people to have biases in favor of wearing seat belts, not overeating, and not engaging in substance abuse. And evidence does not arise from suspension of bias; it emerges from controlled experimentation that absolves researchers from the impossible and even damaging goal of lacking a passion for their ideas. Science does not do itself a service by trying to brand itself as driven by robotic disinterest, and the history of scientific advance is replete with examples of mavericks that achieved success by relentlessly pursuing their biases and savaging their competition.

Another harmful consequence of demonizing bias is the marginalization of expertise. Experts acquire biases toward certain products and procedures based on their experience, justifiably defined as evidence. For example, surgeons and cardiologists will likely emphasize different approaches to heart disease relying on their honestly acquired familiarity with their respective disciplines. How could a "disinterested" arbiter lacking such familiarity better promote heart disease patients' care than the competing recommendations of experts. Patients can address the biases of their physicians by soliciting different opinions.[22]

Another example of expertise marginalization by the conflict-of-interest mindset is its call to prevent "conflicted" experts from giving advice to regulators or participating in clinical practice guidelines. FDA regulation requires that panelists convened by the Agency to advise it regarding product approvals have no financial ties to product manufacturers, but the Agency has made exceptions by granting a limited number of waivers to such panelists when it wanted particular expertise. The conflict-of-interest movement has objected to the FDA's utilization of such waivers. But when the medical arm of Public Citizen reviewed voting patterns of panels and the FDA conducted further analyses, neither found evidence that committee members with ties to manufacturers were more likely to vote in support of those interests.[23] Nevertheless, the FDA has, under political pressure, made waiver conferral so onerous that many review panels have unfilled positions.[24]

Controversy haunts research, and scientific disputes may fester for years before resolution occurs. Sometimes it never does. The antagonists in such polemics all have biases. The obsession with disclosing biases and demeaning them as inconsistent with objectivity debases honest disagreements.

Scare-Mongering About Public Trust

Conflict-of-interest narrative tracts and conflict-of-interest policy justifications routinely claim that financial conflicts of interest—or the appearance of conflicts of interest—endanger "trust" and that regulation is therefore mandatory to prevent such endangerment. In fact, conflict-of-interest movement promoters confidently declare that public trust has already declined.[25]

The reason I enclosed "trust" in quotation marks above is that trust is a complicated concept that has received serious attention from philosophers and economists. Compared to such scholarship, the conflict-of-interest movement's treatment of trust is superficial and muddled. The Nobel Prize–winning economist Kenneth Arrow pointed out that not only does trust enable governments to function with reduced coercion but also facilitates economic transactions.[26] Ironically, Arrow and others who have analyzed the role of trust in societies have emphasized that trust makes economies more efficient by *reducing* the need for monitoring and regulation.[27] Only by claiming that trust has eroded or will erode can the conflict-of-interest movement make a case for *more* such monitoring and regulation.

Measuring trust relies on survey methodology, and answers to survey questions depend heavily on how the questions get framed.[28] As this book shows, physician and academic financial relationships with industry are far from simple or straightforward, and it is unlikely that the public at large is well positioned to assess such relationships knowledgably, especially if surveys pose leading questions. A survey of 1,250 "representative" subjects performed by *Consumer Reports* reported a high level of "concern" if physicians received payments from industry. Another survey concluded that respondents who disapproved of physicians receiving industry payments had less "trust" of the health care system. Which of these two opinions was cause and which effect could not be determined?[29] A summary review of 20 medical journal articles that had surveyed patients or physicians reported a wide range of responses. Between a quarter and a majority of respondents claimed that they wanted physicians to disclose financial ties with industry and that such relationships decreased their confidence in research results or willingness to participate in research studies. [30]

Nevertheless, other research results do not support the straightforward assertions regarding loss of trust. The introduction of polio vaccination in the 1950s brought the medical profession to its highest historical public image. [31] It was so high that it could only go in one direction—down. The descent occurred two decades later when the arrival of managed care raised concerns about medical rationing, but in fact, public esteem of physicians and medical researchers has remained steady since then—and at the top of all professions, as assessed by Gallop and other surveys. [32] Research!America, an advocacy organization for the NIH, conducts surveys consistently showing that a majority of individuals polled believe researchers and industry should work together and that it is acceptable for researchers to profit from discoveries. [33] Two studies have shown that most patients participating in clinical trials were not concerned about whether their physicians running the trials had financial interests in companies sponsoring the studies. [34] Another survey concluded that most research subjects did not consider financial disclosures to be useful or likely to influence their decision making. [35]

Considering the nonstop demonization of the medical products industry by the conflict-of-interest movement and news media, the lack of public concern is noteworthy. Billed as an exception is a study published in *The New England Journal of Medicine*. [36] The researchers performing the study asked internal medicine specialists to read three summaries of the results of fake clinical drug trials supposedly published in medical journals and then record the enthusiasm with which they would prescribe the study drugs for their patients. The faux clinical trials concerned drugs for three different clinical problems and consisted of a mix of low, medium, or high rigor clinical trial designs and were billed as having corporate sponsorship, NIH sponsorship, or no sponsorship. The respondents stratified the trials in accord with their quality but based on the responses, significantly discounted them, irrespective of quality, if they had commercial sponsorship. The authors of the study and an editorial accompanying the article written by *NEJM*'s editor expressed concern that physicians might not prescribe useful products because of their suspicions regarding the validity of industry-sponsored clinical trials. [37]

At face value, this study seems to point to a lack of "trust" in industry-related research by practicing physicians. A problem in drawing this conclusion with confidence, however, is the fact that each physician surveyed received only three study summaries. Making a reliable assessment regarding *one* comparison set—different clinical trial sponsors—when *nine* variables were scattered throughout the clinical trials (three levels of study quality, three different sponsors, three different disease areas) is questionable. Even if one accepts that the statistical manipulations employed by the surveyors sorted these issues out sufficiently to warrant the article's conclusion, the study's authors and the editor—prolific contributors to the conflict-of-interest narrative—blamed the discounting of industry-sponsored research on media accounts of alleged industry malfeasance associated with large off-label promotion settlements. Chapter 14 explains how the media distort these stories, and the authors of the survey article and *The New England Journal*'s editor made no reference to their own complicity in promoting the alleged lack of trust by their own opinions. If trust by physicians in industry-sponsored research has eroded as this and another survey suggest[38] has occurred, the conflict-of-interest movement is to blame.

7

FLAWED AND DAMAGING POLICIES

Most if not all of the research regulations enacted by the conflict-of-interest movement and described in chapter 3 are subject to objections. No evidence supports improved medical innovation or patient care stemming from the restrictions on activities. In fact, they slow progress. This chapter explains why.

REMUNERATION RESTRICTIONS

As summarized in chapter 2, payments to physicians or medical academics from industry include reimbursement for consulting or speaking, payments for licensing of inventions and for milestones achieved during development of a licensed invention, and royalties from sales of FDA-approved products. Another source of payment is stock or stock options.

Financial reward limits imposed on various industry-related activities by conflict-of-interest regulations at academic centers are often arbitrary. References in conflict-of-interest policies, for example, to what is "academically appropriate" remuneration have no inherent frame of reference. The payment amounts allowed by these policies would never raise the incomes most employees of universities or health care systems to the levels of their top institutional administrative leaders who impose the rules.

Very few faculty members have the opportunity to profit handsomely if their inventions help patients. Prior to the imposition of reward limits, great value emerged without adverse complications. For example, Kenneth Murray (1930–2013) was a professor of microbiology at the University of Edinburgh and scientific cofounder of the early biotechnology company Biogen. Biogen supplemented Murray's usual research activities enabling him to investigate in his academic laboratory the virus causing the common liver affliction, hepatitis B. Hepatitis B is debilitating, often lethal, and is the most common cause of cancer in the world because it leads to liver malignancies. It is especially prevalent in the Far East. Biogen's research sponsorship enabled Murray to perform this work without compromising his mainstream research on other topics. This subsidy helped in the development of a vaccine for hepatitis B. Biogen reaped profits, and Murray and the University enjoyed returns of appreciated stock options as well as royalties. Murray donated substantial sums from these proceeds to establish a trust to support the research work of young biologists.[1] Murray continued his academic research, was elected to the prestigious Royal Society of London, and was knighted by Queen Elizabeth II. Most importantly, Murray's work will eventually help eliminate hepatitis B and its lethal complications. The value of his accomplishments to humankind vastly surpasses his personal financial rewards.

If conflict-of-interest regulations at some universities forbidding concurrent equity and sponsored research existed at the time of Murray, it is doubtful whether the hepatitis B vaccine story would have developed at that time and place. Given a choice between performing uncompensated research that might yield medical advances but most likely will not or pursuing projects that more reliably afford academic advancement and consistent research funding, most university researchers will take the latter. The prohibition concerning equity and sponsored research has been in force for a quarter of a century, despite the fact that no case is on record of an investigator falsifying or spinning research results to prop up a company's stock. Nevertheless, Harvard's most recent (2009) conflict-of-interest policy forthrightly pronounced:[2]

> It is highly unlikely that the decision of any one individual to retain a personal financial interest rather than pursue research would result in research not being conducted. In fact, if a technology is truly valued by an individual's colleagues and the scientific community, there will be interest beyond the relevant individual.

A rudimentary understanding of the history of science or medicine shreds these confident statements. "Colleagues and the scientific community" routinely reject important discoveries that are inconvenient or threaten the status quo, for instance, antiseptic methods took decades to spread through the surgical community and hand-washing compliance remains modest today, more than a century after its introduction.[3]

Moreover, even the Harvard conflict-of-interest rule's token concession, to allow faculty to have sponsored research from a company if the equity does not exceed a minimum ($10,000) amount, stipulates that the stock must be from a "widely traded public company." This restriction defeats the very reason for stock grants from the types of companies most likely to license faculty research. These start-up enterprises lack the cash possessed by established pharmaceutical, device, and biotechnology companies and don't have publicly traded stock. Most projects fail, and the stock of companies sponsoring the failures never appreciates in value. Even stranger is the fact that the limited amounts allowed are the *sale price* of the stock, not the size of the stock grant. The purpose of stock grants is to provide incentives for grantees to make the stock appreciate as the product proceeds through development; the rule precludes the stock value from appreciating above the stipulated value.

Academic institutions have also limited fees previously allowed for milestones in the development of licensed inventions. Such milestones include FDA permission to begin clinical trials. The purpose of such payments is to reward inventors for moving an invention forward, even if it does not succeed in achieving final FDA approval. The payment restrictions are based on the same theory for reducing fees and limiting equity, namely that an investigator will misrepresent research results to obtain such profits. But the FDA oversees the steps that garner milestone payments. This oversight is one of the principal reasons no evidence for such misrepresentation exists. Because the majority of medical product development projects fail (all for reasons other than "misrepresentation"), these restrictions deprive creative inventors of just rewards for facilitating the difficult innovation process.

MEDICAL JOURNAL RESTRICTIONS

In a 2000 editorial announcing the imposition of the special requirement that commercially sponsored research papers must include an analysis of reported data by an independent academic statistician, the *Journal of the American Medical Association* (*JAMA*) editors imposing the rule denied that industry-sponsored papers contained deliberate misrepresentations.[4] But in the absence of such misrepresentation, which would constitute research misconduct, the rule made no sense. The number of papers with industry sponsorship published by *JAMA* declined by over 40% after the special requirement for independent statistical review went into effect, a decrease not seen in two other top-tier journals analyzed (*The New England Journal of Medicine* and *The Lancet*).[5] This fact arguably was the principal reason that in June of 2013 a *JAMA* editorial (a new editor in chief had replaced the one who imposed the regulation) announced termination of the requirement for independent statistical analysis and admitted that such analyses had never changed the conclusions of trials in submitted publications. The editorial announcement did not mention the published decline in *JAMA* papers with industry sponsorship.[6]

MANAGEMENT OF CONFLICT OF INTEREST IN CONTINUING MEDICAL EDUCATION

Conflict-of-interest movement promoters have claimed that the Accreditation Council for Continuing Medical Education's (ACCME's) "firewalls" are inadequate to prevent corporate control of continuing medical education (CME). Senate hearings examined the adequacy of ACCME's oversight over CME, and the Office of Inspector General publicly declared that his office has an interest in "limiting commercial influence on CME" and insinuated that physicians participating in commercially sponsored CME activities might be subject to legal action.[7]

Allegations that CME is simply corporate propaganda persist despite the facts that physicians voluntarily participate in CME, and four surveys involving hundreds of thousands of physicians revealed that a vanishingly small percentage perceived any commercial bias.[8] The author of one of these surveys interpreted these findings as evidence that physicians are *incapable* of perceiving industry bias that *must* have been present.[9] The criticism that dependence of CME on industry sponsorship affects educational topic choice is certainly consistent with reality: insulin manufacturers, for example, will support CME concerning diabetes but not that regarding depression or back pain. Nothing, however, is stopping well-heeled sponsors of the conflict-of-interest movement—owners of profitable medical journals, the Pew Charitable Trust, or the American Board of Medicine Foundation—from funding CME courses on topics industry is unlikely to support, such as dietary interventions, end-of-life decision making, and communication skills.

The ACCME plays both ends against the middle. On the one hand, it is at the forefront of hand-wringing about "commercial bias," thereby promoting its (expensive) services as a bias sanitation mechanism. On the other hand, it fights the idea that its vetting services are inadequate, a conclusion that if taken to ultimate action would eliminate commercial support of CME and the need for the ACCME's—well remunerated—interventions.

RESTRICTION OF RESEARCHERS WITH FINANCIAL INTERESTS FROM PARTICIPATION IN PATIENT-RELATED RESEARCH

At face value, this restriction, codified by the AAMC, is reasonable. For example, discoverers of drug candidates are generally not experts in clinical trials, and their participation in designing and conducting the trial is, therefore, unnecessary. Moreover, demonstration of the efficacy of a drug or device by independent clinical investigators promotes its credibility. In some circumstances, however, particularly with respect to complex drug or device regimens, an inventor with financial interests in the invention might possess expert knowledge and skills necessary for optimal testing of a product and could bring knowledge, energy, and passion to promote product development in the face of formidable obstacles. The existence of such exceptional cases presumably underlies the "rebuttal" disclaimer in the recommended policy.[10] Nevertheless, that financial interests put subjects at risk and threaten trust is unsupported and debatable, and the report made no mention whatsoever that its recommendations might *impede* progress.

RESTRICTED FINANCIAL SUPPORT OF
ACADEMIC MEDICAL ACTIVITIES

Prior to conflict-of-interest regulations forbidding it, companies funded the lunches for academic conferences and other gatherings. What information do we have as to whether attendees were aware of it or, if they were, knew to any extent what products the companies manufactured? None. If the enticement of a free lunch meant that a physician or medical student attended an educational event, it is more likely that some patients benefited from what the attendee learned than suffered from any warm feelings the attendee developed toward the company that provided the meal. Likewise, I am unaware of any evidence that physicians and researchers in training who received competitive fellowship awards provided by companies are less competent at medical research or clinical care due to loyalty to the sponsoring companies than those who did not.

When I participated on a panel at the American Orthopedic Association concerning conflicts of interest in June of 2012, a fellow panelist who is an orthopedic surgeon, ethicist, and a committed conflict-of-interest enthusiast expressed contempt that surgeons rely on device company representatives to learn complex techniques. Rather, he claimed, they should educate themselves concerning such use through academic courses. In response, a member of the audience commented that many small hospitals had limited budgets and could not easily afford to pay for such training. When the moderator asked for a show of hands, nearly everyone present was in favor of education from the companies. Having reps do the training at one's own institution is more convenient for surgeons, who do not have to travel, and allows for repeated interactions that ensure optimal practices.

RESTRICTED COMMERCIAL SUPPORT OF
PROFESSIONAL SOCIETIES

My principal current professional society affiliation is with the American Society of Hematology (ASH). ASH was founded in 1958 to promote research and education concerning blood and blood diseases. I attended my first ASH meeting in December of 1970. Several hundred mostly American physicians doing research on blood and treating patients with blood disorders gathered over a weekend at a beach-front hotel in San Juan, Puerto Rico. There they attended concurrent sets of a few hundred 10-minute scientific presentations, followed by audience questions. The presenters had submitted research abstracts some months before, and a committee chose about a quarter for open discussion; the rest were accessible in an abstract book provided at the meeting. In addition to attention to research presentations, some participants organized research collaborations, and others, particularly young members, met with other attendees to broker job opportunities. Many of the attendees brought family members to the meeting and during breaks joined them for recreation on the beach, meals at restaurants, or sightseeing. Except for a few medical book sellers sitting outside the meeting halls with demo textbooks, the commercial presence was minimal.

Forty-three years later, the ASH meeting I attended bore some similarities with my first encounter but differed in many ways. Twenty-two thousand attendees, physicians, non-physician researchers, corporate research, and marketing personnel, about half from outside the United States, occupied over 40 hotels, and the meeting activities took place in a large convention center. A selection process similar to that of 43 years ago stratified submitted research abstracts into a few hundred 10-minute talks and several thousand poster presentations. A thousand or so more of them were relegated to the abstract tome, now as big as the Manhattan telephone book. In addition to the extensive sharing of research, the meeting featured education lectures on diverse topics and sessions honoring research leaders with prizes and young researchers with fellowships, and provided local high school students with an introduction to blood science. Intensive press coverage reported novel findings emerging at the meeting.

The immense increase in size and scope of the ASH meeting over my professional lifetime is almost entirely due to contributions of the medical products industry. This presence is manifest in the enormous exhibit hall populated with company (as well as nonprofit) booths. Physician and researcher attendees mingle with company marketing personnel at the booths—often accepting offerings of coffee, snacks, and marketing materials—unless they are from Minnesota, Massachusetts, or Vermont, whose "gift bans" preclude taking these amenities. Signs at the booths announce that physicians from those states should not take the samples or other giveaways. A day of company-sponsored ACCME-accredited education symposia preceded the formal meeting. Ubiquitous signage and an

ASH newspaper that appears at the attendees' hotel door daily bear corporate logos and advertisements, reflecting the sponsorship of these materials.

The meager corporate presence at the 1970 ASH meeting reflected that there was nothing to sell. Hematologists could manage a few blood diseases with vitamins and minerals, crudely treat hemophilia with plasma transfusions, employ two types of anticoagulants ("blood thinners") to address pathological blood clotting, and use a few chemotherapy drugs to temporarily slow the fatal course of blood malignancies (leukemias and lymphomas). Industry contributions aided by academic- and physician-industry partnerships have radically improved the available treatments: anemias and coagulation disorders are more manageable, with a wide choice of effective medications, and patients with blood cell malignancies achieve prolonged remissions and cures thanks to others. The intrusion of industry has been an adaptive response to amazing opportunity, not a corporate conspiracy.

Thanks to corporate subsidy, adjusted for inflation, the registration fees charged for attendance have hardly changed, and this support has accommodated the expanded scope of ASH activities. Non-physician researchers and hematologists-in-training can afford to attend the meeting. The vast increase in attendance reflects that companies have offset travel and subsistence expenses of non-U.S. attendees, who, receiving far lower salaries than American physicians, could not otherwise attend.[11] The high attendance reinforces America's position at the hub of hematologic science exchange and education, with benefits for the entire world. This confluence makes for efficient research relationships between companies and hematologists. The annual ASH meeting epitomizes a vibrant *market*. This market has made major contributions to blood research and education, with enormous salutary effects on longevity and life quality.

Even if we turned the clock back to 1970, that meeting in San Juan included perfectly justifiable social amenities and pleasant surroundings that lubricate networking, constructive scientific partnerships, and efficient education. I am unaware of any evidence suggesting that such surroundings and amenities compromise learning. Nevertheless, cowed by critics, ASH and other professional societies have mandated formulaic "disclosure." At the annual ASH meeting every oral presentation must now feature a slide shown for at least 30 seconds summarizing the presenters' corporate financial relationships as well as a warning if the presentation includes discussion of off-label uses of products. Signs grace the halls containing poster presentations at ASH admonishing viewers to report commercial "bias or unreported conflicts." Volunteers selected by ASH management to root out bias at oral presentations receive a free night's lodging. Several years of such surveillance at ASH meetings featuring thousands of presentations hasn't unearthed *a single allegation* of inappropriate promotion due to commercial sponsorship.

ASH's approach to management of industry relationships is representative of many other professional societies. A more extreme example is the policies of the American Society of Clinical Oncology, the leading organization for cancer specialists. Cancer treatment has benefited enormously from cooperation between academics, physicians, and industry. Nevertheless, the ASCO policy makers decided that disclosure of corporate relationships was inadequate and imposed a system of censorship that precludes individuals with industry ties from having leadership positions in the organization, presenting original research at the Society's annual meeting, or authoring research articles in its medical journal.[12] Justifying these draconian exclusions are the usual conflict-of-interest narrative allegations and the results of a survey of the Society's membership, to which only 1% of ASCO's tens of thousands of members responded.[13] An additional astonishing feature of the new ASCO regulations is that they relegate industry-sponsored researchers to a second-class status:

> Individuals who are free of these [industry] relationships should play a key role in the authorship of original research submitted to ASCO meetings. . . . Although the contribution of every author is important, ASCO looks to these individuals primarily to ensure the balance and objectivity of the research presented.

We have come to a place in which Gertrude Elion and George Hitchings, who won the Nobel Prize for discovering drugs that became cancer treatment mainstays, could not discuss their results at ASCO because they were employees of a pharmaceutical company.

The sole exception to the general capitulation to restrictions in professional societies has been the American Association of Clinical Endocrinologists (AACE). As explained in chapter 15, AACE shows that resistance to the conflict-of-interest movement is possible.

DEMONIZING KEY OPINION LEADERS

In contrast to conflict-of-interest movement instigators, summarized in chapter 3, key opinion leaders (KOLs) are often the physicians who are at the cutting edge of innovation. They include physicians who have worked with companies to help create devices, develop drugs, understand the best uses of products, and conduct clinical trials. Such physicians existed even in the conflict-of-interest movement's purported golden age of medicine uncontaminated by commerce.[14] A compelling example of the value of such KOLs is how "clinical champions" have been essential for catalyzing the useful clinical application of drugs. Thanks to such individuals, chemical compounds that existed in the 1940s were later shown to be useful for treatment of leukemia, organ transplantation, and virus diseases associated with HIV/AIDs.[15] These KOLs have traditionally been revered and have always been remunerated for their valuable services. They epitomize the most learned, talented, and energetic academics' and physicians' important intellectual, experiential, and research contributions of use to industry innovation. But conflict-of-interest movement promoters deny the need for such expertise. For example, a reporter complaining about physicians with industry ties participating in practice guideline panels stated that:[16]

> [i]t's hardly impossible to find medical experts without financial ties to industry, however, according to research. A survey of academic researchers, for example, showed that 36 percent of full professors at medical schools report no financial connections to the industry in the previous year. The idea "that every *expert in the field* has industry relationships is not supported by the data," said [a medical professor] [emphasis added].

But the 36% of "full professors" who don't have industry connections are not necessarily "experts in the field." The surveyor cited, for example, is a full professor but is neither a physician nor qualified to serve on a clinical practice guideline panel in any specialty. The fact that such individuals populate over a third of medical school faculty positions doesn't automatically make them capable of advancing medicine.

Prior to the emergence of the conflict-of-interest narrative, KOLs appropriately considered working with industry to be a reflection of their value and an asset to their reputations. The conflict-of-interest interest movement's rhetoric has succeeded in hounding some talented physicians out of collaborating with industry.[17]

DEMONIZING USE OF PROFESSIONAL WRITERS

The allegations of ghostwriting by the conflict-of-interest movement go as follows. To promote sales, medical products companies hire professional writers to author articles for submission to medical journals. This strategy is part of a publication planning effort that starts early during the development of products and persists through their approval and postmarketing brand life. The articles may be accounts of research such as clinical trials or review pieces discussing a medical field relevant to company products. The company then commissions academics after the fact, preferably experts in a field to lend their names, possibly paid to do so, to the papers as authors. According to the conflict-of-interest narrative, these individuals are faux authors who may have had nothing to do with either the collection of original data or scientific analysis of information. The actual authors remain anonymous. A variation on the ghostwriting criticism theme is to allege that physician or academic authors of papers describing industry-sponsored clinical trials do not have access to all trial results and therefore cannot determine that professional writers employed by the sponsoring company have spun the results to emphasize benefits and downplay risks.[18]

"Honorary authorship" of scientific articles—a more appropriate definition of the first alleged transgression—has certainly occurred. For example, a physician who committed research misconduct also persuaded eminent physician-scientists who had made no contributions to the experimental work to attach their names to articles, hoping their cachet would encourage peer reviewers to judge them favorably.[19]

Attempts to document the prevalence of such honorary or ghost authorship have involved surveying selected authors of published papers as to their opinions regarding the contributions of their co-authors. One such survey claimed that 18% of articles in six medical journals had honorary authors and 8% ghost authors. These percentages were somewhat lower than in earlier compilations of this nature, leading the surveyors to conclude that conflict-of-interest movement publicity concerning this problem may be having salutary effects. They lamented, however, that the persistence of ghost and the high prevalence of honorary authorship are compromising "responsibility, accountability and transparency in authorship" and the "integrity in scientific publication."[20] Such surveys, however, purporting to document unacceptably high rates of honorary authorship and ghostwriting are essentially worthless because they collect subjective opinions of *one* author about co-authors without allowing the alleged honorary authors to rebut the charge.

Ghostwriting is, in fact, the conflict-of-interest narrative's most ill-defined target. University conflict-of-interest policies routinely contain a statement prohibiting ghostwriting but do not define precisely what the term means. In fact, professional writers are a perfectly legitimate profession consisting of individuals who write for the medical products industry or other clients. They belong to trade organizations with codes of ethics.[21] In the past, the contributions of these writers may not have been adequately acknowledged in medical publications, and they deserve to be.

But *litigation* rather than stealth marketing energizes the inquisition against industry ghostwriting. Plaintiffs' attorneys suing manufacturers whose products allegedly caused harm or, as discussed in chapter 14, prosecutors claiming companies engaged in off-label product promotion hope to influence litigation by insinuating that the companies used devious marketing practices. When extensive trolling of company documents during legal discovery unearths evidence that professional writers participated in composing medical journal publications, the ghostwriting charge emerges. Medical journals have published compilations of such discovery materials assembled by academics that served as plaintiffs' witnesses in the anti-industry litigation.[22] Other journals have even published articles *authored* by attorneys advocating criminal litigation as an antidote to ghostwriting.[23]

One reason companies may seek out academics to serve as authors on their papers is that they have experienced arbitrary rejections of articles they submitted bearing only names of industry employees.[24] In that case, medical journals bear some responsibility for promoting the ghostwriting practice they allege is so prevalent and worthy of condemnation.

That academic authors actually engaged in honorary authorship—the unacceptable activity in which an author has made no contribution to published research—is unclear. In contrast, the ghostwriting insinuations arise from a rigid definition of authorship, an unrealistic view of responsibility for research results, and a romanticized concept of writing motivation. Utopian definitions of authorship are easy to concoct.

These positions impose impractical and largely impossible conditions. In practice, authorship of papers is highly nuanced and often contentious.[25] Sideline theoreticians may assert that authors must take responsibility for design, execution, and writing of papers, but in reality, for example, trainees or junior colleagues who appear as first authors of publications describing laboratory research results usually contributed in a purely technical capacity, and their mentors, who may have had little or nothing to do with execution of the work, write or edit the papers. As biomedical research has become increasingly complex and multidisciplinary—a phenomenon reflected by the large number of individuals listed as authors on publications—the idea that any one of the authors can be intimately familiar with all or even most of the material in a research paper is fantasy.

The following comments epitomize the quality of ghostwriting criticism:[26]

> [T]he opinion leaders who work with pharma are actually the least bright. They are the ones that it occurred to pretty early on that they're not going to get the chair at Harvard or Yale, but who do enjoy the lifestyle of being courted by industry, and having your articles written for you, of having articles in *JAMA* or *NEJM*, which you wouldn't otherwise have—these guys get made by industry.
>
> And industry can pick the people, based on their psychology and things like that to suit their needs. They pick the kind of people who would like to have on their CV [list of publications] that they have written eight hundred articles. When in fact they have written ten or twenty, and the other seven hundred and ninety have been written by medical writers.

These fantastic allegations—that academics actually exist with CVs listing 800 articles mostly created by industry ghostwriters and published in prominent medical journals—defy credulity and beg for evidence.

The most important question is whether authors are willing to take responsibility for what papers bearing their names *say*, implicitly expressing sufficient trust in the honesty of their co-authors. The ghostwriting alarmists have not provided evidence that such responsibility is lacking.[27]

PRODUCT SAMPLE BANS

As is the case with detailing in general, the idea that providing samples increases a doctor's likelihood of prescribing those medications or prohibiting them reduces such prescriptions is intuitively obvious, as is the fact that sampled products are on patent and therefore more expensive than generics.[28] If physicians who receive samples subsequently prescribe more of those drugs than indicated, they, not industry, deserve the blame.

But discussions demonizing samples never *mention* obvious values they provide. One is that making samples available is simply good customer service: what is wrong with making it easy for patients to start using products immediately and giving them leisure to follow up at the pharmacy later? Considering the very low compliance rate with essential medications, getting patients started on drugs that if they make them feel better could in theory improve compliance. More importantly, if a patient shows up in a physician's office with raging hypertension, an asthma attack, or an anaphylactic reaction, having medication available to address it immediately could be life saving. Having devices in the office—inhalers, epinephrine auto-injectors, diagnostic monitors, injection kits—and being able to instruct patients how to use them is simply good patient care. Accounting for samples and storing them properly, an activity physicians supposedly have not done well, is easily addressable with instruction, a remedy far more appropriate than outright bans.

Providing samples for poor patients, the only concession the conflict-of-interest movement makes about samples, is probably the least defensible reason for their existence. Academic centers have permitted samples for this reason, provided physicians give the patients vouchers that they are to present to the pharmacy. The follow-up rate for such vouchers is arguably low.

PEER-TO-PEER (PROMOTIONAL) SPEAKING BANS

The arguments directed by the conflict-of-interest movement against promotional speaking are easily rebuttable. Peer-to-peer speaking, a better term for this activity than promotional speaking, is popular: physicians like to learn from other physicians and have voted with their feet by frequently attending speaking events. Academics have a particularly valuable role to play because they have often participated in the innovation that led to products under discussion. However, nonacademics who are effective teachers can also provide useful product information. Speaking can benefit medical practices and academic institutions by generating patient referrals for care or participation in research studies.

The lifesaving treatment of my patient Grace with the drug eculizumab exemplifies the importance of peer-to-peer speaking. Her condition—and other rare diseases treated with that drug—is sufficiently rare that most physicians have never encountered it. If they do, they are poorly equipped to manage it and may be unaware of the availability of a highly effective treatment. The obscurity of such diseases means that they do not routinely receive discussion in academic courses, hospital rounds, or professional society conferences. By engaging physician specialists to educate physicians about these diseases and their treatment, the drug's manufacturer improves physician awareness and saves lives.

The intimate nature of peer-to-peer speaking sessions enables practitioners to interact with the speaker and discuss specific cases, a benefit absent at large hospital conferences or professional meetings. Moreover, hospitals now employ full-time physicians known as "hospitalists" to care for patients admitted by community physicians. As a result, the community practitioners do not spend time at hospitals and therefore are less likely to attend educational offerings in that setting.

As is the case with all forms of product information communication by companies, the FDA regulates informational content. During formal presentations related to products, the speaker may not mention anything the FDA has not approved regarding the product. The concerns raised by the fact that some physicians profited substantially from speaking reflect the media's misplaced interest in the money. These critics need to prove that payments are not commensurate with educational value or that the highly paid speakers are not good communicators.

Arguments applied by academic authorities to justify banning peer-to-peer speaking by faculty are arrogant: that such speaking isn't consistent with the academic mission because it represents marketing.[29] Or, it is reprehensible that companies often prepare the teaching materials, thereby violating the academic imperative for originality. But for academic institutions that aggressively advertise their clinical services to condemn marketing is hypocritical. Companies want to control content to protect against litigation for off-label promotion (discussed in chapter 14). The anatomy instructor who lectures students is not using original material—the information is hundreds of years old. And the conflict-of-interest movement repeats the same messages regularly.

Finally, conflict-of-interest defenders denigrate many speakers as not being leading educational authorities—a charge we will revisit in chapter 15. But nearly all physicians completing training undergo certification by general and specialty medical boards. Physicians typically are intelligent, highly educated, and well trained. Therefore, despite the fact that only a minority of physicians engage in research or formal education, most physicians are capable of participation in teaching activities, such as peer-to-peer speaking, particularly after training from a sponsoring company.

8

MISUNDERSTANDING INNOVATION

Many industry critics cited in this book acknowledge that medical innovation is difficult and expensive. But their attacks on the economics of medical-industry partnerships reveal profound misconceptions. To gain a better comprehension of those economics and partnerships, let's start with some fundamental definitions necessary to comprehend medical innovation.

Research is the pursuit of knowledge. Research, if successful, generates *discoveries*. Discoveries include theories to explain natural phenomena susceptible to empiric testing, unearthing of previously unrecognized entities, or recognizing and proving the validity of causal relationships. *Inventions* are discoveries with the potential to become practical technologies. In medicine, such inventions might be potentially useful for clinical diagnosis or treatment. *Innovation* occurs only when inventions achieve practical clinical use. The common misapplication of the term "innovation" to represent *anything* new muddles these important distinctions.

Solicitations for medical research funding from foundations and academic institutions imply that discovery research efforts flow seamlessly to invention and subsequently to innovation. But a very inefficient track record for delivering treatments and cures—medical innovation—illustrates how difficult it is to convert inventions in the laboratory into innovations at the patient's bedside.

INNOVATION INERTIA

Medical innovation has never been easy, but it's gotten more difficult with time. Although the *number* of new medical products approved annually by the FDA has remained fairly constant over the past half century, the *cost* to obtain each approval has increased over 100-fold. In fact, average drug development costs roughly doubled every nine years from 1950 through 2010. This hyperinflation is the inverse of the history of the electronics industry in which the power of transistors rose exponentially, yet over the same time their cost fell by the same magnitude. This phenomenon, predicted by Gordon Moore, came to be known as Moore's Law. By contrast, the disheartening pharmaceutical experience has been dubbed "Eroom's Law," "Eroom" being Moore spelled backward. This staggering rise in cost has occurred despite the facts that research has generated vast amounts of information about biology and that technological advances have enabled obtaining such data thousands of times faster and more cheaply than in the past. [1]

Most analysts agree that a major cause of innovation difficulty has been the growing stringency of the FDA's requirements for product approvals. Since the 1960s, the Agency has demanded more and longer clinical trials, increasingly restrictive criteria for enrollment of trial subjects, and stricter monitoring of clinical trial sites. These demands have lengthened the times necessary to complete trials, reduced patient enrollment in such trials, diminished funding for individual trials, and increased the amount of documentation required for new product approvals. [2]

Development failures conspire with increased regulatory burdens to raise the cost of innovation. Nine out of ten drug candidates that enter human trials fail to obtain FDA approval for their specified indications. More than 30% of drug candidates drop out after Phase I trials, 70% of the survivors perish after Phase II, another 40% fail in Phase III, and almost 20% of those submitted for regulatory approval are rejected. Late stage failures are attributed to lack of product efficacy (65%), safety issues (21%), financial concerns (7%), or unknown reasons (6%). [3] When products succeed in early development only to fail in Phase III trials or thereafter, the cost of such failures are much higher than the ones that appear earlier in the development time line. These failures have become more expensive over time because longer and more complicated clinical trials are more expensive to perform.

Shrinking therapeutic windows also compound the risk of failure and its contribution to cost. Consider cardiovascular disease. Fifty years ago, when the mortality rate from cardiovascular disease was twice what it is today, demonstrating that a drug, say a beta blocker, would affect cardiovascular outcomes was much easier. As cardiovascular disease has become better controlled, the magnitude of improvement that any given drug can produce becomes smaller. These smaller improvements are harder to see and therefore require larger and more expensive clinical trials to demonstrate efficacy.

Similarly, few drug development paths are simple and straightforward. For example, the next chapter explains how the gastrointestinal cancer drug that saved my brother-in-law Patrick's life was unusual, enabling a near cure with surprising ease. The drug Patrick took eradicated his cancer by controlling just a single cellular reaction affected by his disease. Most common cancers, such as those affecting breast and lung, have dozens of deviations in their cellular machinery, and addressing just one or two will be of little help.

Whatever the reasons for the staggering increase in the expense of medical product approval, development and marketing strategies and product pricing must keep pace. In at least one case, one company decided that prescription medical product development was too risky, and it abandoned that business to focus on nonprescription consumer products.[4] Other companies have responded with corporate mergers and acquisitions. In most cases, the goal of merging is to build up the product development pipelines of the combined companies, although inevitably the merger results in layoffs and jettisoning of research projects. In some cases, the mergers focus more on acquiring products with brisk current sales rather than on acquiring risky research.[5] Analysts argue that these maneuvers backfire, because the disruption of corporate structure by the mergers demoralizes the workforce and the sheer size of the combined entities creates confusion and poor internal communication.[6] Some blame too much top-down planning in the industry, while others say there is not enough.[7] One recent reaction to the dismal economics of medical product development has been for companies to swap and combine specific competency areas in hopes of concentrating on the ones with which they have been most successful. For example, Novartis bought oncology products in GlaxoSmithKline's pipeline and established a joint venture with Glaxo involving over-the-counter products. At the same time Novartis sold its animal health business to Eli Lilly.[8]

Small start-up companies attempting to develop novel products, some invented by physicians or academics, are less bureaucratic but have limited resources. They constantly struggle to obtain investment, the prospects of which rise and fall with fluctuations in the general economy. They often survive at the mercy of venture capitalists who may exploit barely surviving companies by imposing draconian investment terms. Except for a handful of very profitable biotechnology companies, the industry as a whole is barely profitable.[9]

Failure presents opportunities. A new entrepreneurship promises—for pay—to solve the medical product productivity impasse. This effort, which I label the "innovation management industry," comes emblazoned with an alphabet soup of acronyms. It convenes meetings, holds webinars, conducts courses, and writes position papers.[10] But you can't learn to play a musical instrument by listening to lectures. A few federal agencies provide funding for product developmental projects. Those dedicated to promoting innovation in military medicine and defense against catastrophic events or bioterrorist attacks have considerable resources and can substantively assist company development efforts. Others are marginally endowed, such as the NIH, which has recently diverted some funds it has traditionally provided for academic discovery research into supporting research efforts to determine whether old drugs have new uses. An older NIH program awards grants to small businesses collaborating with academic researchers. Any and all funding can be crucial, and the networking opportunities these enterprises provide may yield dividends, but otherwise the net substantive value of these activities is unclear. Although I hope I am wrong, I am skeptical that most of them transcend much beyond idle "innovation chitchat."

These innovation cheerleading exercises all articulate the benefits of cooperation between academe, physicians, and industry. In some cases, big pharmaceutical companies have made major financial donations to universities and research institutes for discovery efforts. Unfortunately, the managers from industry and academe who preside over these collaborative efforts out of political correctness focus entirely on fostering collaborative research. They avoid rebutting the policy issues that continue to threaten the viability of innovation, such as the marketing criticism advanced by the conflict-of-interest movement. These managers appear not to perceive the contradiction that should the donations of the pharmaceutical companies to universities actually result in discoveries that become products, thanks to the recipients' conflict-of-interest regulations, the companies that have spent billions to develop the products may not be permitted to market them in the institutions where the discoveries originated!

Conflict-of-interest critics have no doubt about the cause of the low medical product development success rates: bad industry intentions. These critics' straightforward solution is for academics and the government to play a greater role in innovation.[11] They accuse industry of having resorted to making trivial modifications of existing products. They charge that aggressive marketing of such noninnovative—and—supposedly unnecessary "me-too" products has supplanted investment of research and development of new and important ones. According to one critic, "There is very little innovative research in the modern pharmaceutical industry, despite its claims to the contrary."[12]

In addition, this critic alleges that industry influence has degraded university research, bringing it down to the current mediocrity that characterizes industry's. Academic medical centers supposedly used to undertake scientifically important, nontargeted basic research into the causes, mechanisms, and prevention of disease funded by taxpayers through NIH grants. But now:

> [i]ncreasingly, industry is setting the research agenda in academic centers, and that agenda has more to do with industry's mission than with the mission of the academy. Researchers and their institutions are focusing too much on targeted, applied research, mainly drug development, and not enough on non-targeted, basic research into the causes, mechanisms, and prevention of disease.

The rest of this chapter challenges these assertions. They misrepresent history and reflect a lack of understanding of research, invention, and innovation.

INDUSTRY, NOT ACADEME IS THE MAJOR ENGINE OF MEDICAL INNOVATION

What scientifically important research is supposed to be done in universities? And does scientifically important research really lead to medical innovation? In the late 19th and early 20th centuries, discoveries made in universities and research institutes did contribute to health advances. At that time, research done by the faculty of a few universities and institutes involved studies of the organs and physiological systems of experimental animals, human volunteers, and patients with various diseases. The researchers' intentions were to identify disease causes, treatments, and cures. For example, Banting and Best discovered that a lack of the hormone insulin was the cause of the then lethal condition of diabetes. The first successful insulin replacement treatments took place at the University of Toronto where they worked. Others discovered that vitamins could help cure diseases brought on by a lack of certain deficiencies.

In the 1950s, academic researchers began to follow the lead of scientists trained in physics who began to glean deep insights into the structure of body cells and cell components. The research agenda in academe now turned away from studies of animals and humans to molecules and cells often unrelated to specific diseases. In one sense, this trend increased the pace of research because experimental systems involved fewer variables and were therefore easier to control. In another sense, however, these efforts were further removed from the clinical reality of intact organisms. The march into reductionism created an academic obsession with hypothesis-driven basic research, rejecting the opportunistic research that had led to the early disease treatments described above. Such research depended more on trial and error or on following leads from accidental discoveries emerging from simply observing and describing the behavior of sick patients. In addition, the motivation of biomedical researchers began more closely to resemble that of academic scientists in general, an abstract search for "truth" rather than emphasizing ways to understand diseases and help patients.

Subjectivity in science is pervasive. What constitutes important scientific research is what influential scientists *decide* is important. One prominent aspect of this subjectivity is a worship of novelty for novelty's sake and of experimental elegance and virtuosity.[13] Michael Polanyi, a prominent chemist and philosopher, declared that the importance of research results depends on *accuracy* (meaning others can apply theories to make predictions or reproduce experimental findings), *intrinsic interest*, and *general relevance*.[14] According to Polanyi, scientists judge as intrinsically interesting and generally relevant those discoveries that bring previously disparate matters to a defined order or open up a field to exploitation by others. But innovation was not on his list of criteria for interest and relevance. Indeed, a discovery may have a large effect in terms of *technical value* to other researchers—for example, a biochemical journal article describing a method for measuring protein concentrations was for many years the most highly cited publication in biomedical science[15]—but lacking virtuosity, such contributions usually do not afford eminence to their discoverers. Academe's obsession with novelty for novelty's sake fuels the conflict-of-interest movement's criticism of incremental innovation that yields useful and important derivative medical products as "me-toos." Chapter 9 addresses this criticism.

Most historians and sociologists of science agree with Polanyi in discounting the importance of invention-seeking or innovation-motivating researchers. They argue that scientists seek the approval of influential peers for elegant solutions of previously unsolved scientific puzzles such as providing simple explanations for natural phenomena.[16] Attesting to biomedical researchers' relative disinterest in practical implications of their work is their documented failure to *mention* such implications in the vast majority of research publications in top-tier biomedical journals.[17] Even when academics do participate in commercial enterprises, professional reputation dominates other reasons for this participation, including financial rewards.[18]

As a result of these historical and cultural developments, although some discoveries that arise in universities and other nonprofit research institutions qualify as inventions, private industry delivers far more inventions and nearly all innovation as defined above. Estimates place the industry contributions to innovation around 85% of the medical product pipeline.[19] The preponderance of not only industry's financial investment but also scientific contributions leads to clinically useful products.[20]

Industry bears the vast majority of the rising costs of FDA product approval mentioned above. Academic institutions lack the financial resources and diverse skill sets required to translate inventions into innovation. With the exception of clinical trials and epidemiology, medical schools provide little or no education concerning the myriad activities required for FDA approval. "Pharmacology" courses taught in medical schools solely concern the mechanisms by which drugs are thought to work. They do not teach the nonlinear processes leading to the development of drugs and the economic challenges of those processes.

Although academic biomedical research has focused more on basic laboratory problems, its justification for funding remains the promise of practical results for medical care. For example, every component institute of the NIH, with the exception of the National Institute for General Medical Sciences, identifies with specific diseases or disease sets. But even as academic researchers take the NIH money based on promises of disease cures, the writers of grant applications or their colleagues reviewing them pay little attention to the claims as to how studies on molecules and cells would surely lead to advances against disease, knowing that such accomplishments are unlikely in the near term. Two decades elapsed before the riveting discovery that DNA is the basis of heredity (*discovery*)[21] led to practical procedures for diagnosing and treating genetic diseases (*innovation*). Researchers working on problems far removed from specific clinical matters fear earmarking of funding for relevant research and repeatedly make special pleadings for the long-term benefits of basic research, the practical implications of which usually become obvious only in hindsight.[22] Because biomedical research is far more expensive than other scholarly disciplines, academics have to seek public or philanthropic monies for their biomedical research programs, and understandably these funding sources have finite appetites for open-ended research for research's sake.

Any accusation that academic institutions are now overly committed to "drug development" is empirically false. Even when physicians and academics have participated in the founding of genetic engineering companies or invented devices, these activities do not "set the research agenda in academic centers." In fact, researchers participating in commercial genetic engineering generally continue to maintain strong academic ties and do not flag in pursuing their academic research activities.[23] Such participation yields positive contributions to the academic mission. Relationships between leading university researchers and their companies then provide job opportunities for talented doctoral students following graduation.

The foregoing discussion summarized the cultural reasons most academic biomedical researchers do not focus on innovation. But even if they *wanted* to innovate, economic forces discourage them. Declining government and nonprofit academic research funding in recent years has forced researchers to divert ever more time and attention from *doing* research to convincing granting agency peer review committees to pay for it.

Reduced funds available to these agencies have exacerbated the pathological aspects of such committees. One of these pathological features is the academic obsession with novelty for novelty's sake. Others include the tendency to impress other reviewers with critical acumen, to kowtow to the most prestigious members of the committees who shoot from the hip without accountability, to reason from anecdote, and, most importantly, to exercise excessive risk aversion. To counteract this behavior researchers have increasingly narrowed their project focus. By limiting focus, grant applicants have a better chance of amassing a record of journal publications and preliminary data that maximize the persuasiveness of their research grant applications. This narrow concentration, however, precludes the expansive thinking and risk taking required for medical product invention and innovation. But the overarching reason that committees are poorly equipped to prioritize research projects is the fundamental uncertainty and variability of biological responses discussed in chapter 5. Experts can fairly readily identify errors in someone's experimental treatment of predictable interactions that characterize engineering, chemistry, or physics projects and determine that such projects will not succeed. Foreseeing the outcome of projects related to biology and disease is far more daunting.[24]

Anti-innovative elements also plague industry's decision making regarding what projects to undertake and investors' assessments of what projects to support. Mature medical products' companies employ business development staff to evaluate potential technologies for possible development. The high and expensive failure rate of medical product development puts these individuals at greater risk if they recommend projects that fail than if they reject them, because nobody knows whether they might have succeeded. Industry insiders who conduct evaluations often have pet projects that they defend by recommending rejection of competing ones from outside the company. The frequency of failure also means that project reviewers nearly always find some aspect of a technology under consideration that resembles properties of past failures and use that reasoning to recommend rejection.

Consultants armed with strategic plans and market analyses frequently encourage company managers to kill projects early, thereby preventing financial hemorrhage incurred by late-stage failures. Killing a project prematurely, however, eliminates the possibility that troubleshooting efforts might have made it viable. The "killers" go scot-free, because the potential for success remains forever unknown. Marketing departments weigh in heavily in this culling activity, but companies' science advisers can also be anti-innovative. They may have had distinguished accomplishments, but these are usually rooted in the past.

The following two medical product development stories exemplify how overcoming or sidestepping expertise and oversight sometimes is necessary for success.

The Development of the Proton Pump Inhibitor

Ulcers of the upper digestive tract—caused by the strong acid produced in the stomach to digest food—used to be a major cause of severe stomach pain. Ulcers also often bled, causing anemia and even fatal massive hemorrhages. The standard treatment for ulcer disease was for affected patients to take large amounts of "antacid" medications to neutralize the acid. Attesting to the inadequacy of antacid therapy, however, was a high frequency of surgical operations to remove parts of the gut containing intractable ulcers, and they often caused unpleasant complications. In 1970, researchers at the Swedish pharmaceutical company Astra (now AstraZeneca) developed a drug named omeprazole that reduced the stomach's ability to make the acid. They proposed that the more direct approach of this proton pump inhibitor in preventing acid production would be more effective than buffering accumulated acid with antacids after the fact. The company's science advisory board, sneering at the low profitability of the abundantly available antacids, blocked pursuit of the project. Astra researchers kept the project alive with Swedish government funds and tried to establish a partnership with the American company Abbot for further development. But in 1980 Abbot declined, citing the same objections raised by Astra's science advisers. Nevertheless, Astra finally went on to develop the drug. It was a stunning success. In the 1990s, its sales in the United States topped $2 billion.[25] Now available over the counter, this drug and others like it are the major reason digestive tract ulcers are rare today.

Thomas Fogarty and the Invention of the Embolectomy Catheter

No research grant evaluation committee staffed by academics imbued with the ethos of important science would fund a medical student's trial and error tinkering in his attic. Yet, just such an effort led Thomas Fogarty to develop the most widely used catheter for removing blood clots clogging patients' arteries. While a medical student at the University of Cincinnati, Fogarty was struck by the problem of high morbidity and mortality associated with embolectomy, the procedure then used to remove blood clots from blocked arteries. The procedure had to be performed under general anesthesia. The clogged artery was squeezed upstream of the clot, and forceps were used to remove it through a large incision that had to be sewn shut. Over half of patients so treated died or had major complications. Fogarty wanted a solution that avoided general anesthesia, upstream vessel compression, and large incisions.

In his attic, Fogarty experimented with a balloon-tipped urinary catheter. His idea was that a properly modified catheter would enable a small incision, eliminate the need to squeeze the vessel, and accommodate clot access while reducing vessel trauma. The specific procedure he envisioned was to push the balloon through the clot, inflate it with saline using a syringe, expand the balloon to the size of the artery, and then retract it, withdrawing the clot through the incision.

He cut off the tip of the pinky finger of a surgical latex glove to create a balloon and attached it to the catheter, using fishing techniques he learned as a boy. He found that the balloon often burst when inflated and dragged through glass tubes filled with Jello—the model he used to simulate an arterial clot. Eventually, he determined the type and thickness of rubber firm enough when inflated to extract a clot but flexible enough to move through it without bursting. Fogarty had a workable device before receiving his MD degree in 1960.

Fogarty made the catheter system by hand for himself and colleagues who wanted to try it. During his residency training at the University of Oregon, Dr. Albert Starr, head of the cardiothoracic division, began using Fogarty's balloon catheters and asked one of his acquaintances, Lowell Edwards, an electrical engineer and president of his own company, to consider producing it (Starr and Edwards developed the first artificial heart valve in 1960). In 1969, Fogarty patented his device and assigned it to Edwards Life Sciences of Irvine, California. The Fogarty Embolectomy Catheter—the first minimally invasive endovascular device—became the industry standard. It remains the most widely used catheter for blood-clot removal. It is used in over three hundred thousand procedures every year all over the world. It is estimated to have saved the lives and limbs of millions of patients.[26] Patients who have benefited from the application of Fogarty's catheter would hardly begrudge the generous royalties he has received for his invention.

Although Fogarty spent much of his career at Stanford University Medical School, he left it to start his own innovation institute, precisely because of his frustration with "the evaluation committee syndrome":[27] "There were 12 committees [to deal with]. That's why I left Stanford. It's not conducive to innovation. It is sad. It's dangerous, because people are dying." Fogarty defined a committee as "a group of the unwilling, picked from the unfit to do the unnecessary."

In summary, industry dominates innovation for several major economic and cultural reasons. The long and meandering product development process requires a passion for the journey, obstinate persistence, and a willingness to adapt to unforeseen events. The laws of economics dictate that someone must make risky long-term investments in that journey.

The Real Reason for Innovation Inertia

Having preliminarily debunked the critics' theory that the difficulty and high cost of medical innovation is the *fault* of industry, I return to the most plausible explanation for these problems. They arise from the disproportionate effect progressively more stringent FDA regulation of medical product evaluation has engrafted on the fundamental complexity and variability of human biology. As discussed in chapter 5, this complexity and variability enabled human survival in the face of predators and pathogens. But it also builds unpredictability into outcomes of therapies. Medical innovation, like soccer and hockey, is a low-scoring activity. If one reduced the size of hockey or soccer goals, analogous to increasing FDA regulation, the already low average game score, representative of patients' unpredictable responses to drugs and devices, would fall out of proportion to the reduction in the goal size. The only remedy in that circumstance is for the teams to increase their shots on the shrunken goal.

The more well-aimed shots that are taken, the better the chance of success. The following discussion illustrates these principles.

What Factors Allow Innovation to Flourish? Studies from My Life and Others

The conflict-of-interest narrative generalizes industry as large, global, publicly traded companies with established revenues. While these entities have most of the industry's financial assets, small firms of diverse types—most desperately seeking financial resources to survive—vastly outnumber them. You can't innovate without money to fund your operation. Successful innovators tend to be obstinate, persistent, and adaptable in the face of inadequate financing. Innovators have to *want* to innovate. They must be willing to change course when results fail to support a particular strategy. They have to beg incessantly for funding. When the funds aren't there, they must imaginatively downsize, defer expenditures, and resort to whatever else it takes to keep their lights on until resources can be found. The fact that these financial problems are the norm helps explain why innovation is so hard and lengthy.

Two examples follow describing companies that originated around the same time. They illustrate why innovation does not arise from arbitrary a priori determinations of scientific importance. It emerges by a tortuous and usually unpredictable route requiring adequate investment as an essential ingredient. A third example recounts my personal efforts attempting to turn research results into an invention and to advance the invention to innovation status.

Millenium Pharmaceuticals

As the analysis of the human genome progressed, a group of geneticists founded Millenium in 1993 based on the premise that the ability to rapidly analyze genes linked to diseases would reveal drug targets efficiently and usher in the era of "personalized medicine." In selling that idea, Millenium was in the right place at the right time. Over 20 major pharmaceutical companies established strategic partnerships with the start-up to take advantage of these promises, and it rapidly amassed over $2 billion in funding. It initially used these monies to invest in gene sequencing equipment only to discover quickly that genetic analysis was not going to be the projected fast track to innovation.

Millenium used its now prodigious assets to license FDA-approved products from other companies that treated inflammation and cardiovascular diseases and a promising drug under development for cancer. Sales of the licensed products generated revenues, and the FDA approved the cancer treatment in 2008. That same year the Japanese pharmaceutical giant Takeda purchased Millenium for $8.8 billion. Millenium's initial investors and corporate partners may not have achieved their hoped-for scientific results, but despite their unconsummated infatuation with a current scientific fad, they inadvertently contributed to the establishment of a new global pharmaceutical company making important products and achieved a fine financial return on their investments.

Alexion

A physician-scientist named Leonard Bell left Yale Medical School in 1992 to found Alexion, the company that made the drug, eculizumab, that I used to treat Grace's HUS.[28] Bell was convinced that blocking the body's defensive, but sometimes self-destructing, complement system would treat many diseases caused by inflammation. Within two years, after discouraging results, the company was nearly broke. Then another company interested in creating organs in pigs that could be transplanted to humans gave Alexion $5 million in 1995 to prevent recipients' rejection of the pig organs. With additional funding from the state of Connecticut, the company took a different approach to blocking complement activation, resulting in the production of eculizumab. The capital markets responded to this progress with a $21 million public offering in 1996. But eculizumab did not work in the prevalent inflammatory diseases it was supposed to target. Then an Alexion researcher started to collaborate with a British hematologist, attempting to modify red blood cells of patients with the PNH, the rare disease described in chapter 1, so they would not break down and cause severe side effects. The specific project did not succeed, but the relationship continued, leading to the demonstration that eculizimab, the complement blocker that had failed to achieve usefulness in treating other diseases, dramatically controlled the symptoms of PNH. After two clinical trials, the FDA approved eculizumab for treatment of PNH in 2007 and for atypical HUS in 2011. In 2008, the Galien Foundation awarded Alexion its Prix Galien for eculizumab, recognizing it as the best new pharmaceutical drug that year.[29]

Both PNH and atypical HUS are vanishingly rare, and Alexion has addressed this rarity by charging $440,000 per year per patient treated. This decision has afforded Alexion $1.1 billion in revenues in 2012 and a market capitalization of $20 billion. Insurance companies and single-payer systems abroad willingly pay the costs because the drug effectively controls conditions that produce huge hospital costs and are lethal if left untreated. In addition, the company's profitability allows it to provide free treatment to the uninsured.

MY PERSONAL ODYSSEY FROM RESEARCH TOWARD INNOVATION

My research work, begun 45 years ago, has concerned a type of white blood cell called a neutrophil. By way of background, every day our bone marrow generates over 100 billion neutrophils that circulate briefly in the bloodstream. In a few hours, however, they migrate out of blood vessels into every part of our bodies to find, devour, and kill microorganisms. During this process, each neutrophil moves about an eighth of an inch under its own power: a hundred billion times that distance adds up to more than twice around the Earth. Failure to produce neutrophils (as occurs in certain types of blood diseases) or, more rarely, disorders in which neutrophil migration is impaired, result in an inability to control infections with often-fatal results.

My research focused on this migration behavior. Japanese researchers had recently discovered that cells such as neutrophils (and the amoebas they resemble) crawl using the same machinery as found in our muscles. This muscle machinery consisted of fibrous proteins organized in parallel arrays that slide past one another in response to signals from the nervous system to shorten (or contract) the muscle. Exploiting these insights, I decided to try to analyze crawling movements of neutrophils by under-standing how these proteins worked inside these cells.

The first goal was to isolate the muscle proteins and see how they functioned. This effort revealed that while in some respects these proteins were similar to their muscle counterparts, they did not operate in parallel arrays. Rather, neutrophil fibers organized themselves into a gel-like substance. This was consistent with observations that dated from the invention of microscopes in the 17th century that the crawling movements of cells seemed to involve transitions between liquid and gel states in their internal substance, like the freezing and melting of water. These transformations enable parts of the crawling cells to be sufficiently rigid and coherent to push against resistance yet at times adequately liquid to allow for changes in shape and direction.

Discoveries

In 1974 my student John Hartwig and I discovered what we named "filamin," which we believed was responsible for the gel formation of the muscle proteins, and published the findings in the leading biochemistry and cell biology journals.[30] Five years later, another student, Helen Yin, and I discovered a second new neutrophil protein that together with filamin rapidly and reversibly transforms the cellular gels into liquids. We named this second protein "gelsolin."[31]

These discoveries have stood the test of time. The National Library of Medicine repository of research publications as of October 2014 lists 1,320 published articles concerning filamin and 2,030 about gelsolin.[32] At the same time, a clearinghouse called ResearchGate, which keeps track of citations to researchers' publications, reported that 11,000 such citations referred to mine.[33] I have had continuous grant funding from the NIH since the mid-1970s to do research work related to these proteins. I have won awards, honorary degrees, and election to elite scientific societies in recognition of these efforts. Based on these criteria, I have accomplished what one could reasonably say is scientifically important research. But no one has lived one second longer or become healthier due to *direct* results from my scientifically important research.

My Research Discoveries Unexpectedly Become an Invention

But events *indirectly* related to my research led to a possible invention. In 1981, the unexpected finding emerged that gelsolin is also a protein that circulates abundantly in blood plasma. Cells produce *two* gelsolins—one that resides within them and another that they secrete to the outside world. The latter has come to be called *plasma* gelsolin.

The existence of plasma gelsolin returns us to the fundamental differences between research, invention, and innovation. The identification of plasma gelsolin was a discovery. I intuited that an abundant plasma protein might be medically important and was determined to try to turn this discovery into invention and innovation. But at that point plasma gelsolin's abundance did not guarantee medical importance because I had no inkling as to its function. Because the academic research culture worships hypothesis-driven investigation and research grant review committees reliably turn down proposals they dub "fishing expeditions" or "descriptive" projects, I had little hope of obtaining any grant support to research the question.

The path around this dilemma required adapting with available resources. At the time I was head of the Hematology and Oncology Unit at Boston's Massachusetts General Hospital and ran a postdoctoral training program for young physicians entering those specialties. Research was a mandatory requirement for specialty certification by the American Board of Internal Medicine, and I had acquired an NIH grant that supported the research trainees. Although many of them had little interest in research, they represented a free labor pool and were relatively happy to participate in a project that might have more clinical potential than the basic cell-crawling work that was the mainstream effort in my laboratory.

Because I knew that plasma gelsolin, like cellular gelsolin, binds muscle proteins that are among the body's most abundant, I reasoned that injury might result in plasma gelsolin depletion. Normally, muscle proteins reside only inside of cells, but if the cells' membrane barriers broke, plasma gelsolin could flow into the cells. Plasma gelsolin might also bind muscle fibers released into the blood and help to clear them from the circulation. Measurements of plasma gelsolin in animals and humans subjected to extensive trauma confirmed these theories but did not reveal whether plasma gelsolin depletion might be clinically important. The most plausible theory was that muscle proteins released from injured cells might somehow be toxic and that by removing them, plasma gelsolin had a protective effect.

This theory might explain a common clinical problem. Patients admitted to hospitals for treatment of diverse problems such as trauma, burns, or infections frequently but unpredictably develop a devastating set of complications over the course of hours or days. The affected patient's blood pressure falls so that blood does not adequately circulate and vital organs become dangerously starved for oxygen. The patient's lungs fill up with fluid, which interferes with oxygen transfer from the air to the blood, further compromising organ viability. These so-called "critical care complications" (that sometimes go by the name adult respiratory distress syndrome) require patients to be cared for in intensive care units, where they receive drugs that raise their blood pressure and artificial ventilators force oxygen to their lungs under pressure through tubes inserted into their airways. These measures have side effects, and about a quarter of affected patients die. Others languish for weeks in intensive care. If they survive, they suffer debilitating long-term complications.

If muscle protein released from damaged tissues caused these consequences, and if gelsolin, by mitigating muscle protein toxicity, could prevent these critical care complications, it would be of great medical importance. In the United States, 250,000 patients die annually from critical care complications, and the estimated cost of critical care consequences is $17 billion.[34]

Research over the next decade provided some, although not overly convincing evidence, for the muscle protein toxicity theory.[35] When I pitched to companies the idea that giving plasma gelsolin to patients with low blood concentrations of it might prevent critical care complications, they rightly responded that I had no evidence at all to support that idea. But in 1993, I learned about a protein therapy for the inherited disease, cystic fibrosis. Cystic fibrosis patients suffer progressive lung destruction because their airways fill up with sticky secretions. Scientists know that the stickiness of these obstructions are due to a high content of DNA fibers. The new protein treatment, Pulmozyme, breaks down these DNA fibers when inhaled by patients, slowing their lungs' progressive deterioration.

Anticipating that pathological cystic fibrosis secretions might contain large quantities of muscle protein from dead neutrophils in addition to DNA and that gelsolin might reduce the thickness of that material, we obtained expectorated lung secretions from cystic fibrosis patients. Experiments revealed that cystic fibrosis sputum contained such proteins and the addition of plasma gelsolin reduced the sputum's high stickiness. We reported the discovery in an article in the journal *Science*[36] and filed additional patent applications, and my hospital licensed an invention—to treat airway inflammation with inhaled plasma gelsolin—to Biogen in 1995 for clinical development.

Within three years, Biogen produced large quantities of plasma gelsolin using genetically engineered bacteria, documented its identity with gelsolin isolated from blood plasma, and showed that giving it to experimental animals in large amounts produced no side effects. Instilled into the airways of normal volunteers, gelsolin also caused no untoward complications. Biogen then performed a small clinical Phase II trial administering plasma gelsolin into the airways of patients with cystic fibrosis. The patients that received increasing doses of plasma gelsolin showed a modest improvement in lung functions. But then Biogen decided to drop the project.

The main reason for this decision was that Pulmozyme had recently failed in clinical trials of chronic bronchitis. Chronic bronchitis is an inflammatory disease that predominantly affects heavy smokers and leads to lung destruction. It is far more prevalent than cystic fibrosis. Unless plasma gelsolin was spectacularly superior to Pulmozyme, an unlikely eventuality, competing with an established expensive drug in a small patient population was not economically viable.

Amazingly, the same week that Biogen decided to stop the plasma gelsolin project, a medical journal publication reported that the prognosis of patients suffering from acute trauma could be predicted based on their admission plasma gelsolin levels. All the patients had levels below normal, but the patients with the lowest plasma gelsolin concentrations had a higher probability of critical care complications, consistent with predictions we had made during the previous decade.[37] Over the next several years evidence accumulated that critically depleted plasma gelsolin values precede and predict adverse outcomes in acute and chronic diseases.[38] Additional research revealed that one of plasma gelsolin's functions is to localize inflammation, explaining how it might prevent critical care complications after injuries. Most importantly, giving plasma gelsolin to acutely injured animals reduced their mortality.[39]

In 2005, James Fordyce, an experienced investor, became intrigued with the plasma gelsolin project and started a company, Critical Biologics Corporation (CBC), to move it forward. He recruited an experienced biotechnology executive, Ashleigh Palmer, to run the company. Fordyce, Palmer, and I pitched our story to venture capital firms, racing the clock imposed by the patent costs that Brigham & Women's Hospital was now reluctantly footing. In late 2005, an investment firm based on a Hong

Kong real estate fortune agreed to finance the company with $10 million in initial funding.

Within two years, CBC reproduced the results obtained previously in the academic laboratories documenting that plasma gelsolin level depletion precedes and predicts critical care complications. It then completed a randomized placebo-controlled clinical trial treating acutely ill patients in an intensive care unit with increasing doses of plasma gelsolin. The purpose of the trial was to determine whether it was feasible to increase sick patients' plasma gelsolin levels without causing side effects. Because of the investor's origin, the trial took place at Queen Mary's Hospital in Hong Kong. The study was a Phase Ib/2a trial, because the patients were not healthy volunteers as is the rule in Phase I trials; the Hong Kong regulators did not consider increasing plasma gelsolin levels above normal in healthy individuals to be ethically warranted.

Although the study was too small to reveal any survival differences between treated patients and those given placebo, it showed that even the lowest plasma gelsolin dose increased the depleted levels in the treated patients. The safety board monitoring the trial concluded that the treatment did not increase adverse outcomes, even though, as is the rule for critical care patients, such outcomes occurred. During the trials, we had also filed additional patent applications for treatment uses including kidney, neurologic, and chronic inflammatory diseases.

In early 2008, CBC set out to raise $24 million to conduct a Phase II proof-of-concept clinical trial in the United States to document whether plasma gelsolin measurements and replacement of depleted plasma gelsolin would save lives in critical care patients. The cost estimate was based on having to manufacture additional supplies of plasma gelsolin, obtain regulatory approval, and based on estimates of critical care adverse event rates, enroll, treat, and monitor 400 patients—200 receiving plasma gelsolin and 200 a placebo.

As we sought this funding, the great recession hit, casting a pall over all biomedical investment. Worse, we were stuck between the early stages of funding when investors make relatively modest commitments and the later stages when investments are more substantial, but the start-up is close to providing actual revenues. By early 2010, CBC's money ran out, and Ashleigh had to find another job. The A-round funder wrote CBC off, the company ceased to exist, and the patent portfolio returned to Brigham & Women's Hospital in June of 2010.

As CBC wound down, Dr. Susan Levinson and Valerie Ceva, two former Novartis Company employees, and Steve Cordovano, a retired investment manager, had formed a consulting company named Trivalent Partners. They became excited by the gelsolin technology and volunteered to take it forward. The Trivalent team incorporated a new start-up, BioAegis Therapeutics. As of early 2014, the BioAegis management had raised over $7 million and made several value-enhancing contributions. They convened a panel of critical care physician experts to help design a clinical trial to determine whether detection of critically depleted plasma gelsolin and its replacement will protect patients with pneumonia from complications such as death. The management team hired a contract manufacturer to produce plasma gelsolin and set out to establish a proprietary test to measure plasma gelsolin during the trial and for subsequent clinical applications. They also networked with federal military and bioterror agencies to obtain nondilutive investment. Because trauma and critical care issues are rampant in war, the military relevance is clear. An infection specialist demonstrated that plasma gelsolin helps white blood cells ingest and kill various types of bacteria, including species that terrorists might turn loose to infect populations. Finally, the team identified a number of other diseases in addition to those previously considered that might benefit from plasma gelsolin diagnosis and treatment. Now, the challenge is to see whether better economic times and the advances made in the past few years will accommodate raising the funds to run the critical trial described above.

In summary, the *research* on gelsolin has gone on for over 33 years. NIH and other research grants and partial salary support from my academic employers paid for this effort. A generous estimate is that this investment amounted to no more than $10 million. Some of it can be credited toward the *invention* phase because of the time colleagues and I spent moving the technology forward. But corporate sources, Biogen, CBC, and BioAegis, provided at least six times that amount, illustrating how the financial investment of industry far exceeds that of government and academe in such cases—and these amounts are only funds *spent*, not *opportunity costs* of returns that never came to Biogen or CBC and may never accrue to BioAegis.

INNOVATION, UNLIKE RESEARCH, REQUIRES MORE BRUTE FORCE THAN FINESSE

Few researchers have taken projects all the way from "the bench to the bedside." If plasma gelsolin measurement and replacement becomes an innovation, I will have made that complete journey. My history certainly belies a dismissive conflict-of-interest movement assertion that relationships between physicians, academics, and industry are overblown in importance, because industry-sponsored researchers are simply "testing" technologies that already exist:[40] The critical care physician experts who test my technology bring essential expertise and experience to bear in ways that can troubleshoot problems and promote the likelihood of the project's success.

My experience illustrates how persistence and adaptation in the face of random events is just as important to the innovation cycle as academic purity or the blessings of research evaluation committees. The projects also illustrate the bidirectional flow between bench and bedside—that innovation is just as likely to promote discovery as vice versa.[41]

The companies described in this book that have survived by transforming their business models, merging, taking advantage of other financial strategies, and dropping projects in response to circumstances, and exploiting ever changing opportunities, show that innovation is not the result of an idealized linear progression originating from elegant, "innovative," "early-stage," and "important" research to product development, product sales, and health benefits. A variety of companies accommodate projects of vastly different natures and scale. In my opinion, the only antidote to the failure rate that impedes innovation is to have as many companies as possible taking as many shots on the innovation goal as they can afford. Anything that keeps such companies alive and financially viable contributes to that valuable multiplicity.

CONCLUSION

This chapter discussed how the conflict-of-interest narrative conveys a confused description of how medical innovation occurs. It contrasted the idealized notion of scientifically important research rationally leading to practical inventions that benefit patients—innovation—with real-life examples, including from my own experiences, demonstrating how difficult and unpredictable the path from research to innovation consistently is.

9

ECONOMIC ILLITERACY

Imatinib, the anti-cancer drug introduced in chapter 1 that saved my brother-in-law's life, has been universally recognized as an important breakthrough—and widely criticized for its high price. Such criticism overlooks essential economic realities underlying medical product development. Critics ignore the enormous costs of such development, the staggering risks involved, and the unpredictable nature of the whole process. No one can predict in advance which products will succeed in human trials. Those that succeed must pay for those that fail. The high cost of products is justified because the profits from their sales underwrite the next generation of product development and because a high return is necessary to compensate investors for risking their money in the uncertain world of medical product development. This chapter explores these issues using Gleevec (imatinib) as a case study exemplifying the broader patterns of product development and pricing.

The FDA initially approved imatinib, developed by the Novartis pharmaceutical company, in 2001 to treat a disease called chronic myelogenous leukemia (CML). Leukemias are a form of cancer that develops in our infection-fighting white blood cells. The cause of CML is a genetic mutation that results in the overactivity of a chemical reaction in such cells. This chemical overdrive causes uncontrolled white blood cell growth. Imatinib blocks the leukemia-causing chemical reaction.

In the past, CML was temporarily controllable but uniformly fatal within five years. Rare patients opted for and survived a harrowing chemotherapy regimen that eradicated the leukemia cells. This treatment also destroyed the patient's normal blood cell-producing bone marrow, so survival depended on the patient having a bone marrow transplant. If the patient's immune system did not reject the transplant, it could replace the patient's destroyed bone marrow. This procedure often killed patients. In contrast to prior treatments, imatinib far more specifically attacks leukemia cells and spares normal cells, producing deep and lasting remissions with minimal side effects. How did imatinib come to exist? Not as portrayed by the conflict-of-interest narrative.

For example, a book critical of industry and physician's relationships with it contains a chapter titled—after Clint Eastwood's film—*The Good, the Bad, and the Ugly*. It reverently declares imatinib "the good."[1] According to its account, Novartis's chemists rationally developed the "good" drug by deliberately designing imatinib to target with high specificity the chemical reaction responsible for the uncontrolled multiplication of CML cells. Generations of researchers working in academic institutions had identified this chemical reaction. A Novartis researcher gave imatinib samples to Brian Druker, a hematologist at the Oregon Health and Science University, who then demonstrated that it rapidly killed CML cells cultivated in his laboratory.

Novartis then contracted with Druker in 1998 to administer imatinib to CML patients who were unresponsive to previously available treatments. Testing of drugs in patients with advanced cancers is the usual first step in assessing a new cancer drug and is mainly used to determine its side effects. Although such trials rarely show efficacy, not only was imatinib easily tolerated, but it also impressively reversed the patients' CML. Novartis then mounted a larger clinical trial of imatinib therapy in previously untreated CML patients and obtained stunningly positive results. Imatinib produced durable complete remissions in nearly all of the patients.[2] Imatinib became the great hope for a future of precisely "targeted" drug therapy.

Except for some grousing about Novartis lobbying against efforts to reduce imatinib's selling price, the aforementioned book presents imatinib as an example of idealized medical product development: rigorous academic science identifies causes of diseases, companies develop drugs to target those causes, and these drugs can market themselves for serious unmet medical needs. It bemoans the rarity of such breakthroughs, which would allegedly be the routine if only the medical products' industry and its physician collaborators were less greedy.

The treatment of the imatinib story in another book, *The Truth About the Drug Companies*[3] is far less positive. It correctly reports that CML is a relatively rare disorder with around 5,000 new patients being identified annually in the United States. Novartis was initially reluctant to invest in such an uncommon disease. Druker applied persuasion to overcome that reluctance. But it contradicts *The Good, the Bad, and the Ugly*'s assertion that imatinib development is a tribute to idealized industry innovation. Rather, the author overwhelmingly credits government-funded academic science for identifying the biological target that Novartis merely exploited and resents the fact that Novartis gets the major monetary profits. As a result of this injustice, the public "pay[s] twice." Another book, *Powerful Medicines*, also gives the main credit to the government and academics for imatinib.[4]

I know Brian Druker personally and served on a panel that in 2009 selected him to win the Lasker Award, considered America's Nobel Prize for his contributions to CML therapy. For those reasons, my interpretation of imatinib's development history is far different. It is in keeping with the examples from the previous chapter illustrating that innovation does not simply flow formulaically from scientifically important research.

While true that many years of academic research identified the chemical reaction targeted by imatinib to attack CML, the Novartis chemists did *not* initially look for them. Rather, they searched for chemicals to block a *different* chemical reaction they thought might cause other cancers or promote inflammation. And imatinib *was not specific* for the CML target. It reacted with several other chemical reactions in body cells.[5]

This lack of specificity is what saved my brother-in-law's life. On learning of imatinib's great success in treating CML, George Demetri, a medical oncologist at Boston's Dana Farber Cancer Center specializing in GIST, the cancer that afflicted Patrick, noted that one of the drug's other targets was a genetically altered cell component recently implicated as driving the growth and spread of GIST cells. Demetri obtained imatinib from Novartis and treated a patient riddled with GIST, and the patient had a remarkable recovery.[6] On the basis of this anecdotal success, Novartis organized a clinical trial to test imatinib in more GIST patients. The trial unequivocally demonstrated imatinib's effectiveness in that disease, again with surprisingly minimal side effects.[7]

Druker's persistence between 1993 and 1998 in encouraging Novartis to mount a Phase I trial of imatinib epitomizes the importance of clinical champions outside of industry to encourage product development.[8] However, recall that some drugs that seem to work in test tubes or animals cannot be conveniently administered to humans, and the challenge of drug delivery is known as formulation. A principle reason imatinib finally got into the Novartis clinical development pipeline was because another Novartis drug candidate encountered a formulation problem. Even then, elaborate toxicity testing and dose finding had to be carried out to arrive at an appropriate formulation of imatinib. An intravenous version failed, but fortunately a pill form worked. Thus, touting scientifically straightforward drug targeting as the basis of imatinib's introduction to the clinic does not stand up to the facts. Imatinib's lack of target specificity leaves us unsure as to why it works so well in CML and somewhat less well in GIST, and why its side effect profile is relatively benign when it attacks so many cellular components.

Subsequent efforts to develop imatinib-like "designer drugs" have yielded a few successes and many failures. Most importantly, imatinib's spectacular effectiveness against CML was unpredictable *until* clinical trials were performed. Only *then* was it clear that imatinib would transform a rare, fatal disease into a growing population of medicated survivors who could financially justify Novartis's investment. A positive therapeutic outcome in humans that mirrors effects observed in test tubes or animals is the rare exception rather than the rule.

Furthermore, neither the idealized nor dismissive versions of the imatinib story come close to encompassing the difficult reality of product development. As discussed in the previous chapter, hypothesis-based science certainly contributes to it, but serendipity and brute force backed by large-scale investment have far more to do with the unpredictable, and often unsuccessful, journey from laboratory science to approved product. The fact that Novartis's extensive chemistry effort got to a right answer for the wrong initial reason doesn't matter to the patients who benefited. And the effort to get the drug to the patients was many times as expensive as the underlying academic science.

DANGEROUS DISCOUNTS

Imatinib exemplifies the aggregate value of industry contributions to product development. Economists have made extensive analyses of health care outcomes in many countries over time and have consistently concluded that medical products extend lives, enhance quality of life, and on balance reduce health care costs by preventing unnecessary hospitalizations, surgeries, and other expensive care.[9]

Conflict-of-interest movement promoters, however, challenge these conclusions by nitpicking at the economists' data and conclusions.[10] The economists have formally rebutted the objections of those critics, inviting them to explain why, despite an obesity epidemic, we are living longer and healthier lives.[11] That products developed by industry are mainly responsible for these advances is intuitively obvious to anyone, like me, who has worked on the front lines of medical care for a long time.

The conflict-of-interest movement points to the fact that America spends more on health care compared to other countries and achieves similar or worse health outcomes. They imply that excessive medical product prescribing is responsible for the discrepancy.[12] But many of the transnational longevity differences cited are apples-to-oranges comparisons of very different social and geographic circumstances. They largely disappear if one removes auto fatalities and homicides from the analysis. Moreover, prescribing accounts for only approximately 13% of total health care costs,[13] so prescribing costs cannot explain our higher health care expenditures.

These facts, however, do not keep the media from laying the blame for these disparities at the feet of the medical products industry. For example, a front page story in the August 3, 2013, *New York Times* featured a large photo of a smiling 67-year-old man named Michael Shopenn dressed in a bright red ski suit jauntily snowboarding on a Colorado mountainside. Titled "For Medical Tourists, Simple Math. US Estimate for a New Hip: over $78,000. The Belgian bill: $13,660," the article recounted how the snowboarder needed a hip replacement because of degenerative hip arthritis. Mr. Shopenn had health insurance, but the insurer wouldn't pay for the procedure, alleging that the hip condition resulted from a sports injury—a preexisting condition. So Shopenn consulted a local hospital regarding the cost of a hip replacement if he paid out of pocket. The hospital quoted Mr Shopenn a whopping $78,000 price. Shopenn eventually opted to have the procedure done in a Belgian hospital at a cost of $13,660.[14]

The article blames the medical products industry for this discrepancy. Although the price of the hip implant device quoted at the high-priced U.S. hospital was $8,000, nearly twice the $4,200 cost of the one in Belgium, that differential accounts for a mere 6% of the $65,000 variation in procedure sticker prices. Even if the U.S. hospital threw in the device for free, the difference would still be enormous. Why it this health care cost guilt trip the fault of the device *manufacturers*? What about the roles of the insurance company that wouldn't cover the procedure or the hospital's markup of its price?

"If you are making $3 billion a year on Gleevec [imatinib] could you get by with $2 billion? When do you cross the line from essential profits to profiteering?" This statement was made by none other than my hero, Brian Druker, who prominently contributed to imatinib's development.[15] It appears in a *New York Times* piece reporting on a medical journal article written by over 100 hematologists from around the world who specialize in treating CML. The hematologists demanded that drug companies lower the high costs of drugs that fight leukemia and charge a "just" price.[16] The medical journal article and Druker's quote are testimonies to the lack of economic insight of even the most accomplished medical academics, a hard-wired human animus against markets,[17] and the success of the conflict-of-interest narrative in demonizing corporate profitability. Many of the numerous CML experts authoring the plea to cut prices work with medical product companies to perform their clinical trials. The medical products industry has failed miserably to communicate the rationale behind its pricing practices—even to its clinical partners.

As with most economic transactions, supply and demand affects prices of medical products. In theory, if demand is sufficiently high for something a firm supplies, it can charge whatever does not reduce demand. Moreover, the development cost of a particular product bears no necessary connection to its price, especially in the case of medical products, where rare successes have to pay for past and future failures. And what consumers end up paying for medical products depends on numerous variables other than what manufacturers want to charge, such as insurance plans, negotiated volume discounts, and the presence or absence of competition. All of these factors contribute to price fluctuations through-out the life cycle of products.

As discussed further in chapter 13, however, the conflict-of-interest movement and many physicians deem medicine "exceptional" and differ-ent from other enterprises that function as markets. They argue that medi-cal care is a "right"[18] and that the demand for medical products is, in contrast to automobiles or entertainment, not voluntary. According to them, medical products are goods that should be made available to all, irrespective of ability to pay. In accusing companies of "profiteering," the CML experts likened the selling of costly drugs to sick patients to com-modity price gouging in natural disasters or during shortages. But devel-opment and production costs of drugs are higher than those of most commodities, and price fluctuations, routinely demonized by gasoline purchasers as conspiratorial, are simply responses to supply and demand. The CML experts' notion of a "socially just price" or Brian Drucker's "essential profits" are throwbacks to earlier notions of economics. These notions fail because sufficient information is lacking to inform what such a price should be. This failure is not merely a matter of opinion but a reality documented throughout history.[19]

Critics also demonize certain industry strategies to defend profitabil-ity. One popular target is the development of derivative products that require competitive marketing—pejoratively labeled "me-too" products. The next chapter discusses these products in detail. Another is to obtain patent monopolies for adjustments to existing products that may extend their sales exclusivity. Defined as "evergreening," the success or failure of such extension depends on decisions made by patent examiners and the FDA, and brand and generic companies often litigate the decisions.[20] A related activity is when brand and generic companies negotiate arrange-ments in which the brand company remunerates the generic company for a period of time during which the generic does not come to market, a practice labeled "pay to delay."

The merits and downsides of these practices are legitimate topics for debate, but in its criticism of them, the conflict-of-interest narrative *only* bemoans the temporary delays in product cost reduction afforded by de-layed generic availability. It *never* concedes that they may add net social value. If companies cannot continue to exist, they cannot innovate. Pay-to-delay deals allow brand manufacturers to stabilize their revenues. This income preservation allows companies to invest in research and development. Generic companies, for their part, can plow the delay payments they receive back into their own development efforts, facilitating the creation of more generics.

Critics also point to the fact that medical products tend to be cheaper abroad than in the United States. The reason for this discrepancy is government price controls in single-payer health care systems. Preferring to sell at discounted prices than not at all, U.S. companies accommodate to the price limitations. As a result, most of the world freeloads off of the American marketplace. The prices charged in America are necessary to cover the costs of innovation, and if forced to sell the products in the United States at the discounted prices charged elsewhere, much innovation would become impossible.

A key factor in product pricing is the length of time a company has a sales monopoly. To offset the vagaries of patent protection that may not reflect how long it takes to obtain product approval, regulatory agencies grant companies such monopolies, known as "exclusivity," for arbitrary time periods. The U.S. has the shortest (five-year) sales exclusivity interval following regulatory approval of any country (Canada and Japan allow eight years, and the European Union awards 10). A consequence of this relatively short time of protection is that generic companies aggressively—and often successfully—attempt to invalidate brand manufacturers' patents and obtain early market entry. [21]

The conflict-of-interest movement also demands that American companies give products away to impoverished nations with epidemic medical problems such as HIV/AIDS, tuberculosis, and malaria. It also encourages these countries to invalidate American patents and allow generic companies to sell the products cheaply, as India has done. [22] American companies have responded to international resource inequalities by establishing "tiered pricing," setting prices according to a country's particular socioeconomic status. While unsatisfactory to critics, this is the only approach that economists believe enables the industry to sustain innovation while providing badly needed products to developing nations. [23] One unintended consequence of differential transnational pricing is "leakage." Products cheaply produced in low- or middle-income countries end up being sold at large markups in first-world nations. In addition to the financial corruption, re-importation and leakage (also known as "the gray market") increase the chances of patients ending up with adulterated or otherwise inferior quality products, because both circumvent FDA product inspections.

WHY THE COSTS ARE REAL

Precisely determining what it costs to develop most medical products is probably impossible. Some of the difficulty arises from the fact that as in most circumstances involving competition, firms justifiably want to keep their procedures private. Economists Joseph DiMasi and Henry Grabowski, of Tufts and Duke Universities respectively, and their colleagues have over several decades analyzed anonymized information provided by a subset of pharmaceutical and biotechnology companies. They report an increase from $500 million to now $2.6 billion in investments required to gain FDA approval of a "typical" brand drug or biological product.[24] Follow-up studies by economists at various federal agencies using public information sources have supported their conclusions.[25]

The principal contributors to the expense of medical product development, above the high cost of the research itself, are the long duration between innovation initiation and regulatory approval and as described in the previous chapter, the high failure rate. Both of these circumstances deprive medical product companies of ongoing investment returns that companies faced with lower risk can enjoy. This central issue driving the economics of product development negates several arguments raised by critics concerning the pricing of medical products. One is that the annual profits as a percentage of revenues reported by major medical product companies and compiled in compendia such as The Fortune 500 Index greatly exceed those of most other industries.[26] The problem with this statistic is that it is an accounting artifact. Companies like Wal-Mart or CVS Caremark that have no research and development costs can quickly plough revenues into expansion of their retail operations, and new outlets rapidly contribute to net revenues. Research and development-intensive industries must save revenues for future investment expenses, and these sums, which ultimately may not yield returns, nevertheless appear as net profits on the annual balance sheets. Consistent with this explanation is the fact that energy companies also have higher than average net profits because they must invest in exploration of energy sources.

A second criticism is that the pricing of a particular product may not precisely parallel that product's development costs. Common sense and economic analysis indicate that depending on the circumstances of individual product development programs, large variations will exist within the averaged expenditures.[27] However, the products that succeed, irrespective of their development costs, underwrite the expenses of those that fail. Moreover, analyses of returns on research and development investments concerning drugs in the 1980s and 1990s have shown that only a small number of FDA approvals resulted in significant remuneration, and the aggregate margins only modestly exceeded investments.[28] The emergence rate of competing products has relentlessly shortened, meaning that the length of a company's monopoly with a first-in-class product has fallen.[29] Another distortion affecting medical product profitability is the fact that third-party payers such as Medicare determine reimbursement prices.[30] For example, payments for diagnostics were set at a time in the past when their value was not as appreciated as it is now. Low reimbursement rates discourage innovation in that area.[31]

Critics deny these principles and challenge DiMasi and Grabowski's development cost estimates and those of their endorsers.[32] To the conflict-of-interest movement, it is a given that companies overstate risks, inflate costs, and conceal profits. One of its objections concerns the proprietary and hence not directly verifiable nature of the corporate disclosures available to DiMasi, Grabowski, and other economists. Another is the signature conflict-of-interest movement's logic arguing that the economic analysts receive research support from industry and company trade organizations and therefore are untrustworthy. The objectors discount the supporting conclusions of federal economists as well because they may also have ties to industry. To buttress their accusations, the detractors collect indirect sources of information such as royalty payments to inventors and interviews of former industry employees. But this indirect evidence is just as—if not more—susceptible to selection as the corporate data that supposedly serves industry's purposes.

Data and common sense contradict these criticisms, and the economists have rebutted them.[33] As one example, the critics have used their indirect assessments to question high production expenditures reported by industry for a vaccine that prevents infantile diarrhea. Their estimates were far lower than those reported by the vaccine's manufacturer.[34]

Vaccine production involves producing disease-causing microorganisms and modifying them so they can no longer cause sickness. Four different virus strains cause the diarrheal disease in question. To make the vaccine, therefore, the company must produce each of the four viruses in bulk. Viruses multiply inside animal cells, and different strains grow in different cells and under different conditions. The orchestration and quality control involved in producing the vaccine are daunting. The company must cultivate the different cell types so that they produce the different viruses at the same time, prevent system contamination with extraneous microorganisms, guarantee inactivation of the viruses so the viruses produce immunity rather than disease, and combine the four inactivated viruses into a single widget that physicians can inject. These tasks are unimaginably complex.

Finally, if medical products industry profits are "excessive," where do these "excess" profits go? If this industry were more profitable than others, everybody would invest in it. Yet for the past decade, the market capitalization of the pharmaceutical industry has lagged behind industry averages compiled in various equity indices because investors perceive losses of profitability from patent expirations and the increasing difficulty of getting new products approved.[35] The medical products industry workforce is on average better educated and trained than that of many other industries, and therefore recruitment and retention of the best talent is costly. Annual surveys document that the CEOs of the major medical product companies are well paid—as they should be—but not as much as top executives of energy, telecommunications, or entertainment company leaders.[36] As mentioned previously the majority of biotechnology companies are barely profitable, if at all.[37] Most medical product start-ups, hoping to move innovative ideas and products to the clinic for sales, must fight tooth and nail for elusive investments to survive. Even the *threat* of price controls has alarmingly disproportionate negative effects on investment in medical product research and development.[38]

Ultimately, medical product pricing is a societal choice issue. If we decide that we cannot sustain desired levels of economic prosperity and life quality because of such pricing, then we must impose price controls. But if we do, we must understand that contrary to the critics who allege that product pricing is not coupled to the rate of medical innovation, such controls will slow innovation.

PUBLIC VERSUS PRIVATE INVESTMENT IN MEDICAL PRODUCT RESEARCH AND DEVELOPMENT: DO TAXPAYERS REALLY PAY TWICE?

Conflict-of-interest movement promoters express offense that companies allegedly profit disproportionately from products based on discoveries made in or licensed from universities. They want to expropriate these profits to subsidize NIH funding of academic biomedical research. They also want to adjust pricing of such products to accommodate resource-poor populations. They aver that while it's "fair" for industry to obtain returns on its investment, some profits should return to the NIH.[39]

This criticism reflects a fundamental misunderstanding of innovation in general and biomedical innovation in particular. The "unfairness" of competitive effort is precisely what makes it succeed. Innovation involves risk, and risky investment depends on reward prospects commensurate with the market value of the innovative products, a value undiminished by arbitrary social agendas.[40] Biomedical innovation resides at the leading edge of unpredictable high-risk, high-reward enterprises because it suffers from the inscrutability of nature, depends on serendipity and trial and error, and endures frequent failures. Only rare successes yield financial returns. Expropriating such returns in the interest of fairness or social welfare discourages investment. When critics disparage the novelty of much biomedical innovation, they overlook that even incremental innovations, discussed in the next chapter, involve substantial financial risk.

To demand compensation for all the background academic research contributing to approved medical products makes no more sense than to expect laptop computer manufacturers to compensate the mainframe computer industry that preceded them. The accusation that taxpayers pay twice for medical advances is simply false.

10

MISPLACED CRITICISM OF INCREMENTAL INNOVATION

In fact, the big drug companies now concentrate mainly . . . on producing variations of top-selling drugs already on the market—called "me-too" drugs.[1]

DEMONIZED "ME-TOO" PRODUCTS ARE ADAPTIVE AND NECESSARY

Most innovation is incremental. Thousands of small and a few larger changes gradually converted the Ford Model T into modern automobiles. No amount of wishful thinking and good intentions could have enabled Henry Ford to accomplish that evolution overnight. Similar evolutions govern most areas of technological progress, from washing machines to computer processors.

Medical product innovation often follows this pattern.[2] The conflict-of-interest movement's ideal of revolutionary innovation reflects its Utopian positions.[3] That said, the FDA has given priority consideration to over a third of follow-on drugs in over half of drug classes, implying that from a regulatory standpoint these "derivative" drugs were considered to have important medical value.[4] Over half of the drugs on the World Health Organization's "essential medicines" list were not the first drugs approved in their class.[5] As of 2013, 70% of over 5,400 medications under development in the pharmaceutical industry are considered novel (first-in-class) products.[6]

More importantly, overlapping products are not simply redundant. Subtle differences in chemical structure or formulation of products targeting the same end points can influence convenience of dosing and improve side effect profiles to benefit particular patients.[7] As discussed below, patients with psychiatric problems respond idiosyncratically to different drugs designed for what was originally thought to be the same target.

Even when derivative products must be withdrawn because of late recognition of side effects, they may become successful in different formulations for new uses. For example, Bromfenac, a drug taken by mouth for pain control was withdrawn from the market because of liver toxicity. One critic invoked Bromfenac's FDA approval in the first place as an example of an at the time redundant and therefore unnecessary addition to the then current class of drugs to which Bromfenac belongs.[8] But Bromfenac is now widely and safely applied as a topical formulation to treat inflammatory eye conditions.[9] And even prior to patent expirations, the existence of competing products can lower their costs through competition.[10]

Other chapters, notably chapters 8 and 9, have discussed the fiscal imperatives that the high risk of failure imposes on companies to build more predictably successful products into development programs. Reflecting their misunderstanding of fundamental product development economics, the critics claim that the medical product industry could be more successful by redirecting the funds used for marketing derivative products to more research on novel breakthroughs. In reality, such a financial shift would reduce sales, decreasing company revenues and diminishing the availability of funding for *any* type of research, especially high-risk investigation on breakthrough therapies. In the long term, such a policy would be financially ruinous to any company that tried it and subsequently detrimental to public health. More financially viable companies mean more research, more research means more products, and more products mean more lives saved and suffering averted.

The development of similar products need not, as claimed in the conflict-of-interest narrative, represent copycat behavior. In all fields of endeavor, emerging public knowledge sets development programs in motion, and as communication has become more efficient, multiple competing firms quickly become aware of scientific advances that are ripe for product development. In the capitalist system, different enterprises compete to take advantage of such information. Although socialists deem this competition duplicative and wasteful, central planning management produces little to duplicate and is far more wasteful. Many novel products become labeled as derivative just because a similar one appeared earlier by winning the race to FDA approval. Empiric data support this conclusion. The timing of patent filings and of developmental milestones reveal that most "me-too" products are under development well before the first product in the class is approved.[11]

The discrimination against derivative products reflects the muddled perception in academe concerning innovation discussed in chapter 8. Defined as getting products with demonstrable value to patients, innovation has nothing to do with novelty, important science, or differentiation from previous products. An example of this confusion is a medical journal article reporting that physicians at academic medical centers with more restrictive policies with respect to industry marketing were less likely to prescribe two out of three recently approved drugs for psychiatric conditions than physicians at centers with more lenient policies.[12] The article describing this study stated: "Although the drugs examined in this study vary in their level of innovation, none represented radical breakthroughs in their class and all relied on mechanisms of action already available on the market."

The article did not specify the criteria for "level of innovation," but the main concern is its implication that only "radical breakthroughs" warrant early adoption. I surveyed six prominent academic psychiatrists to evaluate this article. They confirmed, as discussed further below, that psychiatric patients respond idiosyncratically to drugs, irrespective of mechanism. The respondents also reported that they have had experience prescribing the particular drugs included in the study and that these medications helped their patients who previously had not responded to treatment. One of the drugs has fewer gastrointestinal side effects than its older counterparts and can be taken once rather than twice a day. One of the consultants stated: "[I]t should be prescribed regularly." Another of the medications has more rapid action than its precursor, and this property benefits management of psychotic patients. In addition, the fact that physicians subjected to company marketing restrictions prescribed one of the drugs as much as others not so restricted suggests that even they find that drug useful. Absent the marketing restrictions, it might have been appropriately prescribed *more* frequently.

The conceit grounded in a static view of the world that "experts" can predict in advance the value of any follow-on product with sufficient—or indeed any—certainty to justify delaying or preventing its development is absurd. The following examples illustrate why.

Statins

After over a decade of impediment-ridden development, Merck obtained FDA approval for lovastatin, a blood cholesterol–lowering statin drug (brand named Mevacor) in 1987. Pathologists had long observed cholesterol plugs in blocked arteries of heart attack and stroke patients, and epidemiologists had documented high blood cholesterol levels in such victims. But at the time of lovastatin's approval, skepticism remained high as to whether the elevated cholesterol levels actually *caused* the clogging of arteries that produced these problems. Therefore, the FDA only allowed Merck to claim on its lovastatin label that the drug reduced blood cholesterol, leaving prescribing physicians to decide whether doing so would have any clinical benefit. The completion of a large clinical trial in Scandinavia in 1994 eliminated those doubts: heart attack survivors given lovastatin had 30% fewer further attacks compared to individuals on placebo. Although a small minority of treated patients suffered muscle aches when taking the drug, especially at higher doses (or in combination with fibrates), most had no untoward effects.[13] Because vascular disease is the major cause of death and disability in developed nations, statin therapy represented a gargantuan market. As of 2013, seven statins had been developed, all acting on the same target by the same mechanism. Six, five of which are now generic, are now in clinical use.

Following lovastatin, a second statin, developed by Bristol Myers-Squibb, named pravastatin (brand name Pravachol) was approved by the FDA in 1996. Because pravastatin was roughly equivalent to lovastatin in potency, side effects, and price, Bristol Myers-Squibb engaged in aggressive marketing to compete against Merck's statin. But the FDA's subsequent approval of Pfizer's statin atorvastatin (brand name Lipitor) upset this competitive equilibrium. Atorvastatin was more potent than lovastatin or pravastatin, and patients achieved greater cholesterol reduction with it at lower doses than with the older agents.[14]

A cardiologist specializing in clinical trials of drugs for vascular disorders convinced Bristol Myers-Squibb to sponsor a clinical trial comparing the clinical effectiveness of pravastatin with Pfizer's atorvastatin, based on the hypothesis that atorvastatin's ability to lower cholesterol further would not confer additional clinical benefit. Unexpectedly, however, the trial revealed that subjects with previous heart attacks given atorvastatin to lower blood cholesterol levels below normal values had 16% fewer subsequent heart attacks. Contrary to the conflict-of-interest movement's claim that companies bury economically compromising research findings, Bristol Myers-Squibb allowed the research team to publish the study's results in *The New England Journal of Medicine* within weeks of its completion.[15] These events opened the door for a massive Pfizer marketing campaign that helped make atorvastatin the best-selling drug in pharmaceutical history. More importantly, the medical community now knew that blood cholesterol levels previously considered normal had been too high, especially in individuals with documented vascular disease. Since that time the blood cholesterol levels considered desirable by experts for vascular disease prevention have fallen even lower.

Two additional examples of FDA-approved statins support the value of derivative products. One, cerivastatin (brand name Baycol) developed by Bayer and approved by the FDA in 1997 had to be withdrawn from the market in 2002 because of a higher prevalence of muscle damage of greater severity (including fatal outcomes) than encountered with other statins.[16] These complications were uncommon and did not surface in the preapproval clinical trials, only becoming apparent once a larger number of patients received the medication postapproval.

What if, as critics want, once the FDA approved the first product of a particular type (known as a first in class), the agency imposes a higher bar for approval of subsequent products or precluded approval entirely? What if, under such circumstances, the first approved statin had been cerivastatin? The FDA has approved and physicians use many drugs with important and even potentially fatal side effects to treat serious diseases. Had cerivastatin been the only statin available and further statin development had been delayed or prevented, patients with vascular disease would be at greater risk than necessary for the side effects that resulted in cerivastatin's withdrawal. If other, less toxic, statins had not been available, this withdrawal would almost certainly not have taken place. And finally, as discussed below, the statistically small but medically important benefit of statin therapy for persons at relatively low risk for cardiovascular disease would likely have been eliminated.

A second relevant derivative statin is rosuvastatin (Crestor), manufactured by Astra Zeneca. Approved by the FDA for cholesterol reduction in 2003, rosuvastatin is as potent as atorvastatin, but it entered the market long after atorvastatin dominated statin prescribing. Therefore, to improve its market share, Astra Zeneca mounted clinical trials for a new indication to add to the drug's label. By that time, research had yielded new insights as to how high cholesterol blood levels cause the vascular changes leading to heart attacks and strokes. We now know that the deposition of cholesterol into artery walls causes inflammation. Inflammation, often damages our own tissues and organs. In heart attacks and strokes, the cholesterol-laden blood vessels thicken and become obstructed, preventing blood flow to the heart or brain, respectively.

A Harvard cardiologist and epidemiologist generated considerable evidence that persons with elevated levels of a blood protein named C-reactive protein (CRP)—an indicator of systemic inflammation—may be at increased risk of vascular disease, even if their blood cholesterol concentrations were not elevated. In a very large international clinical trial sponsored by Astra Zeneca, individuals with high CRP but normal cholesterol levels received rosuvastatin or a placebo. The trial outcome revealed a stunning 50% reduction in heart attacks and strokes in the statin-treated individuals who would not have qualified for such therapy based on their normal cholesterol levels. [17] In 2010, the FDA approved Astra Zeneca's marketing of rosuvastatin for patients with high CRP levels.

The manufacturers of the older statins had no incentive to spend hundreds of millions of dollars conducting the CRP study. The market competition presented by the existence of similar drugs motivated Astra Zeneca to do so, advancing both medical knowledge and medical treatment. We should be very grateful for "me-too" products!

High blood cholesterol is just one of many factors contributing to vascular disease, and its effect is indirect. Consequently, not everyone with high cholesterol develops vascular complications, and the timing and severity of such complications is unpredictable. As a result of this unpredictability, far more individuals who have had heart attacks receive statin treatment—a strategy known as secondary prevention—than would otherwise have suffered repeat attacks. This uncertainty is even greater when it comes to treating people with elevated cholesterol levels who have not yet suffered a complication, a strategy called primary prevention.

Invoking these concerns, critics claim that statins are overprescribed due to "disease-mongering" discussed further below.[18] Their onus against statins as commercial products blends with moral bullying behavior: physicians should recommend diet modification and exercise before prescribing statins, and patients should comply.[19]

Were it so easy! Although dietary modification can reduce cardiovascular risk,[20] the prestatin era abundantly demonstrated the relative ineffectiveness of diet and exercise alone in critically reducing cholesterol levels, even in willing subjects. The aging population and the obesity epidemic have accentuated these difficulties. And some statin critics are authors of diet books!

The critics have also focused attention on claims that statins may not be as benign as originally thought. In addition to muscle-related side effects, mild reversible cognitive impairment and a small increase in diabetes incidence in individuals with diabetes risk factors have been attributed to statins. Given the huge populations at risk for heart attacks and strokes, however, the benefits probably outweigh these rare and generally reversible harms.[21]

The fact is that the standard clinical practice *is* to recommend diet modification and exercise before prescribing statins and to start treatment, if necessary, with the cheaper, less potent, generic statins. However, this iterative approach does not work well. A study run by the University of North Carolina concluded that while starting a patient on a high potency statin increased drug costs, it decreased total medical costs by requiring fewer patient visits for cholesterol monitoring and medication changes and by reducing hospitalizations for cardiovascular events.[22] In other words, delaying prescribing of high potency statins in order to try dietary changes, exercise, or treatment with less potent statins increases overall health care costs and patients' risks of developing expensive and potentially fatal complications.

The development and dissemination of multiple statins has not only contributed to reducing the morbidity and mortality of one of humanity's major diseases but by increasing knowledge, has afforded physicians and patients rich choices for management.[23] In keeping with the evolution of greater patient autonomy, individuals with relatively few cardiovascular disease risk factors other than high blood cholesterol can decide on their own—advised by their physicians exercising their best clinical judgment[24]—whether to bear the expense and small risk of taking statins. Given the potentially devastating effects of heart attacks and strokes and preferences for prevention rather than invasive treatments, most informed patients will likely elect to take statins when recommended.

Antidepressants

Severe depression is a prevalent and debilitating condition.[25] It interferes with quality of life and can impair patients' ability to comply with treatments for other chronic diseases. The most serious outcome of severe depression is suicide.

Before medication became available, physicians used psychotherapy and electroshock treatments to alleviate depression. The first antidepressants appeared in the 1950s.[26] The onset of action of the first antidepressants was slow, and concerns arose regarding serious side effects due to their interactions with chemicals in certain foods. Therefore, when a new class of antidepressants known as selective serotonin reuptake inhibitors (SSRIs)—the first and most well known being Prozac—appeared in the late 1980s, their use superseded the use of drugs developed earlier.

Depression differs from the conditions treated with statins discussed above, because unlike those disorders, depression presents with subjective behavioral symptoms rather than physical symptoms such as those associated with heart attacks or strokes. No chemical laboratory tests like measuring blood cholesterol can straight forwardly help physicians diagnose depression and monitor responses to treatment. In these respects, depression resembles back pain. Depression and back pain also have in common that many treatment approaches exist, and proof of their efficacy can be hard to pin down. Yet both can be sufficiently debilitating to force caregivers to try *something*.

Especially challenging to assessments of treatment is mild to moderate depression, because it can remit with no treatment or respond to placebos. The conflict-of-interest movement consistently embellishes disputes concerning treatment preferences, and antidepressants figure prominently in accusations that industry overenthusiastically promotes drug benefits and plays down safety concerns.[27]

Here I focus on whether the SSRIs qualify as "me-too" drugs. Michael Oldani, a former Pfizer sales representative who became a professor of anthropology at the University of Wisconsin cited a *New York Magazine* article written by a reporter named Kirkpatrick to suggest they are:[28]

> Kirkpatrick provides a detailed account of gifting and other activities of drug reps within the United States in a journalistic exposé. He focuses on a recently introduced drug called Celexa, a new player in the $6.3 billion market of antidepressants. Celexa is a selective serotonin reuptake inhibitor (SSRI), similar in its mechanism of activity to Prozac, Zoloft, and Paxil. Kirkpatrick started his inquiry wanting to know how a "me-too" drug like Celexa had captured 13 percent of the SSRI market in just over a year and a half. Kirkpatrick cites *The Medical Letter*, a nonprofit newsletter that evaluates new drugs to enter the market, as characterizing Celexa as a me-too (i.e. no benefit over other SSRIs).

The *Medical Letter* to which Kirkpatrick refers specifically brands itself as "untainted by commercial influence" and provides cursory descriptions of newly approved drugs, most of which it declares no better than older products. However, practicing psychiatrists, such as Daniel Carlat, have a less categorical spin on antidepressants that resonate with the uncertainties described in other chapters under which medical care—often successfully—navigates. In a book titled *Unhinged: The Trouble with Psychiatry*, Carlat writes:[29]

> Once you've decided on a category such as the SSRIs, choosing, say, Zoloft over Celexa is a combination of guesswork and personal preference. In making the decision, we might consider whether someone in the patient's family has responded to a given drug, whether there are particular side effects we want to avoid, or whether the patient strongly requests a certain agent, commonly in response to a TV commercial.
>
> Choosing the right medication for a given patient is crucial, but thus far we are lacking the knowledge to make such choices scientifically. Instead, we rely on the "art" of prescribing—a series of rules of thumb with some backup from clinical studies here and there.

Consistent with Carlat's statements, a clinical trial lasting seven years and involving thousands of patients documented that many patients suffering from depression failed to respond or responded poorly to initial SSRI drug treatments. Some of these patients responded to higher doses of the first drugs, but others did better when switched to other SSRIs. The most refractory patients did not respond well, and substituting the SSRI drug with a drug thought to act by a different mechanism did not cause improvement.[30]

One of the main arguments in Carlat's book is that psychiatry became overly confident that it understood the mechanism of depression as the result of alterations in brain chemistry affected by SSRI antidepressants and that this belief, while at least in part erroneous, encouraged the development of more drugs of this type.

Carlat's comments regarding the unpredictable effectiveness of the drugs, however, indicate that we do not fully understand the mechanism by which these drugs work. Therefore, they cannot be considered "me-too" drugs even if they were designed to act on identical targets. In fact, evidence exists that the drugs have other mechanisms of action and are processed differently by different subjects, explaining in part why they work idiosyncratically.[31]

The most important lesson of the illustrations provided above is that medicine is a constantly evolving art that benefits from adaptive behavior informed by as much information as possible and by the judicious and observant application of innovation. Characterizing this progress as "me too" is ill informed and destructive.

NEW IS NEVER IMPROVED?

Unquestionably, older products abound that adequately meet the needs of many patients. Testifying to this reality are over-the-counter drug and device markets, plus the fact that about 80% of all prescriptions currently written in the United States are for generic products.[32] Nevertheless, the conflict-of-interest narrative consistently preaches that older generic products would provide as much medical value and fewer side effects than newer brand varieties with markedly reduced costs. The conflict-of-interest movement views brand products as inconvenient obstacles to an all-generic medical product inventory.

Because older FDA-approved and well-tested generic drugs exist for treatment of many, and because published studies for these will always be more abundant than newer treatments, one might argue that a physician should never recommend a newer—and more expensive—drug. Payers, private and public, understandably find this idea economically attractive.

If cost control trumps clinical outcomes and big data trumps small data, we may find ourselves perpetually tied to therapies of the past.[33] Novel therapies always have this disadvantage, and early promising studies are relatively easy to dismiss when the stack is taller for the alternative. As discussed in chapter 5, certain interests claim that vast amounts of evidence are the only legitimate bases for medical treatments; yet medicine remains an art as well as a science. Indeed, high-level data, or any data in many cases, may never exist for many therapeutic decisions made by health professionals.

About one-third of all adults in the United States have high blood pressure (hypertension), which is the single most common reason that patients make regular clinic visits. The news media touted the "older is better" message in a 2002 report claiming that cheap generic pills dating to the 1950s were as effective as new but far more expensive hypertension drugs. The story was based on the results of a very large clinical trial begun in 1994, sponsored by the NIH and eventually involving over 42,000 patients. Called ALLHAT (Antihypertensive and Lipid-Lowering Treatment to Prevent Heart Attack Trial), the trial compared the effects of four drugs on blood pressure: one, a generic named chlorthalidone, works mainly by causing the kidneys to excrete more water and salt out of the circulation. This effect is known as diuresis, and the drug is a diuretic. The other three, all brand drugs, worked by different mechanisms.

Despite the potential statistical power of the trial afforded by its large size, its execution and analysis proved problematic. Up to 60% of the patients enrolled in the trial did not initially respond to *any* of the treatments with blood pressures lowered to a desired level, and the experimental protocol called for addition of other drugs. Physicians were aware that some of the drugs added to the regimens worked better with diuretics, and as a result, improved blood pressure control ascribed to diuretics was not simply attributable to their use in and of themselves.[34] The principal victims of this study design were the sizable number of African Americans in the trial who suffered a significant excess of strokes associated with receiving treatment with a generic therapy already shown to be relatively ineffective in this group. In addition, while generic diuretic treatment resulted in fewer patients presenting with heart failure, this effect could not be categorically ascribed to the diuretics controlling high blood pressure (high blood pressure contributes to heart failure and heart failure results in fluid retention). Rather, the diuretics may have simply relieved symptoms of equivalently severe heart failure by their fluid-removing effects.[35] Moreover, ALLHAT showed no mortality difference favoring the use of the diuretic.

Due in part to these ambiguities and to some of the other drugs becoming generic, the trial results did not lead to significantly wider adoption of generic diuretics for treating hypertension. In addition, physicians had concerns that diuretics exacerbated diabetes and predisposed patients to gout. Also, because these drugs cause excretion of key minerals as well as water from the circulation, monitoring patients for mineral depletion complicated patient management.

Critics pinned the minimal effects of ALLHAT on clinical practice on foot dragging by the drug companies. They claimed that the companies' marketing power overwhelmed the government's and, in addition, that the companies obfuscated the supposedly inferior performances of their drugs.[36] I would posit that physicians became quickly aware of the issues inherent in ALLHAT's claims and were reluctant to switch patients to a diuretic agent known to promote metabolic problems. Medicine's complexity and nuance confound efforts to obtain definitive answers by brute force of numbers, and science moves faster than unwieldy clinical trials can accommodate.

Another possible reason that physicians did not rush to prescribe diuretics is that the drugs that had replaced them provided unexpected clinical benefits. Captopril, the first of a class of antihypertensive drugs called angiotensin converting enzyme inhibitors (ACE inhibitors), came to market in the early 1980s. This drug, developed by the pharmaceutical company E. R. Squibb, was effective in treating hypertension and, compared with previously available drug classes, far better tolerated. Soon, the FDA approved other ACE inhibitors, including some that had the convenience of being taken once daily compared with Captopril's twice daily dosing. This history further illustrates the medical value of derivative products.

This competition from new ACE inhibitor market entries led Squibb (later Bristol Myers Squibb) to fund a major clinical trial that demonstrated that Captopril could provide significant protection against the progression of kidney disease. Then, to maintain its competitive edge, the company invested heavily in showing that its ACE inhibitor reduced death and other major adverse events in patients with heart failure. Other companies, to maintain their share of the business, contributed to this vitally important research. To this day, ACE inhibitors, as well as angiotensin receptor blockers that followed are the standards of care for chronic kidney disease and heart failure as well as hypertension. Had this competition to produce similar products not occurred, effective lifesaving strategies would almost certainly have been delayed. In addition, each of these product developments involved physicians who identified the new uses for these drugs. This is consistent with data documenting that practicing physicians making field observations accounted for 57% of FDA approvals of new uses for established drugs in 1998.[37]

SOCIALLY UNNECESSARY PRODUCTS?

Economies succeed when they provide people with what they need *and* want. The conflict-of-interest movement values perceived "need" over "want" and presumes to define the difference. According to its tenets, life prolongation measures take precedence over others that improve life quality. Even in the context of life preservation, a puritanical element creeps in: diet and exercise are preferable to pills, and resorting to medication is a moral failure. In this attitudinal universe, the oncologist is superior to the cosmetic surgeon because the former tries to extend life, and the latter merely to improve personal appearances. But oncologists often subject desperate terminally ill patients to futile last-ditch therapies that only have the effect of making the patients' last days more miserable—and expensive. Yet many people embrace cosmetic surgery, and the male population has enthusiastically sought erectile dysfunction drugs. The profits from sales of these drugs can support development of both life-saving and lifestyle products. Most importantly, however, they reflect a satisfaction of human wants and needs without moralistic value judgments.

On the flip side of lionizing "need," the conflict-of-interest movement attacks companies for promoting products we allegedly *don't* need. The term for this promotion is "disease-mongering," coined in 1994 by a journalist.[38] The critics have alleged that rather than develop new and effective products for disorders that require treatment, the industry invents diseases for its existing wares to treat or declares normal states as pathological and therefore deserving (unnecessarily) of therapeutic intervention.[39] One supposed example put forth of a nondisease is a condition called the restless legs syndrome in which people feel a compulsion to move their arms and legs, and the affliction can cause sleeping difficulties.[40] Another example is female sexual dysfunction. The third normal circumstance allegedly transformed into an illness is menopause.

The disease-mongering claim epitomizes the conflict-of-interest movement's characteristic oversimplification. Of course, industry wants more uses for its products, and as discussed extensively throughout this book, large gaps in scientific knowledge accommodate many therapies that may work poorly or not at all. But the facile idea that the industry has the wherewithal to impose inappropriate therapies at will is a fantasy. Patients do suffer discomfort and crave relief. Restless legs syndrome exemplifies conditions, like chronic fatigue or fibromyalgia, that do not have clearly defined causes, outcomes or definitive treatments. And after having been ridiculed as a nondisease, restless legs syndrome came to be associated with iron deficiency and could be mapped to particular genes. The condition, which may have multiple causes, responds to drugs that treat migraine, Parkinson's disease, and nerve pain.[41] Menopause may be universal, but that fact does not make its symptoms, especially if severe, a curse to be stoically endured. A menopausal woman suffering incapacitating hot flashes and told by a moralizing physician to accept it as normal aging is well advised to seek another opinion.

To be sure, not every ache or pain requires a medical intervention. Physicians often perform unnecessary tests and procedures and prescribe inappropriately. One of the most heavily criticized examples is antibiotic prescriptions for diseases caused by viruses that do not respond to such drugs. This behavior occurs because of patients' demands, excess caution, or fear of malpractice litigation. Sometimes these actions not only do no good but cause harm.[42] Industry hardly has a monopoly on selling sickness.

11

RUSHING TO JUDGMENT WITH FALSE PRODUCT SAFETY ALARMS

In an ideal world, we might hope that drugs, biological therapies and medical devices *never* caused harm. Unfortunately, in the real world, maximizing medical product safety presents excruciating difficulties. The same uncertainties surrounding human biology that confound easy success in identifying inventions and developing them for clinical use impact safety. Indeed, approximately 30% of medical product development failures occur because of safety concerns.[1]

This chapter discusses, first, the current procedures in place for medical product safety management as conceptualized from the standpoint of different participants: those involved in their use, regulation, and manufacture and the conflict-of-interest movement. Whereas patients, regulatory authorities, and medical product manufacturers have nuanced approaches to safety risks, the conflict-of-interest movement generally pictures them as consequences of corporate greed. I then review some problematic cases related to safety of drugs and devices, how the conflict-of-interest narrative depicts them, and how the facts surrounding these cases do not support the movement's assessments of them.

THE BENEFIT-RISK BALANCE: ASSESSMENTS OF DIFFERENT STAKEHOLDERS

Patients

The tension between product efficacy and safety is often a difficult balancing act. The balance set points are very circumstance dependent. The medical stories told in chapter 1 illustrate this specificity. The impulse to "do something" in dire circumstances has a way of coloring precautions. The seriousness of my patient Graces's HUS condition justified the risks associated with multiple invasive interventions involved in the therapy she received. The uncertainties and complexities of her illness rendered the drug treatments and device applications by even the most experienced and conscientious medical personnel liable to be ineffective or inflict complications. Fortunately, in her case, the balance worked out favorably. My brother-in-law Patrick was also fortunate in that a relatively benign new drug was available to treat his cancer—and it worked. But many other cancer patients are subjected to potent chemotherapy drugs even though these agents also predictably harm normal body cells. This trade-off is tolerable if the drugs have a chance of achieving a therapeutic effect, and indeed, many patients are willing to endure numerous side effects even when the prospects of success are small.

At the opposite end of the risk spectrum is the story of my colleagues' and my dental work in Zambia. Extracting painful decayed teeth in the remote village of Muchila carries some risk of bleeding and infection, but it is manageable with careful preoperative evaluation, skilled surgery procedure, and postprocedure vigilance. The fact that many hundreds of villagers show up for treatment when the dental team arrives and the community's positive response to it attest to their willingness to take risks for pain relief.

The story of my back pain falls into the middle of the risk-benefit spectrum, and involves much more subjectivity. The duration and severity of pain, the presence or absence of other symptoms, age, level of activity, pain tolerance, and patience all determine risk tolerance. And the risk benefit picture is a moving target. When I was a medical student, *not* treating back pain was viewed as risky, because a prevalent belief was that the bulging discs supposedly responsible for the pain might cause permanent and severe nerve damage. Subsequent clinical experience has modified that view.

The FDA

The FDA is best positioned to address safety concerns. The limitations associated with preapproval safety assessment pale before the magnitude of uncertainty that emerges once a product is on the market. Despite the rigor of FDA review, low-incidence side effects, possibly serious, may be missed, ascribed to chance, or simply not rise to sufficient scrutiny. For most of recent history, most safety monitoring after product approvals has been "passive." The FDA encourages health professionals and mandates product manufacturers to report adverse outcomes.[2] If, as a result of further evaluation after receiving such reports, the FDA determines that problems systemically associate with a product, the Agency responds proportionally to the seriousness of the complications. The most severe action is to demand removal of the product from the market. Short of this extreme is imposition of a "black box" warning on the product label. Written communications to physicians concerning such a warning and the particular product's label literally describe the concerns inside of a black-bordered box. Reporting of possible adverse outcomes, however, is neither reliable nor efficient. Individual physicians often have relatively few patients exposed to a particular drug, and when complications arise, the relationship to that product may not be obvious.

Recently the FDA has begun to institute an "active" surveillance system to monitor data from large numbers of patients seen by physicians equipped with electronic medical records and from insurance companies making payments based on clinical information in addition to companies' clinical trial reports.[3]

A review encompassing 548 drugs approved between 1975 and 1999 reported that 8% of those approved drugs subsequently received black box warnings, and 3% had to be withdrawn.[4] Evidence suggesting that drugs approved by the FDA on a priority basis because of their perceived novelty cause more adverse outcomes than drugs approved on the basis of conventional review has not been consistent.[5] Although the conflict-of-interest movement claims novel products given accelerated approvals have higher complication rates,[6] some of this adverse event reporting is simply a statistical anomaly related to the greater attention physicians pay when prescribing new drugs, a phenomenon named the "Weber effect."[7] The FDA's track record in assuring durable outcomes is certainly superior to the reproducibility of results reported in the published biomedical literature. The conflict-of-interest narrative that older products are categorically safer than new ones is also false.

The Medical Products Industry

To maximize prospects for FDA approval and to keep expenditures compatible with commercial success, medical product companies design clinical trials using subjects not only most likely to respond favorably to treatments but also who are least prone to suffer adverse events that might sabotage product approval. Such preapproval trials do not accurately reflect the messy environment of clinical practice in which patients vary in clinical status and in which the careful monitoring associated with clinical trials is not routinely possible.

But aside from product approval, medical product manufacturers have a deep interest in understanding risks that goes far beyond premarket evaluations of efficacy and safety. Inadvertent errors can lead to product recalls and resulting revenue losses. Therefore companies engage in major quality control efforts—far greater than exist in medical practice or academic research. These efforts have to address complex supply chains with constantly changing players and changing geographic, political, climatic, and myriad other variables that influence the availability and composition of product components. Errors due to negligence invite fines, litigation costs, and possible damage payments.

The industry, compared to other stakeholders, has the most resources to sustain vigilance regarding effects of their products. The networks of investigators who perform their clinical trials or provide expert consultation are directly in contact with patients exposed to those products. For example, Alexion, the company producing eculizumab that my patient Grace received, recognized that a few patients treated with it came down with a severe infection caused by a bacterium that normally is fended off by the system targeted by the drug. These findings led to the recommendation that patients receive vaccinations against the microbe in question.[8]

Further evidence for industry's position in monitoring product safety is the fact that most high-profile safety problems summarized below did not emerge or lead to remedies due to physician, regulatory, or academic vigilance. Rather, they resulted from companies' assessments of product performance in populations different from those in preapproval studies and efforts to identify new uses.

The Conflict-of-Interest Movement

Safety is consistent with the medical product industry's self-interest. However, a persistent claim of the conflict-of-interest movement is that companies deliberately flaunt safety by concealing evidence of adverse outcomes. An article titled "Dangerous Deception—Hiding the Evidence of Adverse Drug Effects" illustrates this view:[9]

> On September 30, 1982, six people in the Chicago area died after taking acetaminophen (Tylenol) that had been laced with cyanide. The tragedy riveted the country's attention for months. We should be able to muster at least a fraction of that concern to address more clinically relevant adverse drug effects that could sicken or kill thousands of patients. How can we capture such interest in less sensational problems of medication safety? A good start would be to make a national commitment to publicly support studies of drug risks so that no company could take possession of critical findings for its own purposes.

This analysis is catchy, but the poisoned Tylenol episode is not an apt model for problems with medical product safety. In fact it differs from it in all respects. In the Tylenol case, an unidentified perpetrator—or perpetrators—deliberately added lethal amounts of cyanide to medication containers, although the medications themselves were perfectly safe. The cause of the tragic problem and its remedies were entirely straightforward and predictably manageable. In contrast, drug and device safety problems are not deliberate and far more opaque, and "critical findings" alluded to above recounting the Tylenol story are often sufficiently ambiguous to render their universal public exposure not just unhelpful but subject to abuse.

Echoing the plea for a "national commitment to publicly support studies of drug risks," critics have called for the establishment of a separate agency, a "drug safety board," to address postapproval adverse events, based on the premise that the FDA has a vested interest in defending its approval decisions.[10] These critics want to terminate the user fees paid by industry to help subsidize FDA reviews, create an entire new bureaucracy, and have the proposed board monitor the safety of *all* new products, not just those, as currently mandated by FDA, given accelerated approvals or requiring safety assessments for use in children. These sweeping demands are economically nonviable. Another unworkable recommendation of this criticism concerns the membership of the proposed safety board: it should be "completely independent of influence from the pharmaceutical industry, biotechnology firms, and medical device manufacturers." In that case, having disqualified the FDA analysts who became familiar with products during their development prior to approval from the postmarketing evaluation, where would the proposed board find qualified individuals to perform the desired safety assessments?

SOME SPECIFIC SAFETY CONTROVERSIES

Vioxx

In September of 2004, Merck abruptly removed its painkiller rofecoxib (brand named Vioxx) from the market. Vioxx had launched with an aggressive direct-to-consumer marketing campaign featuring television clips showing the famous Olympic skater Dorothy Hamill twirling on the ice and extolling how the drug made it possible. The campaign was successful in that many physicians prescribed Vioxx for their patients. The recall occurred after a large clinical study called APPROVe indicated that the drug conferred a small but statistically significant risk of adverse cardiovascular events such as heart attacks and strokes.[11] Data reported by Merck to the FDA and an earlier published study, titled VIGOR, that tested Vioxx's pain relieving activity and side effects in patients with arthritis had also revealed this finding. But the low absolute number of adverse events and the fact that the drug caused less gastrointestinal bleeding than the drug to which it was compared led the FDA to conclude that the benefits outweighed the risks.[12] Without a placebo arm in the clinical trials, which would not have been ethically acceptable in patients suffering from severe joint pain, one could not determine whether the difference in cardiovascular effects resulted from a deleterious effect of Vioxx, a protective action of the comparison drug, or some combination of the two. But when the subsequent APPROVe trial designed to ascertain whether Vioxx prevented growth of precancerous gastrointestinal growths (it did) and that included a placebo arm confirmed the cardiovascular risk, Merck withdrew the drug from further sales.

The withdrawal triggered a legal avalanche. Tort lawyers filed individual and class action "failure to warn" suits on behalf of patients allegedly injured or killed by Vioxx. They also mounted class actions claiming Merck undersold Vioxx's risks, thereby failing to enable investors to predict that the company's stock value would fall when the risks became more widely known. In addition, they litigated academics and medical journals that had respectively participated in and published research on the drug. Pharmacies sued Merck to recover costs of Vioxx supplies they had purchased and could no longer sell. Prosecutors conjured up civil and criminal charges of illegal marketing of the drug. Abetting the legal assaults were academic and media critics who vehemently declared that the Vioxx saga epitomized everything that was amiss in the medical products industry and its regulation. When the first failure-to-warn lawsuit, played out in Texas in 2005, resulted in a guilty verdict and a $253 million award to the widow of a patient who suffered a fatal heart attack while taking Vioxx, the criticisms appeared justified.

Seeming further vindication emerged from the elaborate discovery process fired up by the legal opportunism.[13] Trolling of company files unearthed messages allegedly implicating employees in conspiracies to cover up what they supposedly knew were Vioxx's lethal side effects, distorting information in press releases, using ghostwriters to promote Vioxx in medical journal publications, and intimidating physicians who voiced misgivings about the product.[14]

Built into clinical trials are "data safety monitoring boards," which periodically review the trial results as they emerge. Unlike investigators or sponsors, these monitors either know which subjects are in the treatment or placebo arms of the study, or else, as was the case for the VIGOR trial, the two groups are separated so that the reviewers can detect a benefit or risk in one or the other arm. If either outcome is sufficiently clear cut, the board might recommend stopping the trial. National Public Radio ran a segment titled "Conflicted Safety Panel Let Vioxx Trial Continue," alleging that Michael Weinblatt, the physician (a colleague of mine and a leading expert in the treatment of arthritis) who chaired the VIGOR data safety monitoring board, overlooked the cardiovascular warning signs because he had $73,000 of Merck stock.[15]

An FDA epidemiologist asserted to a congressional hearing and in a medical journal article that Vioxx was responsible for tens of thousands of deaths.[16] Academic statisticians attacked Merck's interpretations of Vioxx clinical trial results published in medical journal articles and testified against Merck in court in the tort cases. *The New England Journal of Medicine* published a "statement of concern" accusing Merck of withholding adverse outcome data from its publication of the VIGOR trial.[17] All of these factors have held up "the Vioxx scandal" to embody corporate corruption of medicine recounted in numerous academic and media articles and books.

When medical science achieved some understanding of how aspirin, discovered in the 19th century, works to control pain and fever, subsequent research based on that knowledge led to more potent painkillers called nonsteroidal anti-inflammatory drugs (NSAIDs). But NSAIDs mirror aspirin's gastrointestinal irritation and bleeding side effects to promote, and they also can cause kidney damage and high blood pressure. When more investigations suggested the possibility of designing drugs related to NSAIDs but different in that they could relieve pain with fewer side effects, pharmaceutical companies competed vigorously to develop such compounds—known as "coxibs"—and a decade later had completed clinical trials of them resulting in FDA approval.[18]

Aspirin was known to cause gastrointestinal bleeding by two mechanisms. One is a direct irritant effect on the lining of the gut. Another is to suppress the function of blood platelets, trillions of which circulate in the blood and clump together at sites of blood vessel injury to stop bleeding. Physicians use this antiplatelet action to prevent heart attacks and strokes by inhibiting blood platelets' obstruction of blood vessels by prescribing aspirin in low doses. NSAIDS were widely thought to have the same effects on blood platelets, although this impression was based on only laboratory tests and not, as with aspirin, by patient outcome studies that correlated reduced platelet clotting functions with more clinical bleeding and a reduction in heart attacks and strokes. In fact, some experts even speculated that coxibs might not only lack aspirin's platelet-inhibiting actions but might have an opposite effect, to *promote* blood clotting leading to vascular complications.[19] But when the VIGOR trial revealed more cardiovascular events in Vioxx-treated subjects, Merck discounted this theory and initially attributed them to platelet inhibition by the NSAID, naproxen, against which Vioxx was compared. In support of this conclusion, a Merck-sponsored academic analysis of all clinical trials involving Vioxx failed to detect an increase in cardiovascular events except in the VIGOR trial comparing Vioxx with naproxen.[20] The subsequent placebo-controlled APPROVe trial however, killed the naproxen platelet inhibition explanation, leading to Merck's decision to withdraw Vioxx from sales.

The Vioxx story has had a long tail. Subsequent to its withdrawal, the FDA held advisory meetings to determine whether other coxibs should also be taken off the market and one was. Even to this day, Vioxx-related lawsuits continue to dribble in. Statisticians persist in mining medical journal publications and other information unearthed by litigation. They interpret their findings to conclude that Merck overstated the drug's benefits and underestimated its risks.[21]

But the reflexive assignment of Vioxx as the icon for medical product industry venality does not stand up to close examination. Some have opined that Merck's withdrawal of the drug was premature and ill advised, depriving pain patients of an effective pain remedy.[22] An investigation led by a former federal judge concluded that Merck's management was not guilty of negligence, cover-up, or fraud but rather beset by ill luck, inadvertent error, and inevitable judgment lapses.[23] No body of research subjected to minute and lingering analysis by committed ideological and legal opponents could escape the kind of criticism directed at Merck. With the drug off the market, Merck employees or their allies had little motivation to devote time to rebutting such attacks.

Media coverage of Merck's behavior was biased and often inaccurate. Persistent journal article and editorial comment even long after the drug's withdrawal confidently asserted that Merck deliberately concealed Vioxx's problems.[24] But the provenance of these statements was newspaper articles citing e-mail messages between company employees, most likely called to reporters' attention by litigators. More importantly, if read carefully, the messages concern internal company *debate* over ambiguous data.[25]

The NPR segment vilifying Michael Weinblatt epitomizes the media's sacrifice of complex nuance to oversimplification. In fact, it was the VIGOR trial's data safety monitoring board that first noted an increase in cardiovascular complications in the Vioxx-treated patients. This increase was not evident in a subsequent review, although when it reappeared a few months later, the data safety monitoring board informed Merck of that finding. However, because this particular complication had not been predicted in advance, the reports concerning it were not "adjudicated." Adjudication means that additional documentation verifies that events mentioned in the clinical records, such as a heart attack or stroke, actually took place. In other words, physicians enrolling patients in a trial might interpret chest pain or neurological symptoms as representing a heart attack or stroke respectively, but without other supportive evidence—such as electrocardiographic analysis, blood tests, or imaging studies—the symptoms might be due to other causes. Only when the data safety monitoring board called its suspicions to Merck's attention was an adjudication process for monitoring cardiovascular complications added to the study. This delay, the very low incidence of such complications, and the fact that they came to light only when the trial was nearly complete explain why the board did not recommend discontinuation of the trial. Indeed, no members of the VIGOR trial data safety monitoring serving under Michael Weinblatt, including those without Merck stock, recommended discontinuation of the trial.[26] In fact, Weinblatt insisted on a more stringent statistical evaluation than Merck originally proposed to assess the significance of the cardiovascular findings.[27]

Merck initially defended itself in court against all the failure-to-warn cases. The Texas guilty verdict with its astronomical damage award was overturned on appeal; Merck won most of the tort cases and eventually obtained a class-action settlement far less onerous than original estimates predicted. Further research has revealed that all coxibs and even NSAIDs confer some cardiovascular risk.[28] A large Swedish study revealed that coxibs do not increase cardiovascular disease incidence of patients of low risk of such complications.[29]

So how should physicians respond to industry marketing of a new product with incremental benefits and unknown risks? Arguably the worst mistake Merck made was to attribute the results of the VIGOR trial showing increased cardiovascular complications in patients on Vioxx to unproven protective effects of the comparison drug, naproxen, which was unproven. But ascribing this error purely to financial motives is arbitrary. The researchers who developed the drug and championed its use were in good company: medical journal articles and medical textbooks at the time of the VIGOR trial routinely declared that NSAIDS impaired platelet function[30] and discouraged the use of NSAIDs in patients at risk of bleeding, and surgeons tell patients not to take NSAIDs preoperatively to this day.

In hindsight, Merck might have marketed Vioxx less aggressively and might act with more circumspection with similar products in the future. But, paradoxically, all parties acknowledge the inherent difficulty of identifying low-incidence adverse effects. Indeed, only wide use of a product may make possible the discovery of such effects. Calls by critics to restrict marketing of new products until they are "proven safe" may actually slow such discovery.

The inflammatory depiction by academics and the media of this complicated problem as a black and white clash of academic science against commercial greed is hardly accurate or helpful. The never-ending mantra that "more research" should precede product approvals and continue post-approval ignores that resources do not exist to pay for such research. And, it was Merck's research attempting to extend Vioxx's uses that finally established its adverse side effects definitively.

Trasylol and Avandia

The blood coagulation system has the challenging task of keeping blood flowing through vessels while stopping it from leaking outside of them when damaged. It does the job through the balanced opposing actions of blood clot formation (coagulation leading to fibrin glue formation) and fibrin clot breakdown (fibrinolysis). This complicated exercise comes under particular challenge in the setting of major tissue damage, and, unfortunately, cardiovascular surgical procedures simulate such injury. During the insertion of artificial heart valves, for example, the surgeon needs to prevent blood clotting in the operative field around the valve, and if the heart is stopped, to keep blood pumping through the patient's circulation via machines. Therefore, the patients undergoing such surgery receive anticoagulants, and, unsurprisingly, may experience considerable bleeding necessitating blood transfusions.

Reasoning that slowing down the breakdown of formed blood clots might alleviate intraoperative bleeding, surgeons experimented with a natural protein inhibitor of fibronolysis called aprotinin, which had been discovered in the 1930s. The Bayer company manufactured aprotinin by extracting it from cow pancreas and brand named it Trasylol. When placebo-controlled clinical trials concluded that Trasylol injections reduced blood replacement requirements in cardiac surgery patients, the FDA approved it for that indication in 1993, and it became widely used for heart bypass surgery.

In 2006, two academic studies reported that Traslyol was effective in preventing bleeding but that it also was associated with higher mortality and with increased heart attacks, strokes, and kidney failure, presumably due to formation of blood clots in vessels serving those organs.[31] In response, the FDA conducted a review of these results including unpublished studies that Bayer had sponsored. Confounding the review was the fact that all the research was observational rather than randomized studies. In an observational study, physicians decide what treatments to select based on the characteristics of their patients rather than randomly assigning patients to different treatments. A statistical manipulation known as the "propensity score" can mitigate some of the large biases inherent in observational studies, but these analyses are far from ideal. Furthermore, only one of the two academic investigations reported a marked increase in cardiac side effects associated with Trasylol treatment, and the unpublished Bayer data revealed no such effects.

The FDA review concluded that Trasylol was not unduly risky based on its assessment of the information available to it at the time. Days later Bayer coughed up more observational results that did point to an increased incidence of adverse cardiac events in Trasylol-treated patients. Needless to say, this late revelation—labeled by Bayer as "a mistake"—irritated the academics participating in the FDA review and prompted publication of the "Dangerous Deception" editorial cited above. Nevertheless, even with this late-breaking news, the inherent limitations of observational studies with the potential for confounding factors left the FDA unwilling to make a firm conclusion declaring Trasylol unsafe.[32]

This impasse seemed to resolve in 2007 when three medical journal articles, including one summarizing a large randomized controlled trial (named BART) comparing Trasylol with two other inhibitors of fibrinolysis strongly affirmed the risks of Trasylol.[33] In response, Bayer withdrew the product from the American market, and Canadian and European regulators suspended its approval. Due to the product withdrawal in the United States, the FDA did not take additional action.

The Trasylol case appeared closed until further reviews and provision of additional data by Bayer led the Canadian and European regulatory agencies respectively to reinstate the drug in 2011 and 2012. The reasons were that even though BART study patients had been randomly assigned to different treatment groups, confounding influences after randomization, such as extent of anticoagulation, procedure complications, and other imponderables, undermined the conclusion that Trasylol in and of itself accounted for worse outcomes than those reported in the BART trial.[34]

A similar episode concerns controversy regarding a diabetes drug brand named Avandia. After a journal article alleged that it caused fatal heart attacks, the FDA ordered the drug's manufacturer to undertake clinical trials to assess that complication, but before the studies' completion required a black box warning on the drug's label in 2007 and imposed restrictions on its use. Avandia prescribing plummeted.[35] But in 2013, based on further analysis of clinical data, the FDA concluded that the heart attack risk did not exist and removed the restrictions.[36] That outcome notwithstanding, like Trasylol, Avandia has essentially disappeared from clinical use.

Erythroid Stimulating Agents

One of the early practical accomplishments of genetic engineering was the production of clinically useful quantities of a hormone called erythropoietin (abbreviated Epo). Epo, the natural version of what has come to be called erythroid-stimulating agents (ESAs), stimulates the production of oxygen carrying red blood cells. Our kidneys play an essential role in maintaining the right number of such cells. A large amount of our blood constantly flows through our kidneys for cleansing purposes, and their constant exposure to blood volumes positions them to sense how much oxygen the blood contains. When the oxygen content drops due to, for example, lung diseases that impair oxygen absorption or a reduction in the number of red blood cells—anemia—the kidneys sense this lack of oxygen and increase their production of Epo. Epo, in turn, stimulates the bone marrow to produce more red blood cells. Once the number of cells is normal, Epo production falls.

Many medical conditions cause anemia. But the one that became the principal indication for Epo therapy was chronic kidney disease. Recall that my patient Grace received dialysis treatments to keep her alive until successful management of the HUS allowed them to recover. But had the treatment not been successful, Grace's kidneys might have been destroyed. This condition, more commonly a result of diabetes, chronic infection, or exposure to toxins and some drugs is known as end-stage renal disease (ESRD). ESRD condemns affected patients to repeated dialysis treatments for the rest of their lives.

Although chronic dialysis can take over much of the blood purification functions of normal kidneys, it does not substitute for other kidney activities such as the production of Epo. Therefore, anemia was a major problem for ESRD patients and a cause of fatigue, light-headedness, shortness of breath, and lack of energy. Physicians treated the anemia with frequent blood transfusions, and although the transfusions alleviated the anemia symptoms, they afforded other complications such as inconvenience, transmission of infectious diseases, and pathological deposition of iron. In addition, blood for replacement is always in short supply, and the growing number of ESRD patients exacerbated this availability problem.

Recognizing the medical necessity, genetic engineering companies vied to be first to produce Epo for therapy of ESRD patients. Amgen, founded in 1980, narrowly won the race, and clinical trials revealed that its Epo powerfully promoted red blood cell production in ESRD patients who received it by injection. The FDA approved Amgen's Epo (brand named Epogen) in 1989. When Amgen's Epo patent approached expiration, the company introduced a derivative version (brand named Aranesp) that lasts longer in the body than the earlier product and therefore requires fewer injections.

Anemia has many causes, some of which are theoretically addressable by ESAs. The indication unrelated to kidney disease most actively pursued was for anemia associated with cancer. Several factors contribute to anemia in cancer patients. Cancers may cause blood loss from body orifices, and cancers also interfere with blood cell manufacture and sometimes promote accelerated red blood cell destruction. Chemotherapy used to treat the disease can interfere with red blood cell production. Aranesp sales for cancer-related anemia became brisk.

Most patients with ESRD and some cancer patients have very profound anemia, and raising their red blood cell counts reliably promoted symptomatic benefits. As the red blood cell numbers approach the range of normal, however, the effect of the actual red cell concentration on the presence or absence of symptoms that are to some extent subjective becomes more difficult to define. Factors such as gender, age, and physical activity affect normal red blood cell numbers and the physical consequences of reduced levels. To address this ambiguity, Amgen mounted clinical trials comparing the outcomes of ESRD and other patients receiving variably aggressive Aranesp regimens. The results were troubling. Not only was documenting any symptomatic improvement at higher red blood cell levels difficult for the reasons cited above, but some of the trials revealed a higher incidence of cardiovascular complications: high blood pressure, heart attacks, and strokes in the most intensively treated ESRD patients.[37] Some of the data suggested increased mortality in cancer patients receiving ESAs.[38] The FDA responded to these findings in 2007 by adding black box warnings to the products' labels. The FDA recommendation was that physicians should not allow patients' red blood cell counts to exceed a certain level.

As with the previous examples, a deeper analysis contradicts allegations that ESA manufacturers flaunted safety considerations. First, no proof exists that ESAs directly cause the complications ascribed to them. Although some laboratory studies suggest that ESAs promote the growth of cancer cells or the production of certain other hormones that stimulate growth, a relationship between these effects and clinical outcomes is far from proven. Second, not all of the clinical trials documented adverse outcomes due to more aggressive ESA treatment, and the evidence that ESAs accelerate the growth of cancers has not held up.[39]

The doses of ESAs associated with complications are not, as in most cases involving drug toxicity, predetermined. Rather, the effect determines the dose, namely subjects receive whatever amounts of ESAs they require to drive the blood cell count to a particular level. Individual patients may need widely discrepant ESA amounts to respond. A large clinical trial administering Aranesp to ESRD patients with diabetes revealed that, in fact, it was the patients who received the highest ESA doses who had the most cardiovascular complications.[40] One might conclude that this result is the smoking gun pointing at the toxicity of ESAs, but another plausible explanation is that it is resistance to ESAs, not ESAs in and of themselves, that promotes the observed adverse outcomes. Chronic inflammation is a factor known to inhibit responding to anemia by increasing red blood cell production and a reason for increased cardiovascular and infectious complications. In addition, even if accelerated tumor progression occurred in cancer patients receiving high doses of ESAs for anemia, the reason could well be that the most aggressive cancers cause the most inflammation.

Anemia occurs in diverse pathological conditions involving inflammation, including infections, rheumatoid arthritis—and cancers. Diabetes, a common precursor to ESRD, is considered an inflammatory state, and such inflammation predisposes to its cardiovascular complications and susceptibility to death by infection. Hence, ESAs may have gotten an undeserved bad rap for the ravages of inflammation. A test of this theory will require the development of means to treat inflammation more effectively than is presently possible and determine whether it reduces both resistance to ESAs and the complications ascribed to them.

Class II (501[k]) FDA Devices

Devices present somewhat different challenges than drugs. Some complicated drug regimens require unique knowledge and experience, but in general the administration of drugs is relatively simple. In contrast, the competent operation of devices requires special training and skill. An added element of risk enters when devices are implanted, such as joint replacements, dental prostheses, artificial eye lenses, or machines that deliver electrical impulses to modify heart, brain, or intestinal functions. Patients' immune systems may attack implanted devices and damage surrounding tissues. This complication and the wear and tear of long use present hazards that may not surface until many patients have been harmed. And unlike simply discontinuing to take an offending drug, defective devices often require surgical procedures for removal. Do device manufacturers address these challenges responsibly?

> Medical devices, by their very nature, are intended to offer patients substantial benefit. An inescapable reality is that medical devices have the capacity to inflict significant harm in the event of inappropriate performance or outright failure. The way a company addresses highly complex R & D questions and ambiguous, or even contradictory answers that arise, is an exercise in critical thinking and ethical behavior throughout the bench to bedside continuum.[41]

This statement by a retired Medtronic executive declaring that companies do try to behave in patients' interests, rings hollow if one believes the allegations made by the conflict-of-interest narrative.

Despite the FDA's demonstrable superiority to academic analysis in general and medical journal coverage in particular, critics fault the FDA's approach to medical device safety. Currently, the FDA requires extensive premarket analysis of Class III devices, deemed potentially high risk, such as implantable pacemakers, and only demonstration to FDA's satisfaction that the objects are safe and effective results in their approval for clinical use. Class I devices associated with absent or minimal risk, throat swabs or bandages for example, need not undergo any review. In between are Class II devices that the manufacturer must convince FDA are "substantially equivalent" to a "predicate" preexisting device. Based on the statutory definition for the review process of such devices, they carry the designation "510(k)."

In 2011, the Institute of Medicine released a report concluding that the present 510(k) system is inadequate to assure product safety and effectiveness and recommended that FDA completely scrap it in favor of significantly more prospective clinical trials to determine product risk profiles.[42] The FDA summarily rejected IOM's recommendations, although it recently instituted more stringent evaluation of devices that were already on the market in 1976, when device regulation began.[43]

The current failure rate of products cleared to market by 510(k) is quite low, even after implementation of mandatory adverse event reporting in 2000.[44] When events occur, the FDA and manufacturers work together to resolve them rapidly, including by issuing recalls.

Nevertheless, the calls for more stringent device regulation continue unabated, focusing primarily on a class of hip implants called "metal on metal." Three different manufacturers recalled such devices between 2008 and 2012, because many of them caused inflammation and required surgical removal.[45] An article criticizing the "equivalence" criteria that justified FDA approval of some of these devices states:[46]

> This pathway, called the 510(k) process, instead involves evaluation of "substantial equivalence" to previously cleared devices, many of which have been assessed for safety and effectiveness and some of which are no longer in use because of poor clinical performance.

But the article made no specific reference to any products "no longer in use" as having been subject to an FDA recall. Over time, most products are replaced through evolution by newer and better products. The article implied with no evidence that rogue products were removed from the market because of defects. Products under the 510(k) system are classified based on a determination of "substantial equivalence"—not identical features. Even identical twins, who share a common genetic heritage, are only substantially equivalent, not actually identical.

12

DEMONIZING MARKETING IS FALSE ADVERTISING

Like all things designed to suit the taste of the masses, advertising is repellent to people of delicate feeling. This abhorrence influences the appraisal of business propaganda. Advertising and all other methods of business propaganda are condemned as one of the most outrageous outgrowths of unlimited competition. It should be forbidden. The consumers should be instructed by impartial experts.[1]

In contrast to conflict-of-interest movement *instigators'* denial of the medical product industry's research and development accomplishments, *enablers* generally afford grudging, or occasionally enthusiastic, admiration of these contributions. But the enablers agree with the instigators' claims that industry's sales efforts, especially personal interactions known as "detailing," between company marketing representatives and physicians are corrupt and that medical students should not be exposed to such representatives.[2]

This chapter first challenges the evidence the conflict-of-interest movement claims supports the negative effects of the medical product industry's sales efforts. It then rebuts two broad criticisms of corporate marketing: that marketing is not education and that it does not convey scientific evidence. The chapter then critiques the alleged superiority of commercially independent education and argues that limiting industry promotion is far more likely to promote ignorance than patient benefits. It also points to the hypocrisy of private practices and university clinics aggressively marketing their services while demeaning industry's promotional activities. The next chapter debunks the conflict-of-interest movement's claim that physicians are corrupted by and incapable of resisting industry's devious marketing maneuvers.

CRITIQUE OF THE CASE AGAINST INDUSTRY MARKETING

If true, the following declaration from the 2006 Brennan *JAMA* article would more than justify the conflict-of-interest movement's animus against company sales practices. It would also provide support for the policies limiting or banning sales representatives from academic health centers and private practices: "The systematic review of the medical literature on [industry] gifting by Wazana found *that an overwhelming number of [marketing] interactions had negative results on clinical care* [emphasis added]."[3]

The "Wazana review" is a 2001 article titled "Physicians and the Pharmaceutical Industry: Is a Gift Ever Just a Gift?" also published in *JAMA*. The conflict-of-interest narrative has prominently cited this reference as revealing industry marketing's influence on medical practice. The review summarized 29 articles published in medical journals concerning the marketing-based relationship between physicians and pharmaceutical industry representatives and "its impact on the knowledge, attitudes and behavior of physicians."[4] The data reviewed on "knowledge, attitudes and behavior" predominantly derived from surveys. Most of the relevant articles assessed medical students' or physicians' attitudes. Few addressed "clinical care," and none did so directly. In fact, the article's author explicitly stated that "no study used patient outcome measures," which are the ultimate metrics on which to judge clinical care.

Critiques of that paper point out that it provided no evidence that marketing harmed patients and erred in its conclusions.[5] The presentation of findings in the articles it summarized mirror the one-sided negative interpretations of effects of physician-industry relationships characteristic of medical journal articles.[6] To mention one of many examples, a 1981 article claiming that detailing causes "nonrational prescribing" reported on therapeutic choices of Dutch general practitioners given a series of hypothetical cases with prespecified criteria for "appropriate" prescribing. Pharmacists analyzed the "rationality" of the medications selected by the subjects. The results showed considerable variability, and physicians' age was as important a factor correlating with "irrational" choices as was their using pharmaceutical representatives as information sources. In fact, more extensive use of general medical journals by the physicians surveyed also correlated with nonrational prescribing.[7] No causality pertaining to detailing can be inferred from this study.

In fact, a more recent summary of 59 studies concerning effects of industry detailing and gift giving on physicians, despite being critical of those activities, honestly admitted: "The limitations of the studies reported in the literature . . . mean that we are unable to reach any definitive conclusion about the degree to which information from pharmaceutical companies increases, decreases, or has no effect on the frequency, quality or cost of prescribing."[8]

In addition, these types of analyses do not address subtleties related to marketing of various product classes to different types of prescribing physicians. A circumstance in which only a single brand product exists is radically different than one in which brand products compete with each other or with generics, including products available without prescription. Furthermore, the knowledge and ability to access new information by generalists and specialists differ widely. In some clinical situations, such as cancer patients requiring chemotherapy, only specialists provide treatment. In others, like diabetes or depression, patients are more likely to receive treatment from primary care providers than from endocrinologists or psychiatrists.

That marketing activity enhances prescribing of products is intuitively obvious and empirically validated by an extensive analysis of the prescribing behavior of tens of thousands of physicians. The study showed that contact with company sales representatives increased the rate and extent of prescribing a newly launched diabetes drug. Such contact also diminished the rate and extent of prescribing another diabetes drug after it was given a black box warning by the FDA.[9] Enabling this analysis was the fact that a significant number of clinical practices have banned visits from marketing representatives. But despite its superior quantitative analysis, this research still is not informative concerning patient outcomes.

A study to determine the effect of industry detailing on patient outcomes requires controlling for physician, patient, and product properties, arguably an impossible task. But an unanswerable question does not justify inventing an answer. Nevertheless, in violation of this principle, anti-marketing critics arbitrarily recommend that physicians should not obtain prescribing information from sales representatives.

In summary, the conflict-of-interest movement's evidence justifying its pronouncements concerning medical product marketing is weak. The rest of this chapter and the next discuss the tactics employed by the conflict-of-interest movement to divert attention from the fact that they have little substantive evidence that industry marketing has negative effects on clinical care.

One tactic is to characterize industry marketing as "promotion" rather than as "education": "The traditional independence of physicians and the welfare of the public are being threatened by the new vogue among drug manufacturers to promote their products by assuming an aggressive role in the 'education' of doctors."[10]

A related tactic is to claim that industry promotion has little or no scientific validity compared to academic publications in medical journals.

EDUCATION VS. PROMOTION

What is the difference between watching a football game on TV, listening to an academic lecture, and hearing a sales pitch? There *is* no difference. All three convey factual information to observers. Even the TV advertisements during breaks in the game convey facts.

The difference lies is what facts recipients want. Most TV viewers of a sports event are seeking entertainment, but players and coaches of a competing team are intently looking for strategic clues that might be useful in future competition. A lecture attendee may be fulfilling a course requirement or learning about a topic of personal interest. Similarly, a physician may accommodate a company rep because the rep brought lunch for the office staff, because of previous social contacts, or because the physician actually wants to learn what the rep has to say. To the rep, the interaction is promotion, but for the physician it can be education.

The conflict-of-interest narrative does not recognize the overlapping attributes among these communication activities or care what the participants want. Education, the conflict-of-interest narrative claims, is a deadly serious business of conveying absolute truths. Most people's experiences with schooling superficially resonate with this severe mandate: we can all remember feeling bored or intimidated in drab classrooms by demanding teachers.

But getting past these shallow recollections requires little imagination. Children learn to count and read by observing clownish antics on television's Sesame Street and other programs. We recall having been occasionally entertained and inspired by charismatic teachers. In college, we curried favorable test grades by regurgitating pet ideas of our professors.

The medical company marketer is clearly engaged in promotion, motivated by the wish for the prescriber to use the company's products. Such promotion, according to the conflict-of-interest narrative, is by definition inferior to education. This distinction is nonsense. Perhaps teaching multiplication tables or alphabets to children has little to do with promotion, but when the conflict-of-interest inquisitors educate medical students, physicians, and the public through lectures, books, scholarly articles, and media hype, they are unquestionably promoting the ideology of the conflict-of-interest movement. When individuals who are in the *business* of noncommercial physician education justify their activities by criticizing the validity of industry marketing, they are fully engaged in promotion. And, as discussed further below, academic medical centers promote themselves aggressively, without regulatory restraints.

The segregation of education, entertainment, and promotion sidetracks the discussion from what really matters: the factual content. And, as discussed below and in other chapters, the factual accuracy of FDA-regulated product marketing is generally superior to the unregulated content emitted by the conflict-of-interest movement.

DOES INDUSTRY PROMOTION REPRESENT SCIENTIFIC EVIDENCE?

The pledge of the "No Free Lunch" organization opposing industry marketing contains the following statement: "I _____ am committed to practicing medicine in the best interest of my patients and on the basis of the best available evidence, rather than on the basis of advertising or promotion."[11]

The pledge overtly promulgates the academic legend that pharmaceutical promotion is not scientific evidence. Chapter 5 reviewed the ambiguities concerning what constitutes scientific evidence. The following discussion addresses how physicians acquire such evidence.

How Do Physicians Obtain Scientific Information?

Many physicians forthrightly declare that they learn how to care for patients from reading research described in medical journal articles.[12] But common sense indicates that this claim is largely untrue. As chapter 4 explained, journal articles are not physician users' manuals. They are not easily readable, and their subscription costs are high. And, more importantly, many physicians simply do not have time for such reading. One explanation for what I consider an overselling of the importance of medical journals is the influence of the academic establishment. Students graduate from medical school with the belief that medical journal articles contain the truths that define proper practice. Throughout their curriculum, they hear faculty and postgraduate physicians in training spouting information from journal articles in conferences and on patient rounds and when reviewing clinical topics in "journal clubs." Lacking practice experience, they come to believe that all wisdom resides in such texts. They have no basis to comprehend the diverse sources of information that define practices, some of which go unacknowledged.

Physicians treat patients based on many inputs, and the conveyance of new information is haphazard. Even if they look at medical journal articles, physicians, due to lack of time, interest, or competence, do not evaluate them critically.[13]

The adage "watch one, do one, teach one" aptly captures how physicians acquire competence with medical procedures, many requiring devices, and with complex drug regimens required to treat some infectious diseases and cancers. Representatives of the companies making the devices or designing the treatments are arguably best equipped to participate in such teaching.[14]

In many respects the information-gathering activities of practicing physicians resemble those of corporate CEOs.[15] Both must integrate vast amounts of ever changing data. Contrary to academic legend, physicians, like CEOs, lack the time to process voluminous written materials or scientifically assess conflicting evidence. Rather, they both rely heavily on face-to-face encounters with numerous information sources, including, in the case of physicians, their patients, to arrive at decisions that benefit patients or companies respectively. Guiding the path to decision making are their innate intelligence, education, training, experience, and—as was evident for the research described in chapter 8—intuition and luck. At the end of the day, some perform these daunting evaluations better than others, but arguably no better metric than track records measure such performance.

What Physicians Learn from Company Representatives

One might predict that a mirror image of physicians' stated claim to rely on medical journals or other academically endorsed sources for information would be to articulate suspicion or dislike of company representatives who lack their professional credentials. But, to the contrary, the conflict-of-interest movement despairs over the fact that surveys have consistently reported that medical students, physicians, and paraprofessionals frequently interact with industry marketing representatives, have positive attitudes toward them, and believe they provide useful information, despite perceiving representatives' biases.[16] These critics, who are contemptuous of physicians' failure to "see the light," *never* concede *even the possibility* that the medical students, physicians, and paraprofessionals may have it *right*: they benefit from their industry marketing interactions *and* are skeptical. Rather, critics *insist* on trying to purge these individuals of their supposed "cognitive dissonance."

Business scholars study detailing with the goal of informing the industry as to the effectiveness of its marketing procedures rather than to assess its social value. Stripped of ideological agendas, the business literature finds that detailing may contribute to early adoption of new products[17] and that the marketing content is often more informational than persuasive.[18] Informational impact is defined as a change in chemical-specific prescribing and persuasion as an effect on brand prescribing. The overall impact of detailing is modest compared to what physicians learn from mentors and colleagues, initially during training and later while in practice.[19] Also, the effectiveness of detailing varies for a given product over time.[20] One study suggested that the success of marketing is proportional to how compelling the scientific evidence is regarding a product's efficacy,[21] and another documented that detailing far more effectively drove prescribing of a well-regarded ACE inhibitor–diuretic drug combination than did publication of the same information in a medical journal.[22] Finally, the extraordinary complexity and dynamic nature of the medical product industry renders simple conclusions about the effectiveness of its marketing practices suspect.[23]

Quality of Promotional Information

The conflict-of-interest narrative points to the billions of dollars industry spends on marketing while discounting the value clinicians find in marketing information.[24] But by FDA law, this information must conform to what the Agency has approved—what goes on the product label. As discussed in chapter 5, the FDA's assessment involves an extensive review of a large information package concerning the research that went into product development. After a thorough review, the Agency convenes panels of experts to provide advice regarding the risks and benefits of the product in question. These panels review the evidence and the FDA's evaluation of it and then undertake a nonbinding vote for or against approval. While far from perfect, label content, the information distilled from the arduous FDA review process, is as scientific and trustworthy as any in medicine. On first principles, therefore, the confident assumptions underlying the pharm-free pledge cited above are wrong.

EDUCATION ABOUT PROMOTION

As indicated by the numerous surveys discussed above, physicians continue interacting with sales representatives and find value for patient care in the experience, despite relentless demonization of industry and the imposition of regulations. Because studies indicate that physicians' comfort with sales representatives correlates with frequency of contact,[25] the increasing trend toward restricting such representatives from academic medical centers and clinical practices may change these attitudes. Physicians' migrations from individual or small group practices into large health systems, in response to financial pressures, are contributing to such restrictions because these systems have incentives limiting the number of physicians contacted by company representatives. In addition, active indoctrination efforts introduced into medical schools reportedly convert students' viewpoints toward a more negative direction.[26]

For example, the number of medical students reporting disapproval of pharmaceutical representatives in the learning environment took a large uptick following a former drug rep's presentation, a faculty debate, and a Web-based course sponsored by the AMA at four American medical schools.[27] The disapproval sentiment was higher at schools with more restrictive policies. The course was heavily biased against industry. The webinar featured former drug representatives rendering testimonials describing their devious sales techniques and anti-industry critics expounding their opinions. The presentation did not contain a *single* pro-industry background reference nor one word about the *value* of products.[28]

The sedulous criticism of industry has already spawned generations of misinformed physicians poorly equipped to incorporate rapidly emerging innovation. Now, with the help of organized medicine, it is becoming institutionalized in medical education. Education about conflict-of-interest has become a growth industry for entrepreneurial ethics instructors.[29]

ACADEMIC DETAILING

This chapter's critique of the conflict-of-interest movement's demonization of industry marketing does not lead to the conclusion that such marketing is problem free—only that it is a prevalent, regulated, and effective educational modality. Moreover, the complaint that the heaviest marketing surrounds products that are equivalent or incrementally different is valid. The key questions are whether some mechanism for reducing the promotion of brand and increasing the promotion of generic products would improve patient care and whether such a system is feasible.

Academic detailers (also called counter-detailers) propose to introduce noncommercial, evidence-based prescriber education through written, online, or personal contact with physicians.[30] Considering the challenge for busy physicians to absorb and evaluate new information, such an enterprise has potential value. However, academic detailing brands itself as a preferable alternative to what it characterizes as harmful commercial promotion of medical products.[31] Earlier parts of this chapter argued that commercial promotion has not been shown to either improve or worsen patient outcomes. Similarly, the available evidence demonstrates that academic detailing leads to prescribing changes but not whether these changes improve or worsen patient outcomes.[32]

One assumption underlying academic detailing is that industry detailing results in physicians prescribing brand drugs when generic equivalents are available and are appropriate for patients. However, insurance plans and states have distanced what physicians prescribe and what prescriptions patients actually receive at the pharmacy. As a result, generic prescriptions dominate brand prescriptions by more than twofold. In many cases, unless physicians go to extra lengths, pharmacies automatically substitute brand prescriptions with generic equivalents.

Academic detailing enthusiasts assert that governments, insurers, and pharmacies have purer motives than medical product manufacturers. A few states have funded academic detailing programs, and the program managers claim that their activities have reduced inappropriate prescribing practices, defined as inadequate prescribing of generic products.

Both public and private insurers, benefit financially when physicians prescribe generic products or benefit managers switch brand prescriptions to generic ones. When states or insurance companies pay for such educational operations, they do not *make* money through the effort, but they *save* it, which increases their bottom line. Less well known is that pharmacies also gain financially from generic prescribing. The lower costs of generics mean that pharmacies are out less cash after purchasing them compared to brand products. A large proportion of prescriptions never get filled. Compliance failure has adverse medical consequences but also affects the economics of pharmacies that bear the costs of unsold inventories. Increased generic use has saved costs of insurers,[33] but pharmacies also make greater—double—profit margins from selling generics, because markups on cheaper generics are less obvious to consumers than those on expensive branded products.[34] The greater profitability of selling generics translates into greater corporate profit margins for pharmacies, as clearly stated in Security and Exchange filings of CVS Caremark and Walgreen Corporations, two of the nation's largest pharmacy chains.[35]

Not surprising, therefore, are alliances between insurance companies, pharmacies, and academic detailing operations. The stated objectives of these relationships revolve around optimal patient management, but the financial benefits to the participants are real as well. The Aetna Insurance Company and CVS Caremark have participated in such sponsorship, and its employees have co-authored with academic detailers articles in medical journals promoting the benefits of generic products.[36] CVS Caremark has established a partnership with an academic detailing enterprise.[37]

Financial motivation aside, a key question is whether medical product educators exist who can impart to educated and trained physicians, who receive multiple inputs of data, information superior to that conveyed by narrowly trained company representatives. Academic detailers claim to educate physicians broadly concerning disease management, beyond the use of specific products. Increasingly, however, medical product manufacturers and other companies supported by them provide such management education to help physicians keep up to date with other needs and desires of patients, including use of monitoring devices, participation in wellness programs, and networking for illness support groups.

The ability of academic detailers to improve physicians' prescribing behavior also rests on the assumption that relevant published medical information they use for their education efforts is up to date, accessible, and meaningful. For the reasons discussed regarding scientific evidence in chapter 5, this assumption is often questionable, especially concerning disorders for which management is uncertain or controversial. This concern also applies to the management of rare and complicated diseases like my patient Grace's HUS. Nevertheless, because the academics who promote academic detailing focus on the introduction and use of medical products, neglected topics in medical schools and medical practices, they do make useful contributions.

PRINT AND DIRECT TO CONSUMER (DTC) ADVERTISING OF MEDICAL PRODUCTS

The previous discussion focused predominantly on face-to-face contact between company marketers and physicians (detailing). Television viewers receive a steady diet of medical product commercials, and medical journals often include print advertisements for such products. The televised direct-to-consumer ads have been controversial since their introduction 20 years ago, and the antipathy to them is largely emotional. The frequency of erectile dysfunction advertisements during televised sports events offends some, while others who think all health-related communication must be serious take offense at tacky imagery associated with a drug or device. Advertising has the minimal goal of attracting attention, however, and if it gets patients remedies for sometimes stigmatized problems they know about—or don't—it performs a useful task.

Many medical journal managers who reject that industry detailing has educational value sell expensive advertising copy in their periodicals to medical product companies. I find it odd that companies pay for such ads, which, the back cover excepted, are unlikely to be seen by readers interested in the primary journal content. The ads are a strange mélange of comic book imagery and unintelligible fine print. The imagery is presumably a publicist's conception of what will attract attention. The fine print, mandated by the FDA, is based on the content of the product package insert. Arguably, despite the fact that analysts have identified what they deemed distorted graphics in pharmaceutical company advertisements in print medical journals (they did not provide comparisons with academic medical advertisements), such distortion, even if true, does not provably influence prescribing behavior. [38]

To test the effectiveness of print advertising, companies could limit direct-to-consumer and journal ads to certain geographic segments and see whether it affects sales in those demographics. Or, they could pull the ads altogether for a period of time. While other factors could obscure the results, I suspect that the reason such experiments don't take place is that the marketing departments of companies don't want to risk having their budgets cut.

ANOTHER VERSION OF ACADEMIC DETAILING

A striking blind spot in academe's dim view of medical product advertising is the promotional behavior of university medical practices and medical journals. Academic medical centers issue press releases advertising research accomplishments of questionable clinical relevance or understated limitations [39] and sport huge banners proclaiming their favorable clinical rankings in *US News and World Report*. Print advertisements (airline magazines are popular locations for them) feature patients with happy faces rendering testimonials regarding their treatment at such and such hospital, or physicians in white coats or scrub suits who work at those hospitals described as "the best." None of this puffery is regulated or supported by evidence. Hospitals have even begun to hire former medical product company reps to detail physicians for patient referrals. [40] *The New England Journal of Medicine*'s website contains illustrated advertisements for its reprints to promote the effectiveness of industry detailing.

In summary, because conflict-of-interest movement promoters misrepresent industry's marketing as lacking an evidence base or adequate regulatory oversight, they resort to unregulated promotion. Medical journals happily accept medical product industry money to prop up their own businesses. By advertising in medical journals, the benefit of which is debatable, industry contributes to its own denigration.

13

THE GIFT SMOKE SCREEN

Gifts may have been what overcame the xenophobia of our remote an-
cestors to allow them to engage in trade: the offering of gifts by one set of
strangers to another presumably preempted attack long enough for the
message to sink in that doing business was more mutually beneficial than
engaging in hostilities.[1] Reciprocity impulses are recognized aspects of
human psychology,[2] and gifting as a mechanism for attracting a potential
customer's attention long enough to examine the wares has become en-
grained as an integral element of human interaction. Small gifts and reminder items—serving coffee at the automobile showroom—are not considered problematic in most of our economy. Even politicians can accept
modest gifts. In medicine, attention-getting amenities are but small counters to physicians' deep-seated aversion to disrupt familiar approaches to
patient care and overcome the inertia to possibly adopt better ones. The
conflict-of-interest movement, however, does not brook this tolerant attitude with respect to the medicine-industry interface: "social science research suggests that feelings of reciprocity and changes in attitudes or
behavior can be induced by even small-value gifts."[3]

Responding to the conflict-of-interest movement's gift aversion, the
most recent industry trade group ethics codes have recommended abolishing all gifting, and the industry has complied. A disingenuous aspect of
this capitulation is that while the conflict-of-interest movement argues
circularly that companies wouldn't spend on gifts if they didn't expect
returns, large companies have happily adopted universal gift bans because they save marketing costs at no competitive disadvantage. In other

words, if the industry really believed that the gifts were essential to maintain sales, they would have fought for them. They did not.

This chapter summarizes the conflict-of-interest movement's arguments as to why gifts, writ large, are supposedly so malign. First, the movement arbitrarily defines all industry payments of cash or kind to physicians as gifts and therefore tantamount to bribery. Second, the conflict-of-interest movement alleges that gifts significantly increase medical costs. Third, the movement invokes altruistic self-denial of gifts and other benefits as a defining component of medical professionalism. But nothing more clearly epitomizes the hubris of the conflict-of-interest movement's assault on gifts than its use of overgeneralized anthropology and psychology research as evidence that gifts are malignant.

GIFTS ARE BRIBERY?

The following example epitomizes this conflation:[4]

> In order to promote sales, drug firms create financial relationships that influence physicians' prescriptions and sometimes even reward physicians for prescribing drugs. Three main types exist: (1) kickbacks, (2) gifts, and (3) financial support for professional activities. The prevalence of these practices has evolved over time in response to changes in professional codes, law and markets. There are certainly differences between these types of ties, but all of them can compromise physicians' independent judgment and rational prescribing.

The author of these comments seamlessly equates gifts, defined as reminder items, meals, and "financial support for professional activities," with "kickbacks." Kickbacks are *quid pro quo* transactions implying contractual obligations. Proving a kickback case requires demonstrating with objective evidence direct causation: that a physician prescribes in response to a specific reward. Kickbacks are unethical and strictly illegal. Yet the author asserts that such kickbacks, cataloged in detail in his article, contaminate a vast array of physician activities ("compromise physicians' independent judgment and rational prescribing").

This article is unencumbered by any quantitative evidence and devotes not a word to the *possibility* that the gift menu might actually add some value to medical care. It epitomizes the conflict-of-interest movement's

rhetorical characterization that any activity at the medicine-industry interface that is not adversarial constitutes a gift that compromises objective
science or patient welfare.[5]

The conflict-of-interest movement's attack on gifts employs clever
rhetorical and ascetic elements. The very triviality of most gifts lends
itself to abuse. If you defend gifts, it must be because you greedily crave
freebies or perks. Gift is an epithet designed to invoke instant alarm,
surveillance, and restrictions. The sheer scope encompassed by gifts
makes a target for opprobrium of any and all paid relationships at the
medical-industry interface.

GIFTS INCREASE MEDICAL COSTS?

> And they [physicians] can bear in mind that the costs of industry
> dinners, trips, and other incentives are passed along to their patients in
> the form of higher drug prices.[6]
>
> Eric Campbell, a researcher at Massachusetts General Hospital
> who specializes in conflict of interest in medicine, said, "It is unique to
> recognize that it's inappropriate to pass on the cost of CME to patients
> in the form of higher drug prices" because of overprescribing. "Doc-
> tors should pay for their own education."[7]

The rebuttal to these statements is simple. Medical product costs are a
minor fraction of the total health care economy. Marketing of the products in general and gifts in particular represent a modest fraction of aggregate health care expenditures.[8] Absent adherence to an ascetic imperative
discussed below, physicians have to "pass on the cost of [their] CME to
patients" in some manner. If industry doesn't subsidize it, the physicians
have to increase their billings. No economic analysis supports the confident assumption that "dinners, trips, and other incentives" directly result
in higher drug prices—or that if they do, the benefits in terms of better
health outcomes and economic productivity do not exceed the speculated
price increases.

GIFTS (BENEFITS) ARE UNPROFESSIONAL (UNETHICAL)?

A conflict of interest movement promoter makes the following statements in a book chapter titled "Solutions Requiring Enhanced Professionalism in Medicine," to argue on ethical grounds that physicians and researchers should eschew financial rewards (benefits) from commercial sources: [9]

> It is much more difficult to detect falsification or spin of research results to suit a company's commercial interests, than for the scientists conducting the research to avoid spin and falsification in the first place.
>
> As a matter of professional integrity, we have asked practitioners to forgo all the personal benefits of drug company gifts. Also as a matter of professional integrity, we similarly ask physician-investigators to forgo such benefits. We are asking these investigators to rise to the ethical level of journalists and judges, and admit that reasonable on-lookers could question the objectivity of their "scientific" judgments if they are known to be accepting cash payments from an interested party.
>
> Even if the individual had the capacity to remain totally objective in the face of cash or other gifts, professional integrity demands more than this. It demands trustworthiness. And trustworthiness demands that one behave in ways that would convince even skeptical onlookers of one's good faith.
>
> The change in momentum could produce an important shift in values within the academic workplace. The shift would in some ways turn the clock back to the era between 1950 and 1970, when academics proudly held themselves above such practices as profiting from discoveries.

The pining for a return to a bygone era of supposedly pious medical asceticism demonstrates striking ignorance concerning research and innovation. As discussed in Chapter 8, productive research introduces discoveries that *reproducibly work*. Such reproducibility has *absolutely nothing* to do with "reasonable onlookers questioning objectivity" or convincing "skeptical onlookers of one's good faith." Journalists and judges do not innovate. They merely report, opine, or rule on occurrences. And journalists hardly "avoid spin." Falsification and spin *never* contribute to medical innovation, and as emphasized in other chapters, most research falsification perpetrators have been academics with *no* commercial relationships. Research competitors have no concerns about each other's "good faith." Rather they ruthlessly fixate on promoting their own interests. This self-interest spurs them on to make and defend discoveries.

The call to reject "benefits" would have deprived leading academic researchers and founders of genetic engineering companies in the 1970s and 1980s of well-deserved rewards. Their involvement in the enterprise provided confidence to investors and in some instances, abetted development of valuable medical products. In either case, their participation was a diversion from the academic activities for which they were paid and that lent them prominence. Compensation for their deviation from their usual pursuits was therefore appropriate. If their contributions resulted in useful products, a rare occurrence, commensurate rewards were also in order. [10]

The demonization of benefits takes energy from a concept known as "medical exceptionalism." Medical exceptionalism, as articulated in 1907 by William Osler, an erudite scholar and famous medical educator, rigidly asserts that medicine is a "calling" and not a business: [11]

> You are in this profession as a calling, not a business. Once you get down to a purely business level, your influence is gone and the true light of your life is dimmed. You must work in the missionary spirit, with breadth of charity that raises you far above the petty jealousies of life.

Medical exceptionalism has durable emotional appeal. A century after Osler's admonition, President Barack Obama echoed it in a speech to the American Medical Association to a rousing ovation: [12]

> It [our health care system] is a model that has taken the pursuit of medicine from a profession—a calling—to a business. That is not why you became doctors.
>
> You did not enter this profession to be bean counters and paper pushers. You entered this profession to be healers—and that's what our health care system should let you be.

Medical exceptionalism is a legacy of medicine's pre-scientific history. Until recently, medical practitioners made no positive contribution to human health. In fact, the pious admonition "Do no harm" ascribed to Hippocrates to the contrary, millennia of medical practice based on his principles concerning human body structure and function inflicted massive harm. [13] Practitioners engaged in bleeding, cupping, and purging. These ineffective and often harmful methods persisted in the absence of demonstrable clinical benefit solely because of the wishful thinking of the sick. In pandering to such vain hopes, one strategy of medical practitioners was to elevate the physician-patient relationship to a mystique. The physician's grave concern, availability, and reassurances to the sick could be given credit for occasional spontaneous recoveries and by predicting failure, the doctor might somewhat alleviate its effect.

Medicine also affected trappings of religion. Physicians adopted priestly affectations such as wearing robes and using Latin and classical Greek to describe body parts, diseases, and (useless) therapies. Although priests never had to prove that their ministrations afforded postmortem salvation, the inability of physicians to cure was all too obvious. Hence, physicians' respectability languished far lower than the clerics they aped. This lowly status persisted despite the gradual accumulation of scientific knowledge about human biology and the causes of disease, because no means existed to translate that information into practical prevention and therapy of disease.

Even when specific medical activities such as vaccination, anesthesia, and antisepsis began to supplement improved housing, nutrition, and sanitation as modalities to preserve and improve life during the late 19th and early 20th centuries, a vast reservoir of untreatable medical conditions and patients' dread of painful medical procedures led them to avoid mainstream medicine and patronize a thriving "patent medicine" industry, which promised more but delivered less. The mail order medications purveyed by this industry were predominantly concoctions of opiates and alcohol. [14] Mainstream medical practitioners' approach to opposing this competition was to condemn the commercial basis of patent medicine promotion, although medical journals survived economically by running advertisements for them. Codes of ethics promulgated by professional societies banned physician advertising and other activities such as hospital insurance and group practice as inappropriate. A contemporary surgeon exposed many of these prohibitions as simply defenses against the erosion of fee-for-service private practice that enriched the framers of these codes. [15]

By mid-20th century medicine could really help patients, and the dictionary definition of a "professional"—a well-educated and trained person with demonstrable competency—was applicable. Yet, medicine retained its archaic impetus to differentiate itself from business and place itself in an elevated moral sphere, even though most medical and dental practitioners prospered in small fee-for-service enterprises. Some explanations for the persistence of this attitude include the appeal of superiority, utility in public relations, and having no compelling reason to change.

The promotion of medical exceptionalism reflects the state of medicine prior to the middle of the 20th century. But circumstances were rapidly changing. The Supreme Court set aside medical guild prohibitions against fee setting, collective bargaining, physician investment, and advertising as violating antitrust laws. [16] For-profit hospitals and other commercial health services, such as dialysis centers and home care companies and procedure referral centers, owned or invested in by physicians emerged. [17] Medical school graduates increasingly entered practice hobbled with staggering education debts. More importantly, technological advances markedly diminished the unpredictability of illness invoked to argue that medicine is not a market. [18] Hospitals in the past were predominantly charitable operations. When hospitalization became more widespread, municipalities and charities ran hospitals as nonprofit enterprises because no profits were possible.

The progressive growth of the health care economy dramatically altered this landscape. Hospitals today, especially urban hospitals, are large businesses managed by highly paid executives that compete and advertise aggressively for patients. Previously ignored amenities such as convenient parking, short waiting times, and pleasant surroundings are now increasingly the rule. Market competition has provided better customer service than saintly aspirations. That medicine could be practiced without what President Obama derided as "bean counting and paper pushing" is inconceivable.

An invidious aspect of medical exceptionalists' definitions of "professionalism" is that failure to comply renders one automatically unprofessional. Because the definition of professional to patients most importantly embodies clinical competence, the insinuations of degraded professionalism border on slander. An example of such conflation of ideological stance with morality is a medical journal article titled "Physician Professionalism and Changes in Physician-Industry Relationships from 2004 to 2009". [19] The article describes results of a survey compiling how many physicians have industry relationships. But no information in that article bears on professionalism defined as competence.

And what kind of "calling" is medicine as averred by Osler and Obama? Is it a calling to a medieval monastic set of vows of poverty? The affluence of most physicians and their concentration in relatively affluent urban settings suggest that medicine is better described by the protestant reformation's claim that wealth is a sign of divinity. [20]

DOES ANTHROPOLOGY REVEAL A CULTURE OF RECIPROCITY?

The conflict-of-interest narrative defines gifts with infinite breadth and assumes that *any* relationship, other than adversarial, between physicians and industry, promotes reciprocity. It mocks the fact that surveys report that physicians maintain in surveys that gifts do not affect their prescribing behavior. The surveyed physicians claim that gifts do not influence *them*—but they report believing that such gifts influence *their colleagues*. [21] This apparent contradiction is amusing but proves nothing.

Michael Oldani, the former Pfizer drug rep turned anthropologist posits the existence of a "gift culture" that medical product companies train sales representatives to nurture with physician customers. [22] That Oldani claims companies train sales personnel to be effective persuaders and reward them with competitive salaries and bonuses if they are successful hardly seems remarkable or conspiratorial. But Oldani's approach to documenting the irresistible power of reciprocity is anecdote dependent. He weaves stories concerning how he succeeded with sales wizardry on skeptical physicians into a broader narrative that exemplifies confirmation bias: gift exchange is the best explanation for behavioral change. He neglects, however, to rule out competing explanations. He cites riveting persuasion *success* stories with no denominator of likely *failures* to convince and change physician behavior.

Oldani's most astonishing argument for the power of reciprocity follows:

> What is most critical to this process is that the opportunity now arises for the rep to talk about other products. The doctor, *of course, is compelled to return the favor*, and at least listen to the rep talk about these other products. Reps at Company X were trained to respond to any request for product information by always presenting the older/ nonrequested products first. You were to hold out, if you will, on the

requested information because you had the upper hand and the physician was forced to be a captive audience [emphasis added].

Why is the doctor "compelled"? If reps must bear gifts to get a busy physician's attention, why suddenly does this physician manifest such groveling gratitude for obtaining requested information so as to tolerate having time wasted on information not initially wanted? Oldani gives no reason. Company X may have trained reps to try this approach, but we need better evidence than testimonials that such training is successful.

Finally, the conflict-of-interest narrative literature frequently cites a chapter discussing the role of reciprocity in persuasion in a book titled *Influence, The Psychology of Persuasion* authored by Robert Cialdini.[23] The narrative, however, neglects to mention that Cialdini explicitly states that customers' recognition of marketing strategies involving reciprocity inducements, such as provision of free samples, completely negates the effectiveness of those tactics. Cialdini recommends that if we feel someone is trying to exploit us in this manner, the appropriate response is not to avoid the encounter but to exploit the exploiter by taking his or her free services, recognizing them as sales ploys, and refusing the request for reciprocation on the grounds that the gift was not a gift, but rather a marketing tactic.

DOES SOCIAL SCIENCE MANDATE GIFT BANS?

The Brennan *JAMA* article summarized the scientific basis for banning gifts:[24]

Social science research demonstrates that the impulse to reciprocate for even small gifts is a powerful influence on people's behavior. Individuals receiving gifts are often unable to remain objective; they reweigh information and choices in light of the gift. So too, those people who give or accept gifts with no explicit "strings attached" still carry an expectation of some kind of reciprocity. Indeed, researchers suggest that the expectation of reciprocity may be the primary motive for gift-giving.

If you bring this topic up with most medical professionals, they express great skepticism that accepting a pen or a meal from a medical product company can possibly compromise their professional integrity. Unfortunately, overriding the common sense of the rank and file medical workforce has been the passionate and confident acceptance and marketing of the "social science of gifting" by apparent authorities. Most physicians lack the time or interest to obtain an understanding of what really comprises the social science being discussed. My experience has consistently revealed that if you ask the authorities, they don't really know what it is either! They simply parrot the conclusions.

The "social science research" cited in the Brennan *JAMA* piece above was the topic of a 2007 symposium on the "scientific basis of influence and reciprocity" convened as part of the Association of American Medical College's commission of conflict of interest in medical education.[25] The symposium consisted of five presentations and four responses to them. The introductory presentation emphasized how the sizeable marketing investments made by the medical product industry *must* mean that the marketing efforts succeed in persuading. The next presentation, by a neuroscientist, reported how sophisticated brain imaging studies reveal predictable responses (the brain "lights up" in specific locations) when subjects engage in contrived transactions involving conferral of gifts. These results, he concluded, provide biological support for the power of reciprocity. Three behavioral economists presented subsequent discussions.

Behavioral economics codifies how individuals often draw predictably inaccurate or inappropriate conclusions concerning matters about which they lack expertise, especially when hurried to respond. The manner of presenting—or framing—problems requiring decisions also affects the conclusions in predictable ways. One contribution to the AAMC symposium was to explain that experimental subjects involved in transactions organized by psychological experimenters cheat in a stereotypic manner and the cheating can be mitigated with moral reminders, such as a reading of the 10 Commandments during the transaction.

A second symposium presentation summarized behaviors of college students recruited to engage in games in which experimenters provide financial incentives for certain outcomes and manipulate the subjects in various ways. One such experiment is to have students estimate the number of coins in a glass jar (a variation on this theme is guessing the number of dots projected on a screen).[26] As part of the exercise, other students serve as advisers to the guessers. The person supervising the experiment offers the advisers monetary rewards proportional to the extent to which they can persuade the guessers to make inaccurately exaggerated estimates. The advisers comply, and the guessers increase their estimates. When the supervisor now instructs the advisers to inform the guessers of this subterfuge, the advisers—supposedly absolved of deception by the confession—ramp up the overestimate advice, and the guessers follow it. The researchers described these findings in publications including one with the catchy title: "The Dirt on Coming Clean." They concluded that their studies reveal that disclosure of conflicts of interest are not only ineffective but make things worse.[27]

A third symposium presentation summarized research findings, primarily involving business and accounting activities, that purportedly reveal how we consistently and subconsciously rationalize deviant behavior.[28]

Even if all the research information presented at the AAMC symposium were valid in its experimental context, is it justifiable to extrapolate the results to physicians' prescribing behavior? The symposium participants thought so:[29]

> From the panel of responders, two key messages emerged. First, the task of convincing physicians, who are selected for their ability to reason, that they are not reliably reasonable is not simple. Second, though people cannot exercise unlimited control of their instinctive behavior, they are capable of imposing some modifications on it. Purposeful structuring of relationships and interactions to diminish potential conflicts of interest reinforces that capability.

The responses to the presentations were consistent with the symposium membership. No dissenting voices were present. Two of the respondents were authors of the 2006 Brennan *JAMA* article. Not surprising, they endorsed the idea that the presentations supported the need for maximizing elimination of conflicts of interest. Another respondent, a physician researcher specializing in infectious diseases, said he had previously been unaware of the extent to which subconscious impulses affect behavior. This reaction is odd, given the long recognition by religious tradition, philosophy, and psychiatry that we have severe cognitive limits and that unconscious impulses affect our behavior.

In any case, the symposium participants seamlessly extrapolated the research findings to the context of physicians' receiving gifts as representing subconscious, reward-seeking behavior—akin to experimental animals pushing buttons to obtain pellets—and they translated these extrapolations into sweeping policy recommendations:[30]

> Because bias induced by monetary interests is unconscious and unintentional, there is little hope of controlling it when monetary interests exist. The implication for industry gifts is straightforward: they should be prohibited.
>
> The only viable remedy is to eliminate conflicts of interest whenever possible—e.g. eliminate gifts from pharmaceutical companies to physicians. This should include gifts of any size, because even small gifts can result in unconscious bias.

However, extrapolating the psychology findings to physicians making far more deliberative decisions based on extensive education and training is highly questionable. *Who cares about the value of a jar full of coins or the number of dots on a screen?* The most glaring discrepancy between the games and real life is that the students employed by the researchers to play the games have been *explicitly incented* to cheat, invalidating the sleight of hand required to infer that physicians who interact with marketing reps cheat subconsciously. No adverse consequences derive from the students' cheating. If, on the other hand, physicians make bad decisions due to accepting gifts or consorting with marketers, their actions do have real consequences. They operate with the checks and balances of second opinions and malpractice litigation. In contrast to the student advising activities that have *no* social value, marketers' information can saves lives.

In fact, other psychological experiments resembling the coin jar exercise have shown that providing feedback to the subjects, more experience with the experimental system, and concerns about personal reputation diminish cheating tendencies, even with a system that explicitly rewards cheating.[31] Indeed, the conflict-of-interest narrative overlooks the importance of reputation despite its obvious role in the ability of physicians to attract patients or achieve academic promotion. Chapter 8 reviewed how researchers' prime motivation is to receive recognition from prominent colleagues. That these powerful forces would be less susceptible to exerting subconscious influence than "small gifts" is unlikely.

The social science researchers have also reported survey results they interpret as revealing that physicians justify taking gifts because they believe they *deserve* them, especially if reminded about having endured long and arduous education and training.[32] They refer to this behavior as "entitlement." But doesn't a diagnosis of entitlement invalidate the case for reciprocity? If physicians accept gifts out of entitlement, then how can gifts exert influence? Entitlement should trump reciprocity impulses. If I'm entitled to a gift, its receipt doesn't obligate me to reciprocate by pleasing the giver.

Other chapters have reviewed how frequently carefully controlled laboratory results concerning chemical reactions that suggest possible drug opportunities do not pan out in animal or human testing. This prediction failure has to be far greater in the realm of experimental psychology. Although psychologists may sometimes accurately document irrational tendencies of human cognition under experimental conditions, invoking this information to make policy recommendations is extreme overreach. Indeed, field tests have also questioned the validity of extrapolating psychology laboratory experiments into real-life settings.[33] If we take seriously that physicians are incapable of transcending the wiles of influence, they will never prescribe based on scientific evidence. The conflict-of-interest movement depends heavily on this social science material to justify relationship regulation because it has so little direct evidence that relationships are harmful or, for that matter, not beneficial.[34]

As discussed in other chapters, asking whether company marketers (or their gifts) impose influence is the wrong question anyway. The right question is whether the resulting physician behavior is good or bad for patient care. Physicians do not help themselves if they deny that gifts and relationships influence them. Even academic detailers bear gifts. The right responses are to be conscious of one's cognitive limitations but, in the end, be able to defend one's prescribing behavior. If being reminded about products or involved in a relationship with or rewarded by an industry representative leads the medical professional to a decision that benefits patients, shouldn't such interaction be encouraged?

14

THE LAWYERS' BALL

In 2011, the *New York Times* featured three articles with very similar titles: "Merck to pay $950 million over Vioxx," "Glaxo [GlaxoSmithK-line or GSK] settles case with US for $3 billion," and "Novartis pays $422.5 million in settlement."[1] All three articles featured numerous phrases such as "this is the latest in a series of crackdowns," "fraud cases," "pleaded guilty to a criminal charge," "illegally introducing a drug into interstate commerce," "civil claims that [Merck's] illegal marketing caused doctors to prescribe and bill the government for Vioxx they otherwise would not have prescribed," and "federal prosecutors said the company [GSK] had paid doctors and manipulated medical research to promote the drug."

Nothing in this reporting explains the legal strategy prosecutors use to obtain these settlements or why the companies always settle. This chapter explains how prosecutors use a creative legal strategy to force the settlements described in the *Times* articles by exploiting ambiguities in federal criminal law and the claims of the conflict-of-interest movement to threaten companies with lethal penalties. The companies submit to onerous settlement agreements to avoid even a tiny risk of incurring a corporate death penalty. The cases never go to trial or obtain judicial review, preventing outside scrutiny of the legal arguments.

THE LEGAL BACKGROUND

The extensive regulatory menu affecting the medical-industry interface lends itself to considerable legal attention. Most medical products must run a gauntlet of regulatory oversight before being released for public use. Patients may bring tort actions against physicians for harm resulting from negligent use of a product or against companies for negligence in manufacturing them. Under current law, patients may also sue manufacturers for harm resulting from failure to warn about potential side effects. Manufacturers receive limited protection against failure-to-warn suits related to side effects listed on the product label, whose content companies negotiate with the FDA, yet they remain liable for unforeseen side effects and those which judges or juries believe were inadequately disclosed.

Some scholars have argued that the FDA's extensive premarket analysis of products should further or fully indemnify manufacturers from failure-to-warn liability. They claim that medical products are too technically complex for medically unsophisticated judges and juries, in diverse jurisdictions, to adequately assess. They aver that legal liability can discourage innovation or encourage overly pessimistic product warnings that result in patients not receiving products that could benefit them.[2] Invoking the stories recounted in Chapter 11 concerning medical product safety, conflict-of-interest movement critics have strongly lobbied in the medical literature against any such indemnification of product manufacturers by regulatory approval and have vehemently reasserted the social value of suing for damages in court.[3]

I am skeptical whether juries and judges wisely evaluate evidence regarding damages caused by medical products. Examples abound of flawed judgments resulting from such evaluations.[4] But as much as I disagree with the arguments conflict-of-interest movement promoters contribute to anti-industry tort and prosecutorial litigation, I concede allowing tort remedies for injured patients may be worthwhile. Judicial opinion has concurred, although some preemptive protection against litigation concerning FDA approved devices exists. This protection stems from *Riegel v. Medtronic,* wherein the Supreme Court set aside a New York State verdict concerning a defective coronary stent, ruling that Medical Device Amendment (MDA) to the Food, Drug and Cosmetic Act trumps state consumer-protection regulations in determining the safety of medical devices.[5] Reportedly, this preemption significantly reduced the number of tort cases against medical device manufacturers.[6]

Tort and criminal cases involving drugs, devices, and biological agents often go forward on the common law principle of strict liability for defective products, and if plaintiffs prevail, they receive compensation for damages. But litigants can go after bigger game by invoking failure-to-warn allegations, which carry punitive fines in addition to personal injury damages.

Recall that critics seized on a high failure rate of metal-on-metal hip implants described in Chapter 11 as evidence for the inadequacy of the FDA's 510(k) approval system based on device equivalence for ensuring safety. The recall of these devices evoked the predictable wave of litigation. The first jury trial concerning a device manufactured by Johnson & Johnson awarded damages on the basis of strict liability to a patient who suffered from such a failure. However, the jury did not rule that the company was sufficiently aware of the device's defects to be liable for the far larger punitive award that would have accompanied a failure-to-warn conviction.

Whereas failure-to-warn allegations concern actual damages, the following discussion describes the use of the conflict-of-interest narrative to persecute industry in a context where *no* demonstrable damages exist.

OFF-LABEL PRESCRIBING AND KICKBACK SETTLEMENTS AND CONVICTIONS

Companies can only *sell* products approved by the FDA for a specific indication and, with minor exceptions noted below, can only *promote* them for the approved uses. The promotional content must conform to the uses specified in the FDA label. However, physicians can, and frequently do, *prescribe* products for nonapproved uses.[7]

A prohibition against off-label promotion was enacted as a compromise through the 1962 Kefauver FDA Amendment between the most aggressive advocates for regulation who wanted the FDA to dictate physician prescribing and organized medicine's efforts to protect physician autonomy. The compromise was unsatisfactory because it embraced the fuzzy rhetorical arguments analyzed elsewhere in this book characterizing education as distinct from promotion and favored the assumption that in the absence of efficacy testing, industry claims for benefits of products were more often false than true.

The growth of off-label product prescribing by physicians combined with product manufacturers' superior knowledge about their products led the FDA in the mid-1990s to draft guidelines enabling companies to transmit truthful information to physicians concerning unapproved product uses. However, such communication is sharply constrained in ways that debatably do not assure conveyance of the best information. The guidelines allow manufacturers to provide physicians with copies of peer-reviewed medical journal articles describing off-label product uses in response to direct, unsolicited requests from physicians. The data in such journal articles cannot have originated from research sponsored by the product's manufacturer.[8] The FDA can address what it considers inappropriate off-label promotion by requesting companies to desist from this activity or even fining them. It can also try to convince federal or state prosecutors to litigate the companies.

Pro-regulation advocates opposed the promotional wiggle room afforded by these off-label promotional guidelines and demanded that the FDA exercise more restrictions on off-label marketing.[9] These demands appeared met when in 2004, the media reported that Pfizer settled a false claims prosecution alleging off-label promotion and paid a $430 million fine. Massachusetts-based federal prosecutors in 2001 had joined a former Parke-Davis (now part of Pfizer) employee named Franklin in bringing a mix of civil and criminal actions against the pharmaceutical company for making false claims concerning a drug named gabapentin (brand name Neurontin).[10] Since then, dozens of such prosecutions against most of the major pharmaceutical companies have resulted in some misdemeanor and guilty pleas, but all have eventually settled for billions of dollars in fines. In 2007, the prosecutors litigated companies manufacturing devices for orthopedic practice, alleging that payments to orthopedic surgeons represented kickbacks. Multiple device companies settled the cases and paid huge fines. Over and above the monetary penalties, the prosecutors inflicted corporate integrity agreements on the settling companies. These agreements stipulate elaborate compliance training, monitoring of corporate activities by the prosecutors, and public disclosure of all payments to physicians. Federal prosecutors have also extracted guilty pleas from individuals charged with off-label marketing. According to the conflict-of-interest movement narrative, these cases are the smoking guns for the fundamental venality of the medical product industry. The companies are, by definition, felons.[11] Critics, while conceding that some off-label promotion may be legal, consistently deem it overwhelmingly lacking in medical value.[12] They have weighed in prominently against industry in the prosecutions leading to the fines and legal restrictions on medical product companies.

The *Franklin* case was prosecuted under the federal False Claims Act, which dates back to the Civil War. The law was enacted to punish contractors that fraudulently charged the government for work they did not do. Currently, it is applied to prosecute physicians and hospitals that bill government payers, Medicare and Medicaid, for services they do not perform. From a legal standpoint, only physicians make claims, because only they can prescribe products. Because off-label prescribing is legal irrespective of whether a product approved for some indication has been proven to work in a different unapproved condition, no such claim, defined as a physician prescribing a product that Medicare or Medicaid then pays for, is strictly speaking, "false." A patient claiming a damaging side effect from a product prescribed off label, however, can sue the prescribing physician and use the lack of FDA approval of the product to strengthen a tort case. Conversely, however, cases exist in which physicians were sued for *failing* to prescribe off label when the prescribing was considered standard of care for a disease.

Because prescribing physicians, not the corporate defendants, are actually the ones who made the alleged false claims, the prosecutors must prove that industry promotional sales techniques led to the act of off-label prescribing. To make this case, the prosecutors invoke two tenets of the conflict-of-interest narrative. One, discussed in Chapter 12, is that even *on-label* promotion is misleading or false. The second, discussed in Chapter 13, is that physicians are cognitively incapable of resisting industry's clever and deceptive persuasion techniques.[13] The prosecutorial indictments liberally refer to gifts, payments (benefits), ghostwriting, KOLs, and other platitudes and epithets of the conflict-of-interest narrative.

That proving company sales reps *coerced* physicians to prescribe off label could be a viable court case is almost unimaginable. But such trials *never* materialize. The reason is that the government has a lethal weapon, should it, however improbably, win in court: a punishment imbedded in false claims law known as *debarment*. A company debarred as a result of being convicted of such banned off-label advertising cannot sell *any of its products* to the government (i.e., Medicare, Medicaid, State Children's Health Insurance Program [SCHIP], or the Veterans' Administration). This punishment is so economically severe that no company is ever willing to risk conviction. The prosecutors cram as many indictments as they can conjure up into these prosecutions to increase the risk that a jury will buy at least one. And it only takes one to impose the debarment penalty. As a result, the prosecutors always obtain settlements and marginal guilty pleas from which they extract huge fines. Merck's withdrawal of the drug Vioxx unleashed a legal feeding frenzy, yet the company won the majority of tort cases against it. However, when it came to a false claims prosecution, my presumption is that Merck settled the case because of the debarment risk, even though the evidence for intentional marketing misrepresentation was weak.

Unlike FDA enforcement, false claims cases can reward whistleblowers (also called relators) who file the civil actions—like Franklin in the Parke-Davis case—by awarding them a third of financial proceeds from the case (the legal term for this incentive is *qui tam*). In addition, upon settlement or conviction, false claims actions can arbitrarily triple fines estimated from amounts of alleged inappropriate sales (treble damages). The proceeds from such prosecutions can therefore be—and are—enormous. Some of this windfall from the civil cases goes to the lawyers specializing in dealing with whistleblowers, and these lawyers aggressively solicit them.

The *New York Times* coverage cited above exemplifies how the news media cover this legal activity, avoiding mention of its ambiguities and referring to it baldly as convictions for "health care fraud." But its treatment in medical journals is no better. One medical journal article, for example, declared the staggering fines insufficiently painful to the companies' bottom lines and called for directly fining company executives. It predicted that company behavior would deteriorate again as soon as the corporate integrity agreements expire. And the article, even though written by an attorney, failed to *mention* relators' profits.[14] Another medical journal article claimed, based on interviews with relators, that these individuals' motivations are dominantly altruistic and that their participation in the litigation was personally stressful. It did not consider the possibility that personal grievances unrelated to the cases might motivate relators and made no effort to compare the relators' litigation-related stress with everyday stresses endured by the general population. The take-home message implied by the article was that greater rewards and less personal strain should accompany whistleblower activity.[15] Both articles defined the settlements as straightforward "health care fraud." Neither alluded to the underlying debarment threat nor the exoneration at trial documented below of indicted individuals—none of whom receive whistleblower spoils or compensation for legal costs. Their life stresses are certainly as great or greater than those of the opposing relators. None of the many media or medical journal articles' discussions of the false claims prosecutions ever mentioned the *possibility* that they incur opportunity costs.

Yet this legal activity is arguably the most damaging aspect of the conflict-of-interest movement. The settlements and corporate integrity agreements extorted by these prosecutions have arguably caused significant industry retrenchment recounted in the next chapter in payments to physicians for product research and development relationships. They have compromised physician education and, most importantly, diverted resources from research and development to legal compliance. With billions of dollars in fines at stake, companies now go overboard to ensure that gifts to physicians, previously construed as merely tacky, do not now result in bribery charges with gargantuan price tags.[16]

Off-label promotion false claims cases often concern treatments for difficult medical conditions with limited treatment options. As mentioned above, nerve pain is a prime example germane to much of the off-label prescribing in the *Franklin* case. Nerve pain is a condition for which primary care physicians mostly prescribe off-label medications,[17] and, ironically, the FDA subsequently approved one of the off-label uses (nerve pain after shingles infections) that Parke-Davis allegedly illegally promoted.

Although many legal scholars have criticized the FDA's information conveying restrictions in general and their application to false claims prosecutions in particular, the fact that all the cases settle means that the legal actions have not been subject to judicial review.[18]

Companies ensnared in these prosecutions have sometimes pushed the promotional envelope too far, for example, marketing a sedative not approved for use in children to pediatricians.[19] On the other hand, many allegations, for example, concerning the promotion of an inhaled drug for asthma patients, are more ambiguous. The FDA approved such a drug for severe asthma. The prosecutors claimed that a company promoted it for use in patients with mild or moderate asthma. Unfortunately, the rigorous criteria used to assess asthma severity in clinical trials are too time consuming and complex to be employed in routine clinical practice.

Related to the foregoing discussion and belying the conclusion that the settlements are straightforward proxies for deliberate industry misbehavior is the fact that individual company employees indicted in some of these false claims suits have defended themselves, because the debarment penalty is not a death sentence for them and they wanted to protect their reputations. They have, in such cases, won at trial or on appeal.[20]

Even the Massachusetts prosecutor who originated the false claims strategy against off-label prescribing, who now defends targeted companies, has publicly admitted that the settled false claims prosecutions do not represent punishment for any proven damages.[21] In addition, he has criticized the fact that these cases involve allegations of activities that took place in the remote past and languish for years in sealed indictments that the defendant companies cannot see.[22] Presumably the delay adds to the spoils, because the longer off-label sales go on, the greater the fines and penalties that accrue to the prosecutors, other lawyers, and whistleblowers. Furthermore, defense lawyers gag defendants from reacting to accusations leaked to the press, preventing a balanced public discussion.

STATES AND INSURANCE COMPANIES BELLY UP TO THE FEEDING TROUGH

The success of false claims litigation in extracting large fines has encouraged states and private insurers to use discovery material from the federal false claims cases to pursue similar litigation, with mixed success. Under the aegis of consumer protection laws, state prosecutors have accused companies of false and misleading advertising. For example, the Louisiana attorney general sued the Janssen Pharmaceutical Company, a subsidiary of Johnson and Johnson, for claiming that its antipsychotic drug Risperidal had fewer metabolic side effects than its competitors, a claim the FDA challenged in letters to the company. In October 2010, a jury fined Janssen $275 million, based on statutorily stipulated fines for 35,542 alleged individual marketing violations. The companies appealed the fines, but in August 2012, a state appellate court upheld the verdict. In doing so, it rejected Janssen's arguments that it had compelling scientific evidence to support its claims.[23] But in January 2014, the Louisiana Supreme Court reversed the decision, ruling that the prosecution's use of FDA letters alone did not constitute valid evidence for misleading marketing.

A FOOT IN THE DOOR? RECENT LEGAL CHALLENGES TO THE PROHIBITION OF OFF-LABEL MARKETING

The murky nature of appropriate branding comes up against the First Amendment right to free speech. If a company employee or physician believes, based on available evidence, that a product is appropriate for a nonapproved use, the First Amendment arguably permits truthful expression of such opinions. On this basis, two recent legal cases represent the first potential challenges to the prosecutorial extortion activity against off-label promotion. In one, the U.S. Supreme Court in June 2011 overturned a Vermont law prohibiting selling "data-mining" results to patent-protected drug makers. Data mining facilitates companies' access to physicians' prescribing records and helps them identify physicians most likely to use their products. Information processing companies like IMS Health, which brought the suit challenging the Vermont Law, buy information from pharmacies about what prescriptions were filled at that location along with the prescribing physician. Drug companies in turn purchase this information scrubbed of patients' identities to determine which physicians will be most interested in a particular product. The AMA sells physicians' identities to the data-mining companies.[24] The practice allows the companies to economize marketing costs by avoiding wasteful effort on physicians with little interest in their product. Data mining has the potential to particularly benefit small companies with modest detailing resources.

Data-mining companies had sued Vermont in federal court for violating their First Amendment right to free commercial speech guaranteed under the Fourteenth Amendment. The courts have distinguished commercial speech from other forms of discourse such as political communication, giving more latitude to the latter than to the former. But for the government to suppress commercial speech, one of four elements must be present: (1) the messages are untruthful or misleading, (2) the messages concern illegal activities, (3) the government can convincingly prove that the messages undermine the public interest, and (4) suppression of speech is the only mechanism for preventing the undermining effect.

The data-mining companies lost at trial but prevailed on appeal, whereupon Vermont petitioned the U.S. Supreme Court for review. Vermont argued it could suppress information the data-mining companies sell their customers in the interest of maintaining medical privacy and protecting physicians from commercial harassment. Invoking the conflict-of-interest narrative, Vermont claimed that banning data mining improved public health by deterring sales of allegedly unsafe and unnecessarily expensive drugs. The Supreme Court by a 6 to 3 majority upheld the legality of data mining based on free commercial speech considerations, citing that restriction of such speech should be a last resort and not accommodate government paternalism. [25]

Applying similar logic to a case more directly relevant to the misbranding issue, two of three justices of the U.S. Court of Appeals of the Second Circuit reversed a 2008 jury trial conviction of Alfred Caronia, a marketing employee of the Orphan Drug Company (now named Jazz Pharmaceuticals) for promoting Xyrem, a drug approved only for the treatment of narcolepsy (involuntarily falling asleep during the day), for insomnia and other disorders for which it was not approved. [26] In addition to the free speech issues raised by the *Sorrell v. IMS Health* case discussed above, the justices indicated that the FDA could use other mechanisms to regulate off-label product usage, and therefore, restricting commercial speech could not be justified as the only regulatory option.

The dissenting Supreme Court minority in the *Sorrell* case argued primarily on the basis of legal precedents. These concerned what commercial speech the government may legitimately regulate. But it also invoked conflict-of-interest movement narrative elements excerpted from briefs submitted by conflict-of-interest movement promoters in agreeing with the trial court that: [27]

> [s]haping a detailing message based on an individual doctor's prior prescription habits may help sell more of a particular manufacturer's particular drugs. But it does so by diverting attention from scientific research about a drug's safety and effectiveness, as well as its cost. This diversion comes at the expense of public health and the State's fiscal interest.

More physician-specific detailing will lead to more prescriptions of brand-name agents, often with no additional patient benefit but at much higher cost to patients and to state-based insurance programs, which will continue to drive up the cost of health care.

These and other statements in the dissent represent false conclusions and non sequitor logic. First, detailing messages statutorily *must* include "scientific research about a drug's safety and effectiveness." Second, this requirement is true irrespective of whether detailing messages are "tailored to an individual doctor's prescribing habits."

The dissenting *Caronia* judge also argued on the basis of legalistic issues regarding proper jury instructions and concepts of intentionality that the majority had invoked to set the conviction aside. But she also inappropriately likened Xyrem to patent medicines, arsenic, and saw palmetto extract, none of which have been approved for *any* use. Moreover, the dissenting judge stated:[28]

Congress intended the FDA approval process to prevent dangerous products with false or misleading labels from entering the market, and also to provide a base of reliable, objective information about prescription drugs that could help physicians and patients identify potentially misleading claims.

But Caronia's conviction concerned nonapproved, not "misleading and unsubstantiated" claims. The dissenting justice also cited a medical journal article claiming that 73% of off-label drug prescribing—comprising 21% of prescriptions written by office-based physicians—has "little or no scientific support."[29] Other chapters have discussed in detail how scientific support is often tenuous in medicine, and the cited paper's basis for scientific support was a commercial database used by insurers for reimbursement.[30]

The *Sorrell* and *Caronia* decisions are potentially encouraging to companies who would like to see the heavy-handed prohibitions against off-label promotion and the predatory legal opportunism it encourages curtailed. However, the successful intrusion of conflict-of-interest movement ideology into these judicial decisions and the prevalence of judges—or, for that matter—legislators predisposed to such ideology mitigate such optimism. In stark contrast to predominant legal scholarship cited above, the medical literature, accommodated and contributed to by its conflict-of-interest movement–friendly editors, consistently agitates against any moderation of off-label marketing restrictions.[31]

WHERE DO WE GO FROM HERE? BACK TO THE FUTURE

Rampant unregulated physician and health center advertising discussed in Chapter 12 is only one example of inconsistencies in medical information control. In contrast to the close oversight by the FDA over promotion of approved products and the strict limitation of off-label product marketing is the relatively lax treatment of the $20 billion-plus nutraceutical industry selling natural foods, food supplements, vitamins, and natural products claiming to have health benefits.[32] Disclaiming FDA approval and meeting the criterion of being "generally recognized as safe" enable promoters of these commodities to enjoy relatively unrestricted license to advertise them.[33] Nutraceutical advertising is directed at consumers, many of whom are ill equipped to evaluate the claims. Therefore, judicial reluctance to permit companies informing educated and trained professionals about medical products is hard to understand. But, paradoxically, what freely promoted physician and hospital services, nutraceuticals, and the unapproved product uses have in common is a lack of evidence that they cause damages of sufficient frequency or intensity to represent a clear and present danger.[34]

A relaxation of off-label promotion prohibitions could put an end to the parasitic legal false claims crusade and its diversionary costs, but it could have adverse consequences as well. Having repeatedly declared that FDA assessments of product efficacy and safety are the best analytical game in town, I am not in favor of companies resorting to off-label promotion to avoid mounting the clinical studies that currently lead to an FDA-approved label.

The extensive legal scholarship concerning off-label marketing referenced above has suggested other options that Congress and the FDA could mandate to encourage companies to perform the clinical trials leading to FDA approvals. These options include requiring such trials when off-label sales reach a certain volume or providing tax credits or longer sales exclusivity intervals for products subjected to formal approval. The FDA has resisted these ideas based on the argument that they are difficult to put into practice, especially those requiring monitoring company sales or prescribing information. However, devoting resources for the FDA to analyze product sales, likely through a prescription tracking service such as that offered by IMS Health, seems far more useful and cost effective than—as discussed in the next chapter—forcing companies to disclose $10 payments to physicians. Fortunately, evaluating the viability of alternative regulations is beyond the scope of this book. Any productive discussion of alternative regulations must include influential stakeholders who actually understand the myriad details of product development. Critics obsessed with conflicts of interest should be welcome to weigh in, but their views should be considered in light of their credibility, and deliberations should focus on getting the right products to patients that need them.

IV

The Damage They Do, and How to Stop It

15

THE PRICE WE PAY

Previous chapters documented how the conflict-of-interest movement has led to ubiquitous and intrusive policies mandating disclosing, managing, and restricting remunerated relationships between physicians, medical academics, and industry. I have argued that the policies are not based on factual evidence or sound logic. Ultimately, however, what really matters is whether and how these policies affect patient care, medical education, and medical innovation. I have argued that the conflict-of-interest movement's claims that its regulations can lead to more appropriate medical care, more efficient medical innovation, and better medical education—all at lower cost—are rooted in speculation and misrepresentation. Moreover, the conflict-of-interest movement either ignores the expense of its effects or considers them worth the price.

The aging population's need for medical attention, yearning for longer and better survival and for prevention of and cures for dreaded diseases and the energy and creativity of medical entrepreneurship ensure that progress will continue in spite of all the obstacles raised by conflict-of-interest legislation. And one cannot predict accurately what is *not* going to happen.

However, I do believe that one can make a strong case that the conflict-of-interest regulations *slow* medical progress. For patients like Grace and Patrick, timing is everything. In both cases the drugs that saved their lives had only been available for a matter of months. Even if lifesaving drugs and devices are available, unless physicians are aware of them and know how to use them properly, patients do not benefit. Chapters 8 and 9 described how unpredictable failures delay medical innovation and increase its costs, concluding that no easy remedy exists to accelerate innovation. Chapters 12 and 13 reviewed the difficulties associated with physician education. If conflict-of-interest regulation exacerbates the expense of innovation and its dissemination, it is hardly beneficial.

This chapter first summarizes evidence that conflict-of-interest regulation slows medical innovation and compromises medical education. It then reviews the emergence of the conflict-of-interest movement's obsession with mandated transparency. It explains how this obsession is self-serving and has underappreciated costs, principally the leaching of resources from medical product research and development into compliance activities. Finally, the chapter proposes that the conflict-of-interest movement's worst legacy may be the promotion of intellectual dishonesty. By taking superficial analyses conducted by conflict-of-interest promoters at face value, the medical establishment undermines its commitment to the rigorous pursuit of truth. Perhaps worst of all, the narrative has made it acceptable to dismiss scientific research solely on the basis of who funded or conducted it rather than on the merits of the research itself.

COSTS OF CONFLICT-OF-INTEREST REGULATIONS TO MEDICAL INNOVATION

Investors have told me that they would not start companies based on technologies invented by Harvard Medical School faculty because Harvard does not permit its faculty members to hold equity (stock) in a company that sponsors their research. Based on these anecdotes, between March and April 2007, I mounted a survey in collaboration with a British team based at Cambridge University. We used an on-line questionnaire of 4,813 university technology transfer managers and faculty researchers based at the 50 American research institutions responsible with the most patents issue and technology licensed and the highest commercial royalties. The questionnaire asked respondents with technology transfer experience to estimate the extent to which conflict-of-interest issues had affected the licensing of academic technology to companies, corporate-sponsored laboratory or clinical research, or the establishment of start-up companies based on academic inventions. Respondents were also invited to provide specific comments.

The 118 technology officials and 457 faculty researchers who responded to the questionnaire reported that conflict-of-interest concerns had complicated or prevented some of the aforementioned activities over the previous five years, especially company-sponsored clinical research projects and company start-ups. Of 320 respondents who had been involved in licensing discussions, 121 (41%) reported that conflict-of-interest regulations had prevented or complicated one or more of the licensing agreements, and of these, 56 (18%), specified that these issues prevented at least one licensing agreement.

Of 302 respondents involved in negotiating or performing corporate-sponsored laboratory work, 29% indicated that conflict-of-interest concerns had prevented or complicated this activity, with 16% reporting that such issues had prevented sponsorship on at least one occasion. The respondents reported involvement in 3,320 laboratory research agreements over the past five years. Of these arrangements, 77% were not problematic, 3% were prevented, and 21% complicated by conflict-of-interest issues.

In terms of start-up companies, 34% of the responding survey population had participated in attempts to initiate such a company over the past five years, and 63% of those had done so in the last year. Nearly half of the respondents (47%) reported that conflict-of-interest issues prevented or complicated start-up activities, with 14% reporting conflict-of-interest issues as preventing the establishment of at least one company. The respondents reported being involved in 966 company start-up arrangements. Of these 3% had been prevented and 33% complicated by conflict-of-interest issues.

The major reasons reported for the complication or prevention of all these activities were faculty ownership in companies (stock or stock options) or faculty receipt of more than permitted corporate consulting fees in excess of the limits mandated by conflict-of-interest regulations. Respondents articulated being offended by overly zealous conflict-of-interest policy managers who resorted to speculation that payments to researchers were too high and would compromise research integrity or who stepped in to renegotiate previously accepted research contracts.

To our knowledge, this study was the first to ask whether such regulations might have adverse consequences. By definition, delays to eliminate or manage conflicts of interest in technology licensing, corporate-sponsored research, or company start-ups by definition slow the pace of innovation. The documented prevention of technology licensing, corporate research sponsorship, and company start-ups by conflict-of-interest issues is a more definite adverse consequence. Although we did not determine whether scuttled arrangements eventually came to fruition, considering the difficulties in obtaining private investment, it is likely that if any did, long delays would have been encountered.

As mentioned in Chapter 7, participation in industry consulting by NIH intramural researchers has halved since the imposition of a ban on paid consulting in 2005, and the number of material and intellectual property license transfers from NIH to companies fell since 2005. Surveys of academic faculty documented a small but steady decline in the faculty in academic medical institutions receiving research support, serving as consultants and filing patents between 1995 and 2006.[1] Data from the Association of University Technology Managers reveals that the amount of intellectual property licensing from academe to industry has been constant since 2005 after having risen steadily in previous years,[2] but many factors, most importantly the state of the economy, bear on this statistic, and whether regulations have directly affected this activity or the paid relationship data reported above is unknown.[3]

Based on information deposited in websites created by device companies in response to Department of Justice settlements described in the previous chapter, payments from device companies to orthopedic surgeons declined 44% in the three years following the settlements. Because royalty payments from these companies to surgeon inventors presumably were unaffected by the settlements, the declines could reflect diminished ongoing research relationships between orthopedic surgeons and device companies.[4] Conflict-of-interest movement promoters see this decline as salutary, reflecting a decrease in what they claim is bribery masked as bogus consulting. But the same statistics reveal that only 4% of American orthopedic surgeons received corporate funding, belying the notion that such payments truly represented rampant bribery efforts by device companies. Orthopedic surgeons are the highest paid medical specialists, and they can make plenty of money doing surgical procedures. Plausibly, therefore, reduced industry payments quickly arrive at a tipping point at which such surgeons lose interest in participating in device innovation and shift their efforts simply to performing surgery.

Of nine pharmaceutical companies publicly disclosing payments to physicians, seven reported decreases averaging 25% between 2011 and

2012.[5] In Massachusetts, where the 2009 "gift ban law" has required reporting of physician payments since 2010, payments fell by 14% between 2010 and 2012; payments from the top 20 companies declined by 29% over that interval. Payments to the state's top 50 hospitals have fallen by an average of 36% during that period.[6] Because the preponderance of reported payments were for "bona fide research," [7] arguably industry support of clinical research at hospitals has been markedly reduced.

Academic authorities have justified imposing strict conflict-of-interest regulation as a means to ensure the flow of research funding from the NIH to universities.[8] They argue that erosion of the public's and politicians' trust in the integrity of NIH-funded academic research due to conflicts of interest—or the *perception* of conflicts of interest—would diminish congressional appropriations to the NIH. But in the years that conflict-of-interest regulations have stiffened, including those of the NIH itself, such subsidy has remained flat and, in fact, fallen substantially in inflation-adjusted terms.[9] No evidence indicates that conflict-of-interest concerns have affected NIH appropriations or that they would be worse without stricter regulations.

What is clear is that conflict-of-interest rules have increased regulatory compliance costs, although precise dollar amounts are not known. Until recently, my employer, Partners Healthcare, handled industry relationship issues such as patent filing, intellectual property licensing, and industry-sponsored research through the technology transfer offices of its constituent hospitals. Separate bureaucracies handled the contractual aspects of industry-sponsored clinical trials, oversight of research on human subjects, the humane treatment of animals in research, and management of nonindustry research grants and contracts. With more conflict-of-interest rules, my employer created a new Office of Industry Interactions, managed by an augmented staff of attorneys and their ancillaries, to provide compliance education, manage the increasingly frequent and detailed disclosure requirements concerning industry relationships, and respond to the reporting requirements of agencies such as NIH concerning how the institution addresses its employees' "significant financial conflicts of interest."

COSTS OF CONFLICT-OF-INTEREST REGULATIONS TO MEDICAL EDUCATION

Commercial sponsorship of continuing medical education (CME) has decreased by around 30% since a peak in 2006, when half of CME events had corporate subsidy. By 2011, only 21% of CME activities had such subsidies. This reduction in industry funding has been paralleled by a decline in the total volume of CME activities of comparable magnitude. [10] Specifically, industry contributions fell by $94 million, the number of CME providers dropped from 736 in 2002 to 687, and 72,000 fewer physicians attended CME courses. Industry sources of support for educational activities of professional societies and medical schools decreased by 3.5% and 4% respectively in 2011. The onset of the decline in industry support of CME preceded the economic recession by two years and has been constant, suggesting that the state of the overall economy is not the sole or even a major reason for it. Almost certainly these diminutions in corporate subsidy are a result of the off-label and bribery prosecutions and resulting corporate integrity agreements described in the previous chapter. They have arguably made companies very wary of making contributions that prosecutors could use as evidence of influencing physician prescribing.

Payments to physicians from some large medical product companies for peer-to-peer speaking have also declined by nearly half. [11] To some extent these reductions are a result of companies ceasing replacements. The same situation has driven sales force reductions. The layoffs obligatorily reduce the frequency of interactions between physicians and medical product company representatives.

HOW THE CONFLICT-OF-INTEREST MOVEMENT'S MASS CONFESSION MANDATE DOES MORE HARM THAN GOOD

The Conflict-of-Interest Movement's Industry Payment Disclosure Circus

Once biomedical journals and academic institutions required disclosure of industry relationships by authors and faculty, compliance became an issue. One problem is that the purposes of such disclosure vary, depending on the circumstances. For example, Harvard Medical School mainly collected information to document that researchers did not have both equity and sponsored research funding from the same company above stipulated minimum amounts. Another common purpose of university disclosure was to monitor and, if necessary, prevent investigators with financial interests in a product under development from participating in patient trials of that product. Most journals, with the exception of *The New England Journal of Medicine*, which used disclosures to determine eligibility to author review articles and editorials, simply stuck the disclosed information at the ends of articles, ostensibly to let readers, caveat emptor, decide whether it affected their assessments of the validity of research findings or opinions reported. Because in all these cases the disclosure was voluntary, no information was available as to its completeness or accuracy.

In 1996, *The New England Journal of Medicine* published an editorial affirming the necessity to exclude editorialists with industry ties, bemoaning the woeful state of academic medical research that now harbored so many conflicted participants and critical of the authors for having failed to recuse themselves from editorializing.[12] Similarly, *JAMA* editors demanded written apologies from article authors after whistleblowers reported that these authors had omitted industry relationships in their disclosure statements associated with those articles.[13]

Around that time, Iowa Senator Charles Grassley escalated the public profile of allegations regarding physicians' industry payment disclosure lapses. The NIH had ruled in 1996 that grant recipients must report to their institutions all company payments greater than $10,000 per year. Using the power of Congress, Grassley subpoenaed companies and universities for payment records, and in a dozen or so cases, claimed to have identified large discrepancies.

Most findings of universities investigating Senator Grassley's claims of differences between industry payments medical school faculty members disclosed and what industry reported having paid those individuals have not been made public. However, the university disclosure requirements required faculty to report only consulting or speaking fees or royalties. The payments that showed up in Grassley's inquiries may have included many additional payments, such as clinical trial expenses and the travel of investigators to meetings for consulting.

The striking paucity of straightforward adverse incidents or substantive problems ascribable to industry relationships with physicians and medical academics explains why the critics have harped on researchers' and physicians' more prevalent alleged failures to disclose payments from companies. Such negligence, whether deliberate or inadvertent, often resulted from confusion as to what constitutes a *relevant* industry relationship.[14] For example, critics complained that device surgeons did not disclose in published medical journal articles large payments received from companies.[15] But the impressive sums in the reports represented royalty payments for inventions made in the remote past. These inventions preceded by long time intervals the current publications and had no relationship to the surgeons' current research described in the publications.

Neither Grassley nor anyone else has unearthed *any* damages from them other than the adverse publicity that the conflict-of-interest narrative itself generates. Be that as it may, disclosure has morphed into a grotesque caricature known as the Physician Payments Sunshine Act (Sunshine Act). Relevance is no longer an issue: *everything* must be disclosed, and the inquisitors will decide upon relevance.

The Physician Payments Sunshine Act

This final rule will require applicable manufacturers of drugs, devices, biologicals, or medical supplies covered by Medicare, Medicaid or the Children's Health Insurance Program (CHIP) to report annually to the Secretary certain payments or transfers of value provided to physicians or teaching hospitals ("covered recipients"). In addition, applicable manufacturers and applicable group purchasing organizations (GPOs) are required to report annually certain physician ownership or investment interests. The Secretary is required to publish applicable manufacturers' and applicable GPOs' submitted payment and ownership information on a public website.[16]

With passage of this law as part of health reform,[17] the Centers for Medicare and Medicaid Services (CMS) released lengthy draft guidelines in December 2011 as to how it planned to implement it. The cutoff for payment reporting was $500 when the rule was first proposed, but in the final version had dropped to $10—"applicable manufacturers and GPOs" must keep track of payments equal to or greater than $10 and report them when the aggregate value exceeds $100. In other words, from a practical standpoint, *all* payments are covered. The $10 figure symbolizes how effectively the conflict-of-interest narrative has sold the gift smoke screen discussed in Chapter 13. We have nationalized the fiction that even small gifts cloud medical judgment.

Extensive comments submitted to CMS concerning the draft guidelines brought out just how complicated and expensive tracking small payments of money and kind was going to be. As a result of these complications, the law's implementation was delayed. The final rule totaling nearly 300 pages and containing responses to comments submitted concerning the earlier draft appeared in February 2013. The final rule required applicable entities to start collecting payment data in August 2013 and report it to CMS by the end of March 2014. Failure to comply with the rule or submission of inaccurate reports carries fines of $10,000 to 100,000 per instance with total fines being capped at $1 million. The law preempts similar payment-reporting requirements imposed by the states described above.

The Clay Feet of Mandated Transparency

The fact that information is often useful for decision making is what gives superficial plausibility to the Sunshine Act's logic and the virtues of transparency. However, the case for it abruptly ends there. First, the reality is that far too much information exists for us to process and that overload problem is why we pick and choose what's out there, ideally focusing on what our experience, training, and interests warrant. Very few people and especially patients come even close to having the experience or training to comprehend the minute and complex information that will accumulate from the Sunshine Act legislation. Even if they did, the best survey data indicate that patients have few concerns about physicians' industry relationships. The information will be useless for patients. Because it lacks sufficient context, the purpose of payments will be indecipherable. More importantly, the last question anyone should ask her or his physicians is who pays them. The physicians' training, track record, and user friendliness are far more important.

Second, although nowadays we wallow in a lot of useless information, most of it is inexpensively acquired and easily ignored. A prime example is the dense legal gibberish that we must agree to when we download software for our computers. Most of us never read it; we simply scroll down to the "agree" button and click. A software company hid a message in one of these contracts that stated if one clicked on a link, the reader would receive a $1,000 reward. It took months and thousands of downloads before someone took the bait.[18] In contrast to the hundreds of millions of dollars diverted from more productive uses year after year by the Sunshine Act, the costs of most gratuitous information efforts, like the software terms of use cited above, are minimal. Some lawyer simply writes the material for uploading, and it takes only a few seconds for the consumer to ignore it and move on.

Third, the calls for transparency are selective. Medical journal editors, academic administrators, conflict-of-interest movement careerists, and the managers of funding organizations of the conflict-of-interest movement do not seem to be rushing forward to advertise their incomes.

Finally, the most destructive aspect of the Sunshine Act is its false premise that all information is useful and good. Chapter 5 presented the evidence for rejecting the conceit that all medical problems are resolvable by allowing analysts to peruse all available information about them. The fact is that information can serve good or bad purposes. The good outcome the Sunshine Act advocates claim, that transparency will contain medical care costs, is based on the absolutely unproven and arguably false premise that industry payments to physicians drive overprescribing of unnecessary and overly expensive brand products. Products constitute a minor fraction of health care spending. As discussed below, the compliance expenses associated with the Sunshine Act's disclosure will increase medical costs—and will be passed on to insurers—and patients.

Private and proprietary information is important. Success in competition depends on not having all information instantly—or sometimes ever—made public. We cannot predict in advance what transfers of value will ultimately result in success or failure defined in terms of medical progress, and innovators need time to sort out and analyze the information they acquire before inviting others to weigh in. And, finally, enforced transparency has clearly documented dangers. The track record of surveillance exercised by political regimes—that enabled the powerful to promote personal and political agendas—ought to give us pause before embracing wholesale exposure of private information.[19]

Who Really Benefits from Mandated Disclosure?

According to the CMS Sunshine Rule:[20]

> We plan to establish mechanisms for researchers who may want information that is not publicly available. We believe that the data included in the database is primarily for consumers, but understand that it also provides numerous opportunities for research on provider-industry relationships.

The record of how payment data have previously been exploited contradicts the claim that "research on this information is an important benefit." In an effort to preempt the impending Sunshine Act or else comply with conditions of prosecution settlements, medical product companies began to report payments to physicians on publicly accessible websites. This move amplified the population of conflict-of-interest movement promoters who, even without Senator Grassley's subpoena power, could build their careers by getting into the business of trolling for industry payment recipients who supposedly failed to acknowledge such payments.[21]

One example is a media outlet named ProPublica, billed as an "independent, non-profit newsroom" to undertake "investigative journalism in the public interest."[22] In 2011, ProPublica published a compilation of payments to physicians by major pharmaceutical companies for research relationships, consulting, or peer-to-peer speaking. ProPublica cross-referenced the industry payment data with state medical board reports listing physicians who had been reprimanded for various infractions ("Docs on pharma payroll have blemished records, limited credentials").[23] This juxtaposition encouraged stories such as an NPR's "Drug companies hire troubled docs as experts" and a *Boston Globe* item, "Doctors with questionable records earn a lot as drug firms' speakers." ProPublica reported that 250 physicians were reprimanded—out of 17,700 who received industry payments, which comes to 2.1% after correcting for errors in their methodology.[24] In contrast, national statistics reveal a 6.8% prevalence between 2001 and 2011 of disciplinary actions concerning physicians in general[25] compared to the figure reported by ProPublica—a *threefold* difference. Remuneration from industry seems to be a pretty good screen for physician integrity!

The Financial Cost of Mandated Transparency

In its final rule for implementation of the Physician Payments Sunshine Act, CMS estimated that the costs of enactment of the statute in its first year would come to $269 million and that subsequent implementation would cost $183 million annually.[26] Underlying these estimates were many assumptions and omissions of likely additional requirements that will render these guesses far lower than practice will reveal. The assumptions included arbitrary estimates of the number of companies and other commercial entities subject to reporting and of the quantity of physicians, hospitals, and other potential industry payment recipients who will need to keep records. Most importantly, however, the estimates primarily cover salary expenses for clerical employees of payers who compile the data and report it to the government and of payees who check it for accuracy. Missing from the cost consideration was the time spent by company marketing representatives to record what they spend on which physicians. In addition, a collateral industry populated with lawyers and accountants is emerging to provide education, which must be paid for, to the numerous stakeholders affected by the Sunshine Act.[27] Taking these activities into account arguably doubles the annual CMS cost estimate to over $400 million.[28]

Also missing from the CMS estimate are legal expenses. Anyone reading the final report and its elaboration of detailed provisions and responses to comments will be struck by its extensive eye-glazing minutiae. A partial list of such content, in addition to detailed catalogs of types of payments, includes definitions of a "covered entity," of whether a global company has a sufficient U.S. presence to have to report, of the tipping point for exclusion of entities with less than 10% of their business being manufacturing or less than 5% involved in common ownership with other entities, how to estimate device-related payments bundled into hospital charges, how to deal with parsing out individual payments within consolidated reports, and how to determine whether research payments satisfy criteria for a four-year reporting delay because of competitive considerations. Several pages deal with the small details as to how to calculate food provided to physicians. Considerable legal input will be required to navigate these morasses, and the default will be to report more rather than less or avoid the hassle by ceasing payments altogether.

The regulation does preempt state industry-to-physician payment reporting requirements, but it does not invalidate state bans on such payments, and these will continue to require enforcement with concomitant costs. Most importantly, the estimates do not take into account the opportunity costs of diverting resources from research, development, and education to compliance activities. Even the probably low-ball CMS annual compliance cost estimate of $183 million is a sum that would underwrite six of the Phase II proof-of-concept trials for which my company, BioAegis Therapeutics, is trying to raise funds. Once again, smaller companies will suffer disproportionately. One prediction I will venture to make is that in response to the Sunshine Act, companies will increasingly go abroad for research collaborations with physicians. This maneuver will save them reporting costs. But it will also compromise American research centers and deprive American inventors of innovation opportunities.

INTELLECTUAL DISHONESTY

The conflict-of-interest movement has occupied over a quarter of the century during which the medical-industry interface has existed. This time interval presents a more than adequate historical frame to accommodate reasonable conclusions regarding the risks and benefits of those activities. This book has attempted to prove that the predominance of evidence supports that benefits far outstrip risks.

By contrast, the exposure of medical students, medical practitioners, and medical academics to the risk-emphasizing propaganda of the conflict-of-interest narrative qualifies as what the philosopher J. S. Mill characterized as "the tyranny of the prevailing opinion and feeling."[29] This tyranny obstructs rigorous thinking and experimental precision that can resolve uncertainty. The numerous declarations cited in previous chapters make a caricature out of the confident notion that medical opinion and medical practice are evidence based. Perhaps nothing more clearly epitomizes the legacy of such misinformation than the economically illiterate arguments described in Chapter 9 put forth by medically credible and well-meaning physicians for reducing cancer drug prices to levels less unappealing to their emotional taste. If the arguments are heeded, large profitable companies may survive, but struggling start-up enterprises may not.

COSTS OF CONFLICT-OF-INTEREST REGULATIONS: CONCLUSIONS

Unless one is in complete denial, the expense and difficulties of developing new products that benefit patients are crystal clear, as are the equally daunting difficulties and costs of ensuring that physicians receive education that equips them to provide optimal clinical care. How to mitigate these difficulties is uncertain. But maneuvers that erect barriers to innovation and education are unacceptable. If we want biomedical innovation to succeed and medical education to be effective, we must remove barriers to cooperation, not impose them. I propose that the case for serious opportunities wasted is more plausible and empirically supported than the one claiming benefits from conflict-of-interest regulation.

Those with the most to lose are patients with unmet medical needs. A consistent feature of the stories behind lifesaving and life-enhancing products, some recounted in this book, is how tenuous their prospects for success were. The ups and downs of the company Alexion that finally produced eculizumab that helped rescue my patient Grace from her HUS and the unpredictable course of events that led to the availability of imatinib that saved Patrick's life exemplify that fragility. Grace and Patrick were lucky enough to have become ill shortly after these products became available. Many others whose afflictions occurred earlier were not so fortunate. Many sufferers, particularly cancer patients, pray in hope of timely lifesaving discoveries. They should be appalled to realize that abstract ethical speculation, economic inanity, academic and legal careerism, and vested administrative interests are making it harder to develop the next generation of lifesaving products.

16

WHAT IS TO BE DONE?

This book summarized the errors and costs of the conflict-of-interest movement. Its premise is that the movement should be stopped and most of its regulations retracted. Before presenting ideas as to how this goal might be accomplished, however, I summarize what *hasn't* worked.

THE "RODNEY DANGERFIELD" SYNDROME

Lately, I have taken to asking people the following question: "I've been involved in medicine for nearly 50 years. Do you think health care is better, worse, or the same as when I started out?"

Despite the fact that the right answer is unequivocally "better," people hesitate. The responses average, "Well, I guess it's better," but a few people emphatically answer, "Worse!"

I follow up on the former responses with, "Why do you think that is?"

Again, most people hesitate.

So, I continue, "Do you think it's because of doctors, hospitals, the government, or medical schools?"

"All of those, I suppose."

"Did I leave anything out?"

Silence.

"What about industry?"

Answers range from, "Well, perhaps it does contribute some technology," to, "Don't even get me started about pharma!"

To paraphrase comedian Rodney Dangerfield (1921–2004), why is the medical products industry faced with a situation where "I[t] don't get no respect"?[1] Only a deeply disrespected industry could find itself saddled with regulations requiring that it publicly report $10 payments to its collaborators. Unfortunately, as reviewed below, the medical product industry deserves much of the blame for its predicament.

HOW THE MEDICAL PRODUCT INDUSTRY AND ITS ALLIES HAVE FAILED TO RESIST THE CONFLICT-OF-INTEREST MOVEMENT

A surefire formula for garnering disrespect is to passively accept spurious accusations of wrongdoing while allowing others to take credit for your achievements. Recall that Chapter 4 explained how medical journals historically enabled researchers to obtain credit for their accomplishments. Ironically, as also documented in that chapter, the journals now take credit from researchers in general and industry in particular.

When I first started writing and speaking about the errors, intellectual dishonesty, and potential damage of the conflict-of-interest movement in 2005, I naively assumed industry and its trade associations would welcome my efforts with open arms. I was wrong.

At that time, the conflict-of-interest movement was about 15 years old and mainly concerned with regulating research relationships. Otherwise, it principally focused on academic researchers for failing to disclose their industry relationships in journal articles or public presentations. While mildly embarrassing to the attacked academics, it had no immediate effect on the medical products industry per se. Rules prohibiting equity in a company from which an academic researcher received sponsored research or vice versa, or precluding inventors or their institutions from participating in clinical trials affected few academic researchers, and the consequences were difficult to quantify. I tried to interest the Venture Capital Association in documenting whether these rules prevented or delayed start-ups and got no response.

The 2006 Brennan *JAMA* article marked the escalation of the conflict-of-interest movement's assault on industry marketing, gifts, and subsidy of medical education. Shortly after that paper's appearance and *The Wall Street Journal's* publication of my op ed titled "Witch Hunt" in response to it, a large pharmaceutical company invited me to join an academic leadership advisory board designed to help the company forge better relationships with academic medical centers. I assumed that the convening of this board signaled emergence of some resistance to the conflict-of-interest movement—until I learned that the keynote speaker at the first meeting was a co-author of the Brennan *JAMA* piece.[2] The rest of the advisers consisted of medical school deans and some other academics that had participated in company-sponsored clinical trials. The board met six times over two years. The company executives (and the Brennan article co-author) stopped attending after the first meeting. The company board's organizers floated proposals for discussion forums at medical schools, research data-sharing schemes, and other partnerships, not registering that the schools would happily lap up cash offered to them, but without relaxing their conflict-of-interest rules. The advisers recounted anecdotes they believed reflected bad behavior by drug company reps. Little of substance came from the exercise.

My experiences on two more pharma company committees, during a brief consulting relationship with another pharmaceutical company, and presenting at additional pharmaceutical and biotechnology companies, to the pharmaceutical and biotechnology industry trade organizations, and at meetings of professional and other industry groups have similarly accomplished little. Listeners thank me for correcting misconceptions about the conflict-of-interest narrative, and some express interest in helping, but no follow-up action takes place.

As the regulatory ratchet bore down, I received invitations to speak or participate in panels at legal compliance forums. I would start my presentations by congratulating the attendees for being in the right place at the right time, because they populated a growth industry; I just wished it wasn't bad for my patients. And I ended by asking them to consider that because of their efforts when they retired with their profits from compliance management and couldn't remember which hole on the golf course they had just played—and their knees hurt—products might not exist to help them. The audiences were amused but weren't at all interested in the fundamental principles. Their focus was on building an extensive regulatory compliance apparatus.

Even groups that receive consistent abuse from the conflict-of-interest movement haven't responded with constructive action. For example, I spoke or was on panels at gatherings of professional writers and other industry support organizations, such as convention planners. But such brief encounters simply can't convey enough information to people hearing it for the first time to energize groups preoccupied with their day-to-day concerns.

In 2009, I co-founded an organization to oppose the conflict-of-interest movement with a small group of physicians and industry employees. Named the Association of Clinical Researchers and Educators (ACRE), it convened a meeting in July 2009 at my hospital, and several hundred participants attended, about half from industry. The organization's founders spoke concerning the value of physician-industry partnering. Funding for the meeting originated from nominal membership dues and admission fees from industry attendees. The meeting attracted some media attention, and I was asked to testify at a Senate hearing as an ACRE representative.

But all of the ACRE members had full-time jobs as industry employees, clinicians, or academic researchers and sustaining their primary activities precluded their devoting more than token efforts to the organization. In addition, they came from diverse medical disciplines, and their primary allegiances were to the professional groups that represented their major obligations. An antidote to the interference caused by these distractions might have been an administrative infrastructure with full-time contributors to solicit membership and promote the goals of the Association. Such an infrastructure, however, had to be paid for.

Following the inaugural meeting, ACRE's leaders visited several drug companies and the pharmaceutical, biotechnology, and medical device trade organizations (PhRMA, BIO, and ADVAMED, respectively) to solicit financial support. They experienced the same inattention and seeming lack of understanding of the stakes from these parties that I had encountered in my speaking forays. ACRE never raised a nickel from these groups. The organization held one more meeting in New York in 2011 and then went belly up. Its only durable accomplishment is that it connected some like-minded individuals. The solicited companies referred to the "optics" that ACRE receiving industry support would compromise its credibility—standard conflict-of-interest narrative thinking.

WHY THE MEDICAL PRODUCT INDUSTRY AND ITS ALLIES HAVE FAILED TO RESIST THE CONFLICT-OF-INTEREST MOVEMENT

One possible reason for their demurral of support is that most of the solicited corporations are under corporate integrity agreements, as discussed in Chapter 14. I speculate that these companies' lawyers advised their managements that supporting anyone who was exposing the story behind the off-label settlements might invite more prosecutorial persecution. A second more cynical reason may be that large companies simply think they can afford the costs of conflict-of-interest regulation. If the regulation compromises smaller companies lacking resources and time to understand or oppose it, then the big companies reap competitive advantage. The saddest reason for why the medical product industry hasn't supported its defenders may be that some industry employees actually *buy in* to the conflict-of-interest narrative's conviction that *motives* trump *performance* and that *appearances* trump *reality*. That conclusion certainly resonates with the companies that declined support by referring to the adverse optics of underwriting conflict-of-interest movement opposition.

One stark illustration of industry's errant response to the conflict-of-interest movement is a 2012 commentary titled "Ten Recommendations for Closing the Credibility Gap in Reporting Industry-Sponsored Clinical Research" published in a respectable medical journal.[3] Authored by employees of five major pharmaceutical company publication departments, representatives of medical publishing trade organizations, and several medical journal editors, the commentary uncritically aired the conflict-of-interest narrative that "industry-sponsored studies fail to meet the needs of the public and clinicians" and apologetically served up a menu of suggestions for remedying alleged past sins responsible for this negative impression. I co-authored a letter to the journal spelling out the article's errors.[4]

Similarly, the biotechnology editor of an industry-subsidized blog recently bemoaned the degraded reputation of the pharmaceutical industry benchmarked against a 1994 book titled *Built to Last: Successful Habits of Visionary Companies*. This book had declared Merck as one of the most popular businesses at that time.[5] The blogger then proposed a 12-step rehabilitation program to restore the industry to its earlier vaunted status. The recommendations were (1) lower drug prices, (2) share all data, (3) care about patients' problems, (4) support the FDA, (5) do more for global health, (6) discover more great drugs, (7) provide more welfare for employees (e.g., researchers laid off by research program downsizing), (8) stop marketing fraud, (9) invest more in public R&D, (10) stop direct-to-consumer advertising, (11) find creative ways to improve clinical trials, and (12) come up with a moonshot (e.g., cure Alzheimer's disease by 2025).

Leaving aside that the 1994 *Built to Last* also praised Reynolds Tobacco as a "visionary" company and that patients are more concerned about companies providing them with useful products than winning popularity contests, this book has tried to explain why every one of the blogger's suggestions is not factually based, is economically untenable, or is a Utopian fantasy.

Suggestions number one and seven assume the industry has infinite resources and can sacrifice profits without consequences. Chapters 8 and 9 explained the fallacy of that assumption. Recommendation number seven ignores the fact that industry generally takes much better care of its professional employees, financially and otherwise, than academia does. Industry supports the FDA (recommendation four) by paying "user fees" that augment the Agency's congressional appropriation. The conflict-of-interest movement complains that these fees make the regulators and the regulated "too cozy" with one another.[6] More collusion between industry and the FDA would only exacerbate those criticisms.

Suggestion five is unfair, because industry already invests substantial resources in global health and gets little credit for it. For example, Merck receives little recognition for having donated vast quantities of a curative drug (ivermectin, trade name Mectizan) to help eradicate river blindness, formerly a leading cause of blindness, worldwide.[7]

Chapter 14 deconstructed the marketing fraud accusation mentioned in recommendation number eight. Industry repeatedly claims it cares about—and does—help patients (recommendation three). The recommendation overlooks industry-sponsored product discount programs. Moreover, the conflict-of-interest narrative sneers at industry's claims to good intentions for patients. For example, it derides industry's support of patient advocacy groups, such as the National Alliance on Mental Illness, as covert marketing (and it applies the same criticism to drug discount programs).

Regarding recommendation number nine, industry *does* lobby for public research funding, for example by providing substantial financial contributions to the NIH advocacy organization Research!America.

Likewise, industry sponsors both internal and academic discovery research but appropriately focuses the bulk of its funding on projects likely to identify potential products for the treatment or prevention of disease. Further industry subsidy of open-ended research as a public relations exercise would, on a population level, produce minimal goodwill at great cost and would be dismissed as pandering.[8]

Industry supports direct-to-consumer advertising in part based on the presumption that such advertising increases awareness of obscure or stigmatized conditions and appropriate treatment options. Industry perceives such advertising as a win-win in that it encourages patients to seek treatment and boosts sales concurrently. If public relations concerns really override such gains, then industry should discontinue the advertising. But the decision should rest on empiric evidence, not on subjective tastes.

Many analysts inside and outside industry are diligently searching for ways to make clinical trials more effective (suggestion 11), such as applying advanced information technology to reduce the costs of patient monitoring. But, as discussed in Chapter 8, biology has a way of confounding our creative ideas.

Finally, a "moonshot," like the suggested cure for Alzheimer's disease or a malaria or HIV vaccine, sounds like an appealing source of goodwill for industry. But industry is already making efforts toward those goals. Unlike the rocket science that enabled lunar landings, biology renders those vaunted outcomes very tenuous, and thus far most medical moonshot attempts have disappointingly failed. If industry dropped all efforts toward producing more attainable revenue-producing results to concentrate on risky goals, the public's goodwill would quickly dissipate. Neither the blogger nor the numerous laudatory responses to his blog post volunteered any specific ideas as to how to identify "great drugs" or to achieve "moonshots."

Whatever the reasons, industry has failed to address the conflict-of-interest movement's underlying *principles*—its allegations that industry behavior is corrupt and corrupts physicians and academics. Rather, to the extent it has pushed back at all, it has reacted narrowly—and with little success—to *specific crises* caused by the conflict-of-interest movement. To some extent, industry's apparent apathy is explicable. No one company is likely to want to take on the defense of the enterprise as a whole, not to mention of its competitors. Collective action, on the other hand, might invite antitrust litigation. The industry perceives that attacking academic institutions, government, and professional groups that have embraced strict conflict-of-interest regulation as beating up on its customers. If conflict-of-interest regulations diminish or eliminate corporate payments for partnerships with academics and physicians across the industry as a whole, the companies' bottom lines might actually benefit with no competitive disadvantage—until a tipping point is reached at which partnerships become difficult to sustain.

The diffuseness of the conflict-of-interest movement's narrative also allows seemingly more acute specific problems to take precedence. Threats of pharmaceutical price controls or a device tax, for example, are salient and therefore dominate the attention of companies or their trade organizations. With respect to these particular examples, the narrative's denial of necessarily high medical product development costs and its demonization of industry profits, discussed in Chapter 9, underlie the false notion that excessive profitability justifies the demanded price reductions and taxes.

IS RESISTANCE NECESSARY?

In addition to the dreary proposition that the industry behemoths can afford and may even benefit from the disproportionate effects of conflict-of-interest regulation on smaller companies, it is worth asking whether medical innovation and education can thrive if conflict-of-interest regulations persist. After all, in our daily lives, we could reasonably operate on the assumption that the Earth is flat. It looks flat, and we intuitively behave as if it were, even though we know full well it isn't. Only those engaged in long-distance navigation, satellite operation, or interplanetary travel must actively operate on the reality that the Earth is round. Like navigation or satellite operations, however, medical innovation and education cannot rely on superficially plausible, but ultimately inaccurate, conceptualizations; they require complex technical knowledge and an accurate understanding of reality to function effectively.

RESISTANCE IS POSSIBLE: THE AACE EXAMPLE

Endocrinology, the branch of medicine that deals with the body's hormone-producing glands, has had a rich scientific tradition. Discovery research by endocrinologists identified glands and the hormones they generate and introduced clinically important procedures for addressing the clinical consequences of over- or underproduction.

For many years, the principal professional organization for endocrinologists was the Endocrine Society, founded in 1917. In 1991, some endocrine specialists decided to convene a group more focused on clinical aspects of the field and willing to address policy issues. Diabetes, for example, was becoming increasingly prevalent, and matters concerning patient access to treatment and insurance reimbursement for such treatment needed to be confronted. This decision led to the founding of the American Association of Clinical Endocrinologists (AACE). The Association has grown to claim over 6,000 members residing in 90 countries.

At the 2009 annual meeting of the Association, the group's leadership galvanized to push back against the burgeoning conflict-of-interest movement that was insinuating itself into every medical professional society. Most importantly, the Association explicitly rejected the rhetoric of the conflict-of-interest narrative. It purged "conflict of interest" from its policy language, affirming strongly the value of endocrinologist-industry cooperation and referring to that cooperation as "multiplicity of interests." The Association also resisted calls to reduce industry support for its programs and permitted its leaders to maintain their industry relationships. In addition, AACE's repudiation of the conflict-of-interest narrative coincided with the emergence of ACRE, and AACE participated actively in ACRE's short existence. AACE's medical journal, *Endocrine Practice*, published proceedings of the initial ACRE meeting[9] and subsequently a set of ACRE guidelines written by ACRE members concerning physicians' relationships with industry.[10] All of these principled moves occurred and persisted despite objections from members of AACE who espouse the conflict-of-interest narrative.

Why did this one organization at this one time mount resistance that has persisted? The answer is not clear, but possibly the Association's practical clinical emphasis, which contrasts the more basic science orientation of the competing Endocrine Society, is a factor. The Endocrine Society, in contrast to AACE, has dutifully incorporated all the cant about conflict of interest in its policies and, like many other professional organizations, excludes members with industry relationships from leadership positions. Whatever the reasons, the AACE story implies that capitulation is not inevitable.

HOW TO STOP THE CONFLICT-OF-INTEREST MOVEMENT

The plan involves two phases: the first is a preparatory education and planning effort leading to the second, political action.

Phase I: Education and Strategizing

Only industry has the resources to accomplish this goal. But applying those resources will require overcoming the reticence described above that has characterized past industry behavior. The precondition for such transcendence is that someone in industry with decision-making capability "gets it," perceives value in the proposed resistance, and sets into motion specific plans that achieve such value. I identify two target audience sets for education and strategy: one is researchers and physicians; the other is a segment of the general public.

Researchers and Physicians

A key ingredient is to connect *specific* company needs for their relationships with the *specific* physicians and academics that benefit from such relationships. This strategy deviates from ineffectual past efforts, such as ACRE's, that predominantly addressed generalities. Companies know who their actual and potential outside partners are. The companies should recruit as many of these partners as they can, and they should especially seek out individuals with influence in their professional organizations. For the specific conclaves suggested below, however, companies must avoid reflexively defaulting to past collaborators or high-ranking academic advisers. My experience with the various industry boards discussed above and observation of policy deliberations at academic health centers has consistently led to the conclusion that physicians and academics who have either cashed in handsomely from past industry relationships or currently occupy cosmetic—and well-remunerated—company directorships almost never oppose the conflict-of-interest policy narrative and its consequences. They want to have it both ways: keep the money and avoid exposure to adverse publicity.

All of the interactions of the suggested affinity pairs should include thorough education to equip all the parties to rebut the unjustifiable assertions of the conflict-of-interest narrative. Abetting this education effort could be excerpts of this book, webinars, and other presentations concisely conveying the most important messages. The interactions should be programmed and facilitated to produce action plans. Some examples of the specific physician and academic synergies with industry follow:

1. Medical device manufacturing companies that want their technical support personnel to have ready access to practitioners who use the devices and the practitioners who want ready access to those personnel should come together for strategic conversations. The conversations arm the practitioners to advocate strongly at their employer institutions for the value of access and the damages of access prevention. A specific practice to insist on discontinuing is the intentional stigmatization of the company device technicians who train surgeons on new devices by making them wear black scrub suits labeled "VENDOR" in the operating room.

2. Device manufacturing companies and device inventors should meet to discuss how to prevent restrictions on rewards, such as royalties, milestone payments, and consulting fees, from inhibiting or eliminating future device invention partnerships.

3. Companies that manufacture psychiatric, dermatologic, antiasthma, and antidiabetes (and certain other) drugs that believe product samples promote their sales should connect with practitioners who prescribe those products and believe that providing such samples is good for patient care. By focusing on specialties that have traditionally used samples, stronger arguments for samples arise than those in a more general conversation involving, say, surgeons, for whom samples have never been particularly important.

4. Pharmaceutical, biotechnology, and device manufacturing companies that believe detailing (and other marketing practices) encourage prescribing of their products should interact with physicians who believe that industry marketing provides them with useful

information and that academic institutions and clinical practices should not restrict it.

5. Device manufacturing companies that have relationships with high-volume surgical specialists who perform particular procedures utilizing the companies' devices should work with those specialists to rebut media abuse insinuating that the relationships cause device overutilization.[11]

6. Pharmaceutical, biotechnology, and device manufacturing companies that believe peer-to-peer speaking promotes product sales and appropriate prescribing of those products should work with their speakers who are good teachers and enjoy participating in such speaking to rebut the subjective and snobbish arguments mounted by the conflict-of-interest narrative. They should explain the value of such speaking and resist rules that have restricted such speaking and empowered critics to try to embarrass speakers.

7. Medical education companies should caucus with authoritative education leaders of professional groups and academic institutions strapped by extortionate and arguably useless costs of CME accreditation to make the case against the accreditation bureaucracies' monopolies.

The Public: Curing the "Rodney Dangerfield" Syndrome

To regain respect, rather than abjectly submitting to the 10 Commandments or 12-step rehabilitation programs discussed above, the industry needs to reject the conflict-of-interest narrative's diagnosis of greed and take back the recognition it deserves. The message isn't that doctors, medical schools, and journals are *bad* or *don't* contribute to medical innovation; it's that they are important, but they're *not* as important as they claim to be. Conversely, the medical products industry is not unqualifiedly wonderful; but with the cooperation of physicians and researchers it clearly does contribute dominantly to medical progress. Unfortunately, this information is novel to most people. Moreover, the target audience for the message has to have enough at stake to pay attention to it, deal with the confrontation associated with it, and be willing to participate in advocacy to promote it. The groups to focus on are the many people with diseases or whose families have diseases that they want to have prevented, better managed, or cured.

Phase II: It's Politics, Stupid!

Ultimately, whatever emerges from the synergies proposed above has to translate into advocacy. The targets of such advocacy are the institutions that have enacted and enforced conflict-of-interest regulation: academic health centers, professional organizations, states, and the federal government.

As one of the most regulated enterprises, the medical product industry needs to exercise advocacy to protect its interests from political exploitation. But the industry's approach to conflict-of-interest movement allegations has been silence, defensive crisis management, or pleading—with detailed and flashy audiovisual aids—that it does good things. Failing to rebut the conflict-of-interest narrative's allegations and regulations straightforwardly is akin to politely debating that the Earth is round. This strategy will never succeed. It is necessary to vigorously oppose false accusations that not accepting that the Earth is flat is a sign of corruption or sacrilege. Politicians understand the importance of and engage in passionate advocacy. Yet, their acrimonious debates about the role of government in society and how much wealth to redistribute to what social ends are far less grounded in empiric fact and solid logic than the polemics in question concerning the medical-industry interface. Only straightforward and aggressive exposure of the factual and logical errors of the conflict-of-interest narrative will overcome the background noise emitting from the numerous books, medical journal articles, and symposia produced by the well-organized and well-funded conflict-of-interest movement. For the foregoing reasons, the frequency and volume of counter messaging must increase. Paying for message frequency and volume is why political campaigns cost so much.

The public and the medical profession must demand a stop to the damage caused by conflict-of-interest regulations. Throughout this book, I have tried to spell out how the hyperbolic rhetoric, faulty data, and distorted logic of the conflict-of-interest narrative are toxic to medical innovation. It impedes transfer to physicians of important information regarding new options for patient care. It is a force built on shadows and lies. We cannot allow the conflict-of-interest propaganda machine to continue unchallenged.

The medical product industry that provides physicians with tools to save lives and reduce suffering is hardly like "Big Tobacco," whose products inflict pain and death. The only feature these industries have in common is that they expect profits. Yet, despite the vast gulf between the social outcomes of these industries, the conflict-of-interest movement exploits the profit expectation they have in common to conflate them. The conflict-of-interest movement demands that the medical product industry must operate from the nonexistent absolute altruism that it alleges characterizes medical "professionalism." Indeed, all enterprises—even nonprofits—must profit to thrive.

If we limit medical product industry profits, we impair the industry's ability to produce the beneficial tools. If we limit physicians' exposure to information about those tools, physicians may not know about them. But such limitation is the conflict-of-interest movement's agenda. It is sacrificing your future health to its misplaced ideology.

NOTES

INTRODUCTION

1. Pharmaceuticals are chemical compounds—often defined as "small molecules"—that include all prescription and nonprescription medications that are not biologics.

2. Biologics are medications based on naturally occurring body substances, such as hormones like insulin.

3. Medical devices include a broad variety of products ranging from surgical implants and medical-imaging devices to wheelchairs and bandages.

4. Partners Healthcare, "Partners Policy for Interactions with Industry and Other Outside Entities," (2012), http://www.partners.org/Assets/Documents/About-Us/OII/OII_Policy.pdf.

5. TP Stossel, "Free the Scientists! Conflict-of-Interest Rules Purport to Cure a Problem That Doesn't Exist—and Are Stifling Medical Progress," *Forbes*, February 14, 2005.

6. TP Stossel, "Regulating Academic-Industry Research Relationships—Solving Problems or Stifling Progress," *N Engl J Med* 353(2005).

7. TP Stossel, "Mere Magazines," *Wall Street Journal*, December 29, 2005.

I. THE STAKES

1. HUS also is a result of the uncontrolled activity of a basic body defense system called "the complement system." The complement system is a collection of blood proteins evolved to help the body recognize and destroy potentially lethal microorganisms, but when its regulation goes awry it can destroy tissues

and organs. Complement-mediated damage is implicated in diverse diseases (D Tichaczek-Goska, "Deficiencies and Excessive Human Complement System Activation in Disorders of Multifarious Etiology," *Adv Clin Exp Med* 21(2012)). For reasons that are not clear, the Shiga toxin responsible for HUS causes complement to become active against normal body cells, thereby causing destruction of the kidney and other organs.

2. Eculizumab shuts down the unregulated complement activity caused by Shiga in HUS. The first clinical use of eculizumab was in an even rarer condition called "atypical HUS." Atypical HUS is a genetic disease in which affected individuals lack circulating blood proteins that prevent spontaneous activity of the complement system. Atypical HUS patients suffer progressive deterioration of the lungs, kidney, and gastrointestinal system. Eculizumab prevents these complications (C Legendre, C Licht, and C Loirat, "Eculizumab in Atypical Hemolytic-Uremic Syndrome," *N Engl J Med* 369(2013)). It also provides clinical benefit in another uncommon acquired disease caused by the complement system known as "paroxysmal nocturnal hemoglobinuria" (PNH) (Risitano, "Paroxysmal Nocturnal Hemoglobinuria and Other Complement-Mediated Hematological Disorders," *Immunobiology* 217(2012)). Chapter 8 describes the commercial development of eculizumab.

3. http://www.optionsforchildren.org.

4. M. C. Jensen et al., "Magnetic Resonance Imaging of the Lumbar Spine in People without Back Pain," *N Engl J Med* 331(1994).

5. RR Edwards et al., "Symptoms of Distress as Prospective Predictors of Pain-Related Sciatica Treatment Outcomes," *Pain* 130(2007).

6. T. S. Carey et al., "The Outcomes and Costs of Care for Acute Low Back Pain among Patients Seen by Primary Care Practitioners, Chiropractors, and Orthopedic Surgeons," *N Engl J Med* 333(1995); M BenDebba et al., "Persistent Low Back Pain and Sciatica in the United States: Treatment Outcomes," *J Spinal Disord Tech* 15(2002).

7. My son, Scott, has written a *New York Times* best-selling book devoted to anxiety, an affliction he has personally endured his whole life. The book minutely and comprehensively summarizes the murky definitions of anxiety, the competing theories concerning its causes, the diversity of treatments directed at it, and yet how despite the opacity of the disorder, patients can benefit from diagnosis and therapy (S. Stossel, *My Age of Anxiety: Fear, Hope, Dread and the Search for Peace of Mind* [New York: Knopf, 2014]).

2. A PRACTITIONER'S HISTORY OF MEDICAL INNOVATION

1. T. McKeown and R. G. Record, "Reasons for the Decline of Mortality in England and Wales During the Nineteenth Century," *Popul Stud* 16(1962).

2. H. Wang et al., "Age-Specific and Sex-Specific Mortality in 187 Countries, 1970–2010: A Systematic Analysis for the Global Burden of Disease Study 2010," *Lancet* 380(2012).

3. E. G. Nabel and E. Braunwald, "A Tale of Coronary Artery Disease and Myocardial Infarction," *N Engl J Med* 366(2012).

4. American Cancer Society, "Cancer Facts and Figures 2013," http://www.cancer.org/acs/groups/content/@epidemiologysurveilance/documents/document/acspc-031941.pdf.

5. Centers for Disease Control and Prevention, "Rheumatoid Arthritis," http://www.cdc.gov/arthritis/data_statistics/arthritis_related_stats.htm.

6. "Osteoporosis," http://www.cdc.gov/nchs/fastats/osteoporosis.htm.

7. R. J. Wurtman, "What Went Right: Why Is HIV a Treatable Infection?" *Nat Med* 3(1997).

8. Centers for Disease Control and Prevention, "HIV/AIDS," http://www.cdc.gov/hiv/topics/surveillance/basic.htm.

9. T. Dixon et al., "Trends in Hip and Knee Joint Replacement: Socioeconomic Inequalities and Projections of Need," *Ann Rheum Dis* 63(2004); P Cram et al., "Total Knee Arthroplasty Volume, Utilization, and Outcomes among Medicare Beneficiaries," *JAMA* 308(2012).

10. M. E. Bowden, A. B. Crow, and T. Sullivan, *Pharmaceutical Achievers. The Human Face of Pharmaceutical Research* (Philadelphia, PA: Chemical Heritage Press, 2003).

11. JP Swann, *Academic Scientists and the Pharmaceutical Industry* (Baltimore: The Johns Hopkins University Press, 1988).

12. C. Kerr, *The Uses of the University* (Harvard University Press, 1963).

13. F. G. Cottrell, "The Research Corporation, an Experiment in Public Administration of Patent Rights," *J Indust Engin Chem* 4(1912).

14. B. N. Sampat, "Patenting and Us Academic Research in the 20th Century: The World before and after Bayh-Dole," *Res Policy* 35(2006).

15. Academic institutions evolved an arbitrary system in which income from licensing fees, milestone payments, and royalties was divided equally among faculty inventors, the inventors' academic department, and the university administration.

16. M Kenney, *Biotechnology: The University-Industrial Complex* (New Haven: Yale University Press, 1986).

17. JA Greene and SH Podolsky, "Keeping Modern in Medicine: Pharmaceutical Promotion and Physician Education in Postwar America," *Bull Hist Med* 83(2009).

18. Critics of the medical products industry complain about the fact that it engages in extensive political lobbying activity. For example, see M. Angell, *The Truth About the Drug Companies: How They Deceive Us and What to Do About It* (New York: Random House, 2004); H. Brody, *Hooked: Ethics, the Medical Profession, and the Pharmaceutical Industry* (Lanham, MD: Rowman & Littlefield Publishers, 2007). But they neglect to mention that politicization is a direct consequence of government regulation. Exerting political influence is therefore a survival adaptation for any industry as heavily regulated as health care (J. Golberg, *Liberal Fascism* [Doubleday, 2007]).

19. Conflict-of-interest movement critics have a dim view of universities filing patents (M Angell, "Big Pharma, Bad Medicine," *Boston Rev*, May/June [2010]): "Bayh-Dole is now more a matter of seeking windfalls than of transferring technology. Some have argued that it actually impedes technology transfer by enabling the licensing of early discoveries, which encumbers downstream research. I believe medical research was every bit as productive before Bayh-Dole as it is now, despite the lack of patents. I'm reminded of Jonas Salk's response when asked whether he had patented the polio vaccine. He seemed amazed at the very notion. The vaccine, he explained, belonged to everybody. 'Could you patent the sun?' he asked." Salk's memorable statement cited here was part of a 1957 televised response to Edward R. Murrow's question about who held a patent on the polio vaccine he had developed. Salk's answer to the question was indeed, "The people." "Can you patent the sun?" The reality, however, was that both Salk's academic institution, the University of Pittsburgh and the National Foundation (March of Dimes) that sponsored the vaccine development had *tried* to patent the vaccine. Salk's vaccine production used methodology based on previous vaccine technology and was therefore obvious and not patentable (JS Smith, *Patenting the Sun: Polio and the Salk Vaccine: The Dramatic Story Behind One of the Greatest Achievements of Modern Science* (Morrow, 1990); DM Oshinsky, *Polio: An American Story* [New York: Oxford University Press, 2005]). The companies that made the polio vaccines widely available, however, were able to obtain process patents related to scaling up vaccine production. As was the case with the University of Toronto and insulin in the 1920s, the government, the academic institutions, and the charity (March of Dimes) that supported the precommercial vaccine prototype were incapable of creating vaccine supplies accommodating its widespread use.

20. H. M. Marks, *The Progress of Experiment: Science and Therapeutic Reform in the United States, 1900-1990* (Oxford University Press, 1997); P. J. Hilts, *Protecting America's Health: The FDA, Business, and One Hundred Years of*

Regulation (New York: Alfred E. Knopf, 2003); D Tobell, *Pills, Power and Policy: The Struggle for Drug Reform in Cold War America and Its Consequences* (Berkeley: University of California Berkeley Press, 2012); RL Woosley, "One Hundred Years of Drug Regulation: Where Do We Go from Here?" *Annu Rev Pharmacol Toxicol* 53(2013).

21. G. L. Boland, "Federal Regulation of Prescription Drug Advertising and Labeling," *Boston Coll Law Rev* 12, no. 2 (1970); Marks, *The Progress of Experiment: Science and Therapeutic Reform in the United States, 1900-1990*; Hilts, *Protecting America's Health: The FDA, Business, and One Hundred Years of Regulation*.

22. "Food and Drug Amendments Act of 2007," in Pub. L. No. 110-185, 121 Stat. 823, ed. FDA (2007).

23. U.S. Food and Drug Administration, "Small Business Assistance: Frequently Asked Questions for New Drug Product Exclusivity," http://www.fda.gov/Drugs/DevelopmentApprovalProcess/SmallBusinessAssistance/ucm069962.htm.

24. "Orphan Drug Act (Public Law 97-414)," http://www.fda.gov/regulatoryinformation/legislation/federalfooddrugandcosmeticactfdcact/significantamendmentstothefdcact/orphandrugact/default.htm.

25. KA Burke et al., "The Impact of the Orphan Drug Act on the Development and Advancement of Neurological Products for Rare Diseases: A Descriptive Review," *Clin Pharmacol Therap* 88(2010).

26. F. R. Lichtenberg, "The Impact of New (Orphan) Drug Approvals on Premature Mortality from Rare Diseases in the United States and France, 1999–2007," *Eur J Health Econ* 14(2013).

27. G. Mossinghoff, "Overview of the Hatch-Waxman Act and Its Impact on the Drug Development Process," *Food Drug L J* 54(1999).

28. One exception is that a physician can ask the FDA to allow a patient to receive an unapproved product "for compassionate use." This situation arises when a patient has a potentially lethal condition for which a product under development is designed to treat. Companies developing products do not encourage compassionate use out of fear that unfavorable outcomes, possibly unrelated to the use of the product, might prejudice FDA approval.

29. CM Wittich, CM Burkle, and WL Lanier, "Ten Common Questions (and Their Answers) About Off-Label Drug Use," *Mayo Clin Proc* 87(2012).

30. Food and Drug Administration, "PDUFA Reauthorization Performance Goals and Procedures Fiscal Years 2013 through 2017" (2013).

31. P. Huber, *The Cure in the Code: How 20th Century Law Is Undermining 21st Century Medicine* (New York: Basic Books, 2013).

32. *Wyeth, Petitioner v. Diana Levine*, 555 U.S. 555 129 S. Ct. 1187 06-1249(2008).

3. ENTER THE CONFLICT-OF-INTEREST MANIA

1. CD May, "Selling Drugs by 'Educating' Physicians," *J Med Edu* 36(1961); TB Binns and A Smith, "Medical Representatives," *BMJ* 1(1979); J Lexchin, *The Real Pushers: A Critical Analysis of the Canadian Drug Industry* (Vancouver: New Star Books, 1984).

2. R Bailey, "Is Industry-Funded Science Killing You? The Overrated Risks and Underrated Benefits of Pharmaceutical Research 'Conflicts of Interest,'" *Reason*, October 2007; R Bailey, "Scrutinizing Industry-Funded Science: The Crusade against Conflicts of Interest" (American Council on Science and Health, 2008).

3. National Library of Medicine, "Conflict of Interest," http://www.ncbi.nlm.nih.gov/pubmed?term=conflict of interest.

4. PG Gosselin, "Flawed Study Helps Doctors Profit on Drug," *Boston Globe*, 1988.

5. DC Rennie, "Thyroid Storm," *JAMA* 277(1997).

6. J Thompson, P Baird, and J Downie, *The Olivieri Report: The Complete Text of the Report of the Independent Inquiry Commissioned by the Canadian Association of University Teachers* (Toronto: James Lorimer and Company Ltd, 2001).

7. SE Raper et al., "Fatal Systemic Inflammatory Response Syndrome in an Ornithine Transcarbamylase Deficient Patient Following Adenoviral Gene Transfer," *Mol Genet Metab* 80(2003).

8. S Johnson et al., "*Estate of Gelsinger v. Trustees of University of Pennsylvania*," in *Health Law and Bioethics: Cases in Context* (Aspen Publishers, 2009).

9. KAA Fox et al., "Decline in Rates of Death and Heart Failure in Acute Coronary Syndromes, 1999-2006," *JAMA* 297(2007).

10. CD Furberg, BM Psaty, and JV Meyer, "Dose-Related Increase in Mortality in Patients with Coronary Heart Disease," *Circulation* 92(1995).

11. HT Stelfox et al., "Conflict of Interest in the Debate over Calcium-Channel Antagonists," *N Engl J Med* 338(1998).

12. D Willman, "Stealth Merger: Drug Companies and Government Medical Research," *Los Angeles Times*, December 7, 2003.

13. MM Mello, BR Clarridge, and DM Studdert, "Academic Medical Centers' Standards for Clinical-Trial Agreements with Industry," *N Engl J Med* 352(2005).

14. Association of American Medical Colleges, "Protecting Subjects, Preserving Trust, Promoting Progress: Policy and Guidelines for the Oversight of Individual Financial Interests in Human Subjects Research," (Washington, DC, 2001).

15. "Responsibility of Applicants for Promoting Objectivity in Research for Which PHS Funding Is Sought," in 42 CFR Part 50, Subpart F, ed. National Institutes of Health (2011).

16. National Institutes of Health, A Working Group of the Advisory Committee to the Director, "Report of the National Institutes of Health Blue Ribbon Panel on Conflict of Interest Policies," (2004).

17. R Steinbrook, "Financial Conflicts of Interest at the NIH," *N Engl J Med* 350(2004); "Conflicts of Interest at the NIH—Resolving the Problem," *N Engl J Med* 351(2004); "Standards of Ethics at the National Institutes of Health," *N Engl J Med* 352(2005).

18. F Van Kolfschooten, "Can You Believe What You Read?" *Nature* 416(2002); JA Blum et al., "Requirements and Definitions in Conflict of Interest Policies of Medical Journals," *JAMA* 302(2009).

19. "Avoid Financial Correctness," *Nature* 385(1997).

20. P Campbell, "Declaration of Financial Interests: Introducing a New Policy for Authors of Research Papers," *Nature* 412(2001).

21. LE Ferris and RH Fletcher, "Conflict of Interest in Peer-Reviewed Medical Journals: The World Association of Medical Editors (WAME) Position on a Challenging Problem," *Int J Occup Environ Med* 1(2010). The International Committee of Medical Journal Editors has created a template for "disclosure of potential conflicts of interest" "to provide readers of your manuscript with information about your other interests that could influence how they receive and understand your work." International Committee of Medical Journal Editors, "Form for Disclosure of Potential Conflicts of Interest," http://www.icmje.org/conflicts-of-interest/.

22. PB Fontanarosa and CD De Angelis, "Conflicts of Interest and Independent Data Analysis in Industry-Funded Studies," *JAMA* 294(2005).

23. KJ Rothman and S Evans, "Extra Scrutiny for Industry Funded Trials: JAMA's Demand for an Additional Hurdle Is Unfair—and Absurd," *BMJ* 331(2005).

24. C DeAngelis, "The Influence of Money on Medical Science," *JAMA* 296(2006).

25. EA Boyd and LA Bero, "Assessing Faculty Financial Relationships with Industry. A Case Study," JAMA. 284(2000).

26. TA Brennan et al., "Health Industry Practices That Create Conflict of Interest: A Policy Proposal for Academic Medical Centers," *JAMA* 295(2006).

27. To date, more than 40 anti-industry books have been published on this topic, many from major publishing houses. See, for example, M Angell, *The Truth About the Drug Companies: How They Deceive Us and What to Do About It* (New York: Random House, 2004); B Goldacre, *Bad Pharma: How Drug Companies Mislead Doctors and Harm Patients* (London, UK: Fourth Estate,

2012); J Kassirer, *On the Take: How Medicine's Complicity with Big Business Can Endanger Your Health* (Oxford: Oxford University Press, 2004); J Abramson, *Overdosed America* (New York: HarperCollins, 2004); Moynihan and Cassells, *Selling Sickness* (Nation Books, 2006); Healy, *Pharmaggedon* (University of California Press, 2012); Healy, *Let Them Eat Prozac* (NYU Press, 2004); Weber, *Profits before People?* (Indiana University Press, 2006); Strand, *Death by Prescription* (HarperCollins, 2006); Krimsky, *Science in the Private Interest: Has the Lure of Profits Corrupted Biomedical Research?* (Lanham, MD: Rowman & Littlefield, 2003); Mundy, *Dispensing with the Truth: The Victims, the Drug Company and the Dramatic Story Behind the Battle over Fen-Phen* (New York: St Martin's Press, 2001); Bass, *Side Effects: A Prosecutor, a Whistleblower, and a Bestselling Antidepressant on Trial* (Chapel Hill, NC: Algonquin Books of Chapel Hill, 2008); PC Gotzsche, *Deadly Medicines and Organised Crime: How Big Pharma Has Corrupted Healthcare* (Singapore: Radcliffe Medical Press, 2013); R Whitaker, *Anatomy of an Epidemic: Magic Bullets, Psychiatric Drugs, and the Astonishing Rise of Mental Illness in America* (New York: Random House, 2011). The deluge of mutually redundant books on this topic has shown no signs of abating.

In contrast, I am aware of only four books on the other side of the debate: RA Epstein, *Overdose: How Excessive Government Regulation Stifles Pharmaceutical Innovation* (New Haven: Yale University Press, 2006); JL LaMattina, *Drug Truths: Dispelling the Myths About Pharma R&D* (Hoboken, NJ: Wiley, 2009); R Goldberg, *Tabloid Medicine: How the Internet Is Being Used to Hijack Medical Science for Fear and Profit* (New York: Kaplan Publishing, 2010); JL LaMattina, *Devalued and Distrusted. Can the Pharmaceutical Industry Restore Its Broken Image?* (New York: Wiley, 2013).

The scholarly literature is no better on this front. For example, in the fall of 2013 *The Journal of Law, Medicine & Ethics* published a special issue containing 16 articles encompassing 202 pages discussing "institutional corruption and the pharmaceutical industry."

28.   G Harris and J Roberts, "Doctors' Ties to Drug Makers Are Put on Close View," *New York Times*, March 21, 2007. http://www.nytimes.com/2007/03/21/us/21drug.html?pagewanted=all&_r=0.

29.   State of Massachusetts, *Pharmaceutical and Medical Device Manufacturer Code of Conduct.* http://www.mass.gov/eohhs/gov/departments/dph/programs/hcq/healthcare-quality/pharm-code-of-conduct/medical-device-manufacturer-code-of-conduct.html.

30.   State of Vermont, *Prescription Drug Cost Containment. Expenditures by Manufacturers of Prescribed Products.* 18 V.S.A. § 4631a. http://www.leg.state.vt.us/statutes/fullsection.cfm?Title=18&Chapter=091&Section=04632.

31. SD Curi and L Vernaglia, "Industry 'Gift Bans': Massachusetts and Beyond," American Health Lawyers Association's Physicians and Physician Organization Law Institute. February 24, 2010: 1-7.

32. Pharmaceutical Research and Manufacturers of America, "PhRMA Code on Interactions with Healthcare Professionals, Revised," (2005); ADVAMED, "Code of Ethics on Interactions with Health Care Professionals" (Advanced Medical Technology Association, 2008); Pharmaceutical Research and Manufacturers of America, "Code on Interactions with Healthcare Professionals" (2008).

33. American Medical Association, "Report 1 of the Council on Ethical and Judicial Affairs (CEJA Report 1a-08): Industry Support of Professional Education in Medicine" (2008).

34. N Singer and D Wilson, "Misgivings Grow over Corporate Role in Keeping Doctors Current," *New York Times*, June 23, 2010.

35. DJ Rothman et al., "Professional Medical Associations and Their Relationships with Industry: A Proposal for Controlling Conflict of Interest," *JAMA* 301(2009); H Brody, "Professional Medical Organizations and Commercial Conflicts of Interest: Ethical Issues," *Ann Fam Med* 8(2010).

36. NB Kahn and AS Lichter, "The New CMSS Code for Interactions with Companies Managing Relationships to Minimize Conflicts," *J Vasc Surg* 54(3) Suppl (2011).

37. D Morelli and MR Koenigsberg, "Sample Medication Dispensing in a Residency Practice," *J Fam Pract* 34(1992); JM Westfall, J McCabe, and RA Nicholas, "Personal Use of Drug Samples by Physicians and Office Staff," *JAMA* 278(1997); SL Cutrona et al., "Characteristics of Recipients of Free Pharmaceutical Drug Samples: A Nationally Representative Analysis," *Am J Public Health* 98(2008); GC Alexander, J Zhang, and A Basu, "Characteristics of Patients Receiving Pharmaceutical Samples and Association between Sample Receipt and Out-of-Pocket Prescription Costs," *Med Care* 46(2008).

38. D Carlat, "Dr. Drug Rep," *New York Times Magazine*, November 25, 2007.

39. E Katz and PF Lazarsfeld, *Personal Influence: The Part Played by People in the Flow of Mass Communication* (Glencoe, IL: The Free Press, 1955).

40. R Moyhihan, "Key Opinion Leaders: Independent Experts or Drug Representatives in Disguise?" *BMJ* 336(2008).

41. RM Pearl, "Medical Conflicts of Interest Are Dangerous: For Some Patients, What Their Doctors Don't Tell Them Could Be Hazardous for Their Health," *Wall Street Journal*, April 24, 2013.

42. GA Chressanthis et al., "Can Access Limits on Sales Representatives to Physicians Affect Clinical Prescription Decisions? A Study of Recent Events with Diabetes and Lipid Drugs," *J Clin Hypertension* 14(2012).

4. THE MANIA MONGERS

1. W. Faloon, *Pharmocracy: How Corrupt Deals and Misguided Medical Regulations Are Bankrupting America—and What to Do About It* (Mount Jackson, VA: Practikos Books, 2012).

2. IMAP Funding Information, http://imapny.org/about-imap/funding-information/.

3. B. Lo and M. Field, "Conflict of Interest in Medical Research, Education, and Practice." (Institute of Medicine, 2009).

4. "Pew Prescription Project," http://www.pewtrusts.org/en/projects/pew-prescription-project.

5. P Starr, *The Social Transformation of American Medicine* (New York: Harper, 1982).

6. A. Flexner, "Medical Education in the United States and Canada: A Report to the Carnegie Foundation for the Advancement of Teaching; Bulletin No 4" (New York: Carnegie Foundation for the Advancement of Teaching, 1910). Although most historical accounts concerning medical education treat Flexner and his report with reverence (e.g., J. R. Evans, "The "Health of the Public" Approach to Medical Education," *Acad Med* 67[1992]), Flexner was an unemployed schoolteacher with no medical background, poorly qualified to evaluate medical education. He achieved the position of undertaking such an evaluation through personal connections and conducted the study in a cursory manner. The influence of his report depended less on its quality than on the fact that it promoted the agendas of the Carnegie and Rockefeller Foundations and of the AMA to further the dominance of allopathic medicine and by limiting the number of physicians, the economic health of the AMA's members. (M. D. Hiatt, "Around the Continent in 180 Days: The Controversial Journey of Abraham Flexner," *The Pharos* Winter [1999]; M. D. Hiatt and C. G. Stockton, "The Impact of the Flexner Report on the Fate of Medical Schools in North America after 1909," *J Am Phys Surg* 8[2003]).

7. V. A. Harden, "A Short History of the National Institues of Health," http://history.nih.gov/exhibits/history/.

8. L. Thomas, *The Youngest Science. Notes of a Medicine Watcher* (New York: Penguin Books, 1983).

9. J. B. Wyngaarden, "The Clinical Investigator as an Endangered Species," *N Engl J Med* 301(1979); A Schafer, *The Vanishing Physician-Scientist?* (Ithaca, NY: Cornell University Press, 2009).

10. M. Movsesian, "Intramural Conflicts of Interest Warrant Scrutiny, Too," *Nat Med* 17, no. 5 (2011).

11. S. W. Glickman et al., "Ethical and Scientific Implications of the Globalization of Clinical Research," *N Engl J Med* 360(2009).

12. G. Suntharalingam et al., "Cytokine Storm in a Phase 1 Trial of the Anti-Cd28 Monoclonal Antibody Tgn1412," *N Engl J Med* 355(2006).

13. E. Horstmann et al., "Risks and Benefits of Phase I Oncology Trials, 1991 through 2002," *N Engl J Med* 352(2005).

14. K. J. Rothman, "Conflict of Interest: The New McCarthyism in Science," *JAMA* 269(1993).

15. T. P. Stossel, "Regulating Academic-Industry Research Relationships—Solving Problems or Stifling Progress," *N Engl J Med* 353(2005).

16. R. Lesko, S. Scott, and T. P. Stossel, "Bias in High-Tier Medical Journals Concerning Physician-Academic Relations with Industry," *Nat Biotechnol* 30(2012).

17. R. Steinbrook and B. Lo, "Medical Journals and Conflicts of Interest," *J Law Med Ethics* 40(2012).

18. D. J. Boorstin, *The Discoverers: A History of Man's Search to Know His World and Himself* (New York: Random House, 1983).

19. R. K. Merton, "Priorities in Scientific Discovery," *Am Sociol Rev* 22(1957).

20. See R. Smith, "The Trouble with Medical Journals," *J Roy Soc Med* 99(2006), for an exposition of this viewpoint.

21. D. A. Kronick, *A History of Scientific and Technical Periodicals* (New York: Scarecrow Press, 1976).

22. Academics complain about the abuse of journal impact factors (T. C. Ha, S. B. Tan, and K. C. Soo, "The Journal Impact Factor: Too Much of an Impact?" *Ann Acad Med Singapore* 35, no. 12 (2006); F. Hecht, B. K. Hecht, and A. A. Sandberg, "The Journal 'Impact Factor': A Misnamed, Misleading, Misused Measure," *Cancer Genet Cytogenet* 104, no. 2 (1998); American Society for Cell Biology, "Scientific Insurgents Say 'Journal Impact Factors' Distort Science"; ScienceDaily, www.sciencedaily.com/releases/2013/05/130516142537.htm), but even absent their existence, which simply numerically formalizes the prestige hierarchy of journals, the social pecking order is so well entrenched that abolishing the numbers game would have little practical effect.

23. N. S. Young, J. P. A. Ioannidis, and O. Al-Ubaydli, "Why Current Publication Practices May Distort Science: The Market for Exchange of Scientific Information: The Winner's Curse, Artificial Scarcity, and Uncertainty in Biomedical Publication," *PLoS Medicine* 5(2008).

24. L. K. Altman, "The Ingelfinger Rule, Embargoes, and Journal Peer Review—Part 2," *Lancet* 347(1986).

25. H. B. Zuckerman and R. K. Merton, "Patterns of Evaluation in Science: Institutionalisation, Structure and Functions of the Referee System," *Minerva* 9(1971).

26. T. P. Stossel, "Reviewer Status and Review Quality: Experience of the Journal of Clinical Investigation," *N Engl J Med* 312(1985); "Beyond Rejection: A User's View of Peer Review," in *Ethics and Policy in Scientific Publication*, ed. JC Bailar, Jr (Bethesda, MD: Council of Biology Editors, Inc, 1990).

27. J. P. Ioannidis, "Why Most Published Research Findings Are False," *PLoS Med* 2(2005); JPA Ioannidis, "Contradicted and Initially Stronger Effects in Highly Cited Clinical Research," *JAMA* 294(2005); JP Ioannidis, B Nosek, and E Iorns, "Reproducibility Concerns," *Nat Med* 18(2012); V Prasad et al., "A Decade of Reversal: An Analysis of 146 Contradicted Medical Practices," *Mayo Clin Proc* 88(2013); JPA Ioannidis, "How Many Contemporary Medical Practices Are Worse than Doing Nothing or Doing Less?" *Mayo Clin Proc* 88(2013).

28. F. Prinz, T. Schlange, and K. Asadullah, "Believe It or Not: How Much Can We Rely on Published Data on Potential Drug Targets?" *Nat Rev Drug Dev* (2011); CG Begley and LM Ellis, "Raise Standards for Preclinical Cancer Research," *Nature* 483(2012). Chapter 5 contrasts the rigor of FDA evaluations with the relative laxity of journal peer review.

29. J. D. Wilson, "Peer Review and Publication: Presidential Address before the 70th Annual Meeting of the American Society for Clinical Investigation, San Francisco, California, April 1978," *J Clin Invest* 61(1978).

30. Massachusetts Medical Society Form 990, 2011.

31. J. Beall, "Predatory Publishers Are Corrupting Open Access," *Nature* 489(2012); C Haug, "The Downside of Open-Access Publishing," *N Engl J Med* 368(2013).

5. ABUSING EVIDENCE

1. D. Wootton, *Bad Medicin: Doctors Doing Harm Ssince Hippocrates* (New York: Oxford University Press, 2006).

2. T. A. Brennan et al., "Health Industry Practices That Create Conflict of Interest: A Policy Proposal for Academic Medical Centers," *JAMA* 295(2006).

3. A. Schafer, "Biomedical Conflicts of Interest: A Defence of the Sequestration Thesis—Learning from the Cases of Nancy Olivieri and David Healy," *J Med Ethics* 30(2004).

4. E. G. Campbell, "Doctors and Drug Companies—Scrutinizing Influential Relationships," *N Engl J Med* 357(2007).

5. R. Steinbrook, "Financial Support of Continuing Medical Education," *JAMA* 299(2008).

6. W. Stroebe, T. Postmes, and R. Spears, "Scientific Misconduct and the Myth of Self-Correction in Science," *Persp Psychol Sci* 7(2011).

7. B. K. Redman and J. F. Merz, "Scientific Misconduct: Do the Punishments Fit the Crime? What Happens to Researchers after a Finding of Misconduct," *Science* 321(2008).

8. K. L. Woolley et al., "Lack of Involvement of Medical Writers and the Pharmaceutical Industry in Publications Retracted for Misconduct: A Systematic, Controlled, Retrospective Study," *Curr Med Res Opin* 27(2011).

9. P. G. Gosselin, "Flawed Study Helps Doctors Profit on Drug," *Boston Globe*, 1988.

10. R. Bailey, "Is Industry-Funded Science Killing You? The Overrated Risks and Underrated Benefits of Pharmaceutical Research 'Conflicts of Interest,'" *Reason*, October 2007; Tseng, http://www.ocularsurface.com/.

11. J. R. Garber et al., "Clinical Practice Guidelines for Hypothyroidism in Adults: Cosponsored by the American Association of Clinical Endocrinologists and the American Thyroid Association," *Endocrine Pract* 18(2012).

12. M. Shuchman, *The Drug Trial: Nancy Olivieri and the Science Scandal That Rocked the Hospital for Sick Children* (Random House, 2005).

13. Compassionate use waivers allow physicians to treat particular patients with unapproved medications outside of clinical trials. http://www.fda.gov/ForPatients/Other/ExpandedAccess/ucm20041768.htm.

14. FDA News Release, "FDA Approves Ferriprox to Treat Patients with Excess Iron in the Body," http://www.fda.gov/NewsEvents/Newsroom/PressAnnouncements/ucm275814.htm.

15. A. Pepe et al., "Deferasirox: Deferiprone and Desferrioxamine Treatment in Thalassemia Major Patients: Cardiac Iron and Function Comparison Determined by Quantitative Magnetic Resonance Imaging," *Haematologica* 96(2011).

16. R. Horton, "The Dawn of Mcscience, March 11," *The New York Review*, March 11, 2004; C Seife, "Is Drug Research Trustworthy?" *Sci Am*, December 2012.

17. D. E. Zinner et al., "Participation of Academic Scientists in Relationships with Industry," *Health Aff* 28(2009).

18. N. Ackerley et al., "Measuring Conflict of Interest and Expertise on FDA Advisory Committees," Eastern Research Group, October 26, 2007, http://www.fda.gov/oc/advisory/ERGCOIreport.pdf.

19. *Leenan v. Canadian Broadcasting System et al.*, 54 O.R. (3d) 612.

20. S. Johnson et al., "*Estate of Gelsinger v. Trustees of University of Pennsylvania*," in *Health Law and Bioethics: Cases in Context* (Aspen Publishers, 2009).

21. D. E. Zinner et al., "Tightening Conflict-of-Interest Policies: The Impact of 2005 Ethics Rules at the NIH," *Acad Med* 85(2010).

22. M. M. Gottesman and H. Beckerman, "Comment: A Delicate Balance: Weighing the Effects of Conflict-of-Interest Rules on Intramural Research at the National Institutes of Health," *Acad Med* 85(2010).

23. J. Kaiser, "Forty-Four Researchers Broke NIH Consulting Rules," *Science* 309(2005).

24. T Agres, "Senior NIH Researcher Pleads Guilty," *TheScientist*(2006), http://www.the-scientist.com/?articles.view/articleNo/24591/title/Senior-NIH-researcher-pleads-guilty/; V. Sharav, "NIMH Scientist Charged with Criminal Conflict of Interest," (2011), http://www.ahrp.org/cms/content/view/405/119/.

25. E. Mühe, "Long-Term Follow-up after Laparoscopic Cholecystectomy," *Endoscopy* 24(1992); D. A. Osborne et al., "Laparscopic Cholecystectomy: Past, Present, and Future," *Surg Technol Int* 15(2006).

26. J. E. Muller, P. H. Stone, and E. Braunwald, "Let's Not Let the Genie Escape from the Bottle—Again," *N Engl J Med 304* (1981).

27. H. M. Marks, *The Progress of Experiment: Science and Therapeutic Reform in the United States, 1900–1990* (New York: Oxford University Press, 1997).

28. C. V. Phillips, "Commentary: Lack of Scientific Influences on Epidemiology," *Int J Epidemiol* 33(2008).

29. Marks, *The Progress of Experiment: Science and Therapeutic Reform in the United States, 1900–1990*.

30. D. Karpman, "Management of Shiga Toxin-Associated Escherichia Coli-Induced Haemolytic Uraemic Syndrome: Randomized Clinical Trials Are Needed," *Nephrol Dial Transplant* 27(2012).

31. S. Brownlee, "Doctors without Borders: Why You Can't Trust Medical Journals Any More," *Washington Monthly*, April 2004; S. Brownlee and J. Lenzer, "Does the Vaccine Matter?" *Atlantic*, November 2009; "Tamiflu: Myth and Misconception," *Atlantic*, February 19, 2013; J. Lenzer, "Why We Can't Trust Clinical Guidelines," *BMJ* 346(2013).

32. The PLoS Medicine Editors, "A New Policy on Tobacco Papers," *PLoS Med* 7(2010); F. Godlee et al., "Journal Policy on Research Funded by the Tobacco Industry," *BMJ* 347(2013).

33. R. Smith, "Arguments against Publishing Tobacco Funded Research Also Apply to Drug Industry Funded Research," *BMJ* 347(2013).

34. J. Yaphe et al., "The Association between Funding by Commercial Interests and Study Outcome in Randomized Controlled Drug Trials," *Fam Pract* 18(2001); L. L. Kjaergard and B. Als-Nielsen, "Association between Competing Interests and Authors' Conclusions: Epidemiologic Study of Randomised Clinical Trials Published in the BMJ," *BMJ* 325(2002); C. B. Baker et al., "Quantitative Analysis of Sponsorship Bias in Economic Studies of Antidepressants," *Br J Psychiatry* 183(2003); B. Als-Nielsen et al., "Association of Funding and Con-

clusions in Randomized Drug Trials: A Reflection of Treatment Effect or Adverse Events?" *JAMA* 290(2003); TE Finucane and CE Boult, "Association of Funding and Findings of Pharmaceutical Research at a Meeting of a Medical Professional Society," *Am J Med* 117(2004); L. S. Friedman and E. D. Richter, "Relationship between Conflicts of Interest and Research Results," *J Gen Intern Med* 19(2004); R. H. Perlis et al., "Industry Sponsorship and Financial Conflict of Interest in the Reporting of Clinical Trials in Psychiatry," *Am J Psychiatry* 162(2005); A. W. Jørgensen J. Hilden, and P. C. Gøtzsche, "Cochrane Reviews Compared with Industry Supported Meta-Analyses and Other Meta-Analyses of the Same Drugs: Systematic Review," *BMJ* 333(2006); T. Tungaraza and R. Poole, "Influence of Drug Company Authorship and Sponsorship on Drug Trial Outcomes," *Br J Pschiatry* 191(2007); J. Peppercorn et al., "Association between Pharmaceutical Involvement and Outcomes in Breast Cancer Clinical Trials," *Cancer* 109(2007); L. I. Lesser et al., "Relationship between Funding Source and Conclusion among Nutrition-Related Scientific Articles," *PLoS Med* 4(2007); J. Bekelman, Y. Li, and C. P. Gross, "Scope and Impact of Financial Conflicts of Interest in Biomedical Research: A Systematic Review," *JAMA* 289(2003); J. Lexchin et al., "Pharmaceutical Industry Sponsorship and Research Outcome and Quality: Systematic Review," *BMJ* 326(2003); R. V. Shah et al., "Industry Support and Correlation to Study Outcome for Papers Published in Spine," *Spine* 30(2005); J. J. Fenton et al., "Variation in Reported Safety of Lumbar Interbody Fusion: Influence of Industrial Sponsorship and Other Study Characteristics," *Spine* 32(2007); V. M. Montori et al., "Users' Guide to Detecting Misleading Claims in Clinical Research Reports," *BMJ* 329(2004).

35. To address this reluctance, a journal named *The Journal of Negative Results in Biomedicine* was founded in 2002 and publishes what it considers to be compelling findings that contradict dogma or earlier claims.

36. N. A. Khan et al., "Association of Industry Funding with the Outcome and Quality of Randomized Controlled Trials of Drug Therapy for Rheumatoid Arthritis," *Arthritis Rheum* 64(2012); G. M. Bariani et al., "Self-Reported Conflicts of Interest of Authors, Trial Sponsorship, and the Interpretation of Editorials and Related Phase III Trials in Oncology," *J Clin Oncol* 31(2013); A. Aneja et al., "Authors' Self-Declared Financial Conflicts of Interest Do Not Impact the Results of Major Cardiovascular Trials," *JACC* 61(2013).

37. L. Bero et al., "Factors Associated with Findings of Published Trials of Drug-Drug Comparisons: Why Some Statins Appear More Efficacious than Others," *PLoS Med* 4(2007); H. Melander et al., "Evidence-B(I)Ased Medicine— Selective Reporting from Studies Sponsored by Pharmaceutical Industry: Review of Studies in New Drug Applications," *BMJ* 326(2003); M. R. Cunningham et al., "Industry-Funded Positive Studies Not Associated with Better Design or Larger Size," *Clin Orthop Relat Res* 457(2007); M. Wynia and D. Boren, "Better

Regulation of Industry-Sponsored Clinical Trials Is Long Overdue," *J Law Med Ethics* 37(2009).

38. B. Djulbegovic et al., "The Uncertainty Principle and Industry-Sponsored Research," *Lancet* 356(2000); PM Ridker and J Torres, "Reported Outcomes in Major Cardiovascular Clinical Trials Funded by For-Profit and Not-for-Profit Organizations: 2000-2005," *JAMA* 295(2006); A. Del Parigi, "Industry Funded Clinical Trials: Bias and Quality," *Curr Med Res Opin* 28(2012); Khan et al., "Association of Industry Funding with the Outcome and Quality of Randomized Controlled Trials of Drug Therapy for Rheumatoid Arthritis; F. E. Vera-Badillo et al., "Bias in Reporting of End Points of Efficacy and Toxicity in Randomized, Clinical Trials for Women with Breast Cancer," *Ann Oncol* 24(2013).

39. B. Goldacre, *Bad Pharma: How Drug Companies Mislead Doctors and Harm Patients* (London, UK: Fourth Estate, 2012).

40. J. N. Weinstein et al., "Surgical Compared with Nonoperative Treatment for Lumbar Degenerative Spondylolisthesis," *J Bone Joint Surg* 91(2009); K. H. Bridwell et al., "Does Treatment (Nonoperative and Operative) Improve Two-Year Quality of Life in Patients with Adult Symptomatic Lumbar Scoliosis?" *Spine* 34(2009).

41. E. J. Carragee, E. L. Hurwitz, and B. K. Weiner, "A Critical Review of Recombinant Human Bone Morphogenetic Protein-2 Trials in Spinal Surgery: Emerging Safety Concerns and Lessons Learned," *The Spine J* 11(2011); E. J. Carragee et al., "A Challenge to Integrity in Spine Publications: Years of Living Dangerously with the Promotion of Bone Growth Factors," *The Spine J* 11(2011); S. K. Mirza, "Commentary: Folly of FDA-Approval Studies for Bone Morphogenetic Protein," *The Spine J* 11(2011).

42. C. Weaver, "Studies Fail to Back Medtronic Spine Product," *Wall Street Journal*, June 18, 2013.

43. United States Senate Committee on Finance, "Staff Report on Medtronics Influence on Infuse Clinical Studies," 2012.

44. Medtronic, "Medtronic Response to Senate Finance Committee Staff Report on Infuse Bone Graft," http://investorrelations.medtronic.com/phoenix.zhtml?c=251324&p=irol-newsArticle&ID=1771301.

45. R. Young, "Infuse, Parts I and II," *Orthopedics This Week* 7(2011).

46. M. C. Simmonds et al., "Safety and Effectiveness of Recombinant Human Bone Morphogenetic Protein-2 for Spinal Fusion," *Ann Int Med* 158(2013); R. Fu et al., "Effectiveness and Harms of Recombinant Human Bone Morphogenetic Protein-2 in Spine Fusion," *Ann Int Med* 158(2013).

47. C. Laine et al., "Closing In on the Truth about Recombinant Human Bone Morphogenetic Protein-2: Evidence Synthesis, Data Sharing, Peer Review, and Reproducible Research," *Ann Int Med* 158(2013).

48. H. M. Krumholz et al., "A Historic Moment for Open Science: The Yale University Open Data Access Project and Medtronic," *Ann Int Med* 158(2013).

49. R. E. Kuntz, "The Changing Structure of Industry-Sponsored Clinical Research: Pioneering Data Sharing and Transparency," *Ann Int Med* 158(2013).

50. D. Resnick and K. J. Bozic, "Meta-Analysis of Trials of Recombinant Human Bone Morphogenetic Protein-2: What Should Spine Surgeons and Their Patients Do with the Information?" *Ann Int Med* 158(2013).

51. J. M. Barry, *The Great Influenza: The Epic Story of the Greatest Plague in History* (Viking, 2004).

52. T. M. Uyeki, "Preventing and Controlling Influenza with Available Interventions," *N Engl J Med* 370(2014).

53. Centers for Disease Control and Prevention, "Seasonal Influenza (Flu)," http://www.cdc.gov/flu/pastseasons/1213season.htm.

54. US Food and Drug Administration, "Tamiflu (Oseltamvir Phosphate) Information," http://www.fda.gov/Drugs/DrugSafety/PostmarketDrugSafetyInformationforPatientsandProviders/ucm107838.htm.

55. F. Godlee, "Withdraw Approval for Tamflu until Nice Has Full Data," *BMJ* 345(2012).

56. J. Smith, "Point-by-Point Response from Roche to BMJ Questions," *BMJ* 339(2009).

57. T. Jefferson et al., "Neuraminidase Inhibitors for Preventing and Treating Influenza in Healthy Adults and Children," *Cochrane Database Sys Rev.* Apr 10;4:CD008965 (2014).

58. B. Clinch, "Oseltamivir for Influenza in Adults and Children: Systematic Review of Clinical Study Reports and Summary of Regulatory Comments," *BMJ* 348, no. g2545 (2014).

6. BAD POLICY PROCESS

1. P. T. Bauer, *Reality and Rhetoric: Studies in the Economics of Development* (Cambridge, MA: Harvard University Press, 1984).

2. M. Olson, *The Logic of Collective Action* (Cambridge, MA: Harvard University Press, 1971).

3. T. Kuran and C. R. Sunstein, "Availability Cascades and Risk Regulation," *Stanford Law Rev* 51, no. 4 (1999).

4. C. R. Sunstein, "Deliberative Trouble? Why Groups Go to Extremes," *Yale Law J* 110(2000).

5. W. H. Riker, "The Political Psychology of Rational Choice Theory," *Polit Psychol* 16(1995).

6. W. Broad and N. Wade, *Betrayers of the Truth: Fraud and Deceit in the Halls of Science* (New York: Simon & Schuster, 1982).

7. Commission on Research Integrity, "Integrity and Misconduct in Research," 1995, http://ori.hhs.gov/images/ddblock/report_commission.pdf.

8. S. C. Silverstein, "Letter to Kenneth John Ryan, Chairman of the Commission on Research Integrity," (1995).

9. A. Stark, *Conflict of Interest in American Public Life* (Cambridge, MA: Harvard University Press, 2000).

10. M. Angell, "Is Academic Medicine for Sale?" *N Engl J Med* 342(2000).

11. J. Jacobs, *Systems of Survival* (New York: Vintage, 1992).

12. D. Thompson, "Understanding Financial Conflicts of Interest," *N Engl J Med* 329(1993).

13. T. A. Brennan et al., "Health Industry Practices That Create Conflict of Interest: A Policy Proposal for Academic Medical Centers," *JAMA* 295(2006).

14. J. S. Mill, *Utilitarianism* (New York: Oxford University Press, 1998).

15. L. K. Stell, "Drug Reps Off Campus! Promoting Professional Purity by Suppressing Commercial Speech," *J Law Med Ethics* 37(2009).

16. President and Fellows of Harvard College, "Harvard University Policy on Individual Financial Conflicts of Interest for Persons Holding Faculty and Teaching Appointments," 2012.

17. L. I. Lesser et al., "Relationship between Funding Source and Conclusion among Nutrition-Related Scientific Articles," *PLoS Med* 4(2007).

18. M. B. Cope and D. B. Allison, "White Hat Bias: A Threat to the Integrity of Scientific Reporting," *Acta Paediatrica* 99(2010).

19. M. Movsesian, "Intramural Conflicts of Interest Warrant Scrutiny, Too," *Nat Med* 17, no. 5 (2011).

20. L. L. Fuller, *The Morality of Law* (New Haven, CT: Yale University Press, 1964).

21. "Responsibility of Applicants for Promoting Objectivity in Research for Which PHS Funding Is Sought," in 42 CFR Part 50, Subpart F, ed. National Institutes of Health (2011); National Institutes of Health, "Conflict of Interest Regulations," (1995); SJ Rockey and FS Collins, "Managing Financial Conflict of Interest in Biomedical Research," *JAMA* 303(2010).

22. D. K. Jones et al., "Conflict of Interest Ethics: Silencing Expertise in the Development of International Clinical Practice Guidelines," *Ann Int Med* 156(2012).

23. P. Lurie et al., "Financial Conflict of Interest Disclosure and Voting Patterns at Food and Drug Administration Drug Advisory Committee Meetings," *JAMA* 295(2006); N Ackerley et al., "Measuring Conflict of Interest and Expertise on FDA Advisory Committees," (2007).

24. Food and Drug Administration Safety and Innovation Act of 2012.

25. N. Singer, "Stanford Medical School to Expand Ethics Rules," *New York Times*, March 21, 2010; DC Brater, "Viewpoint: Infusing Professionalism into a School of Medicine: Perspectives from the Dean," *Acad Med* 82(2007).

26. K. J. Arrow, *The Limits of Organization* (Norton, 1974).

27. F. Fukuyama, *Trust: The Social Virtues and the Creation of Prosperity* (Simon & Schuster, 1995); KS Cook and RM Cooper, "Experimental Studies of Cooperation, Trust and Social Exchange," in *Trust and Reciprocity: Interdisciplinary Lessons for Experimental Research*, ed. E Ostrom and J Walker (New York: Russell Sage Foundation, 2003).

28. D. L. Philips, *Knowledge from What? Theories and Methods in Social Research* (Chicago: Rand McNally and Company, 1971).

29. D. Grande, J. A. Shea, and K. Armstrong, "Pharmaceutical Industry Gifts to Physicians: Patient Beliefs and Trust in Physicians and the Health Care System," *J Gen Int Med* 27(2011).

30. A. Licurse et al., "The Impact of Disclosing Financial Ties in Research and Clinical Care," *Arch Int Med* 170(2010).

31. P. Starr, *The Social Transformation of American Medicine* (New York: Harper, 1982).

32. J. Jones, "Record 64% Rate Honesty, Ethics of Members of Congress Low. Ratings of Nurses, Pharmacists, and Medical Doctors Most Positive," *Gallop Politics*(2011), http://www.gallup.com/poll/151460/record-rate-honesty-ethics-members-congress-low.aspx.

33. Research!America, "America Speaks: Poll Data Summary, Volume 5," 2004; "America Speaks: Poll Data Summary, Volume 11," 2010.

34. L. A. Hampson et al., "Patients' Views on Financial Conflicts of Interest in Cancer Research Trials," *N Engl J Med* 355(2006); SW Gray et al., "Attitudes toward Research Participation and Investigator Conflicts of Interest among Advanced Cancer Patients Participating in Early Phase Clinical Trials," *J Clin Oncol* 25(2007).

35. C. Grady et al., "The Limits of Disclosure: What Research Subjects Want to Know About Investigator Financial Interests," *J Law Med Ethics* 34(2006).

36. A. S. Kesselheim et al., "A Randomized Study of How Physicians Interpret Research Funding Disclosures," *N Engl J Med* 367(2012).

37. J. M. Drazen, "Believe the Data," *N Engl J Med* 367(2012).

38. P. Kritek and E. W. Campion, "Jupiter Clinical Directions—Polling Results," *N Engl J Med* 360(2009).

7. FLAWED AND DAMAGING POLICIES

1. "Sir Kenneth Murray Leaves Millions in Will," *BBC News Edinburgh, Fife & East Scotland*(2014), http://www.bbc.com/news/uk-scotland-tayside-central-25883640.

2. "Harvard University Policy on Individual Financial Interest for Persons Holding Faculty and Teaching Appointments," 2010.

3. D. Wootton, *Bad Medicine: Doctors Doing Harm since Hippocrates* (Oxford, New York: Oxford University Press, 2006).

4. P. B. Fontanarosa and C. D. De Angelis, "Conflicts of Interest and Independent Data Analysis in Industry-Funded Studies," *JAMA* 294(2005).

5. E. Wager et al., "*JAMA* Published Fewer Industry-Funded Studies after Introducing a Requirement for Independent Statistical Analysis," *PLoS One* 5, no. 10 (2010).

6. The editorial announcing the retraction of the special statistical analysis policy framed the announcement with all of the alleged validity problems that originally prompted the policy, such as publication bias, failure to prespecify outcomes, failure to distinguish between primary and secondary outcomes, failure to differentiate between prespecified and post hoc analyses—and research misconduct. Although the rhetoric implies that these transgressions are unique to industry-sponsored research, they are in fact, common to the medical scientific enterprise generally. The available evidence, reviewed in chapter 4, suggests that most of them arise from pressure to get articles into journals like *JAMA*, with their artificial scarcity. While stepping back from the arbitrary requirement of independent statistical analysis, the *JAMA* editorial articulated a preference for studies evaluated by an academic statistician and that the articles and analyses should be conducted by academics as a rule. The editorial also stated that *JAMA* has "reserve[d] the right to request the entire data set from authors to conduct our own analysis." Chapters 4 and 5 discussed how medical journals hardly have the resources to conduct such an investigation. Their hubris relegates this policy change to a reactive effort to recover lost business without conceding that the ideological justifications for the previous policy were not empirically sound. H Bauchner, "Editorial Policies for Clinical Trials and the Continued Changes in Medical Journalism," *JAMA* 173(213).

7. L. Morris and J. K. Taitsman, "The Agenda for Continuing Medical Education—Limiting Industry's Influence," *N Engl J Med* 361(2009).

8. R. M. Cervero and J. He, "Final Report: The Relationship between Commercial Support and Bias in Continuing Medical Education Activities: A Review of the Literature" (Accreditation Council on Continuing Medical Education, 2008); J. A. Ellison et al., "Low Rates of Reporting Commercial Bias by Physicians Following Online Continuing Medical Education Activities," *Am J Med*

122(2009); MA Steinman et al., "Commercial Influence and Learner-Perceived Bias in Continuing Medical Education," *Acad Med* 85(2010); S Kawczak et al., "The Effect of Industry Support on Participants' Perception of Bias in Continuing Medical Education," *Acad Med* 85(2010).

9. M. A. Steinman et al., "Commercial Influence and Learner-Perceived Bias in Continuing Medical Education," *Acad Med* 85(2010).

10. Association of American Medical Colleges, "Protecting Subjects, Preserving Trust, Promoting Progress: Policy and Guidelines for the Oversight of Individual Financial Interests in Human Subjects Research" (Washington, DC, 2001).

11. In the past, companies subsidized travel and other expenses of U.S. physicians to attend professional meetings as well. Industry trade group codes in the 1990s recommended against this practice, and it ceased, although it persists abroad.

12. R. A. Spence, "American Society of Clinical Oncology: Policy for Relationships with Companies," *J Clin Oncol* 31(2013).

13. "American Society of Clinical Oncology Policy for Relationships with Companies: Background and Rationale," *J Clin Oncol* 31(2013); AC Lockhart et al., "Physician and Stakeholder Perceptions of Conflict of Interest Policies in Oncology," *J Clin Oncol* 31(2013).

14. K. M. Ludmerer, *Time to Heal: American Medical Education from the Turn of the Century to the Era of Managed Care* (Oxford: Oxford University Press, 1999).

15. C. R. Flowers and K. L. Melmon, "Clinical Investigators as Critical Determinants in Pharmaceutical Innovation," *Nat Med* 2(1997).

16. P. Whorisky, "Antidepressants to Treat Grief? Panel with Ties to Drug Industry Says Yes," *Washington Post*, December 28, 2012.

17. W. Eisner, "David Polly, MD—the Rest of the Story," *Orthopedics This Week—Legal and Regulatory*, December 26, 2011.

18. B. Moffatt and C. Elliott, "Ghost Marketing: Pharmaceutical Companies and Ghostwritten Journal Articles," *Persp Biol Med* 50(2007); S. Sisimondo, "Ghost Management: How Much of the Medical Literature Is Shaped Behind the Scenes by the Pharmaceutical Industry?" *PLoS Med* 4(2007); T. Anekwe, "Profits and Plagiarism: The Case of Medical Ghostwriting," *Bioethics* 24(2010); J. S. Ross et al., "Guest Authorship and Ghostwriting in Publications Related to Rofecoxib: A Case Study of Industry Documents from Rofecoxib Litigation," *JAMA* 299(2008).

19. E. Braunwald, "On Analyzing Scientific Fraud," *Nature* 325(1987).

20. J. S. Wislar et al., "Honorary and Ghost Authorship in High Impact Biomedical Journals: A Cross Sectional Survey," *BMJ* 343(2011).

21. International Society for Medical Publication Professionals, "Code of Ethics," http://www.ismpp.org/ethics.

22. Ross et al., "Guest Authorship and Ghostwriting in Publications Related to Rofecoxib: A Case Study of Industry Documents from Rofecoxib Litigation; LJ Hirsch, "Conflicts of Interest, Authorship, and Disclosures in Industry-Related Scientific Publications: The Tort Bar and Editorial Oversight of Medical Journals," *Mayo Clin Proc* 84(2009).

23. S. Sterns and T. Lemmens, "Legal Remedies for Medical Ghostwriting: Imposing Fraud Liability on Guest Authors of Ghostwritten Articles," *PLoS Med* 8(2011); X. Bosch, B. Esfandiari, and L. McHenry, "Challenging Medical Ghostwriting in US Courts," *PLoS Med* 9, no. 1 (2012).

24. Hirsch, "Conflicts of Interest, Authorship, and Disclosures in Industry-Related Scientific Publications: The Tort Bar and Editorial Oversight of Medical Journals."

25. F. S. Southwick, "All's Not Fair in Science and Publishing," *The Scientist*, July 1, 2012.

26. C. Elliott, *White Coat Black Hat: Adventures on the Dark Side of Medicine* (Boston: Beacon Press, 2010).

27. One *New York Times* report, however, insinuated such a lack of author responsibility. The news item concerned results of a clinical trial published in *The Annals of Internal Medicine* in 2003 (J. R. Lisse et al., "Gastrointestinal Tolerability and Effectiveness of Rofecoxib versus Napoxen in the Treatment of Osteoarthritis," *Ann Int Med* 139(2003)). The *Times* article quoted the first listed author of the *Annals* paper, an arthritis specialist at the University of Arizona, as stating (A Berenson, "Evidence in Vioxx Suit Shows Intervention by Merck Officials," *New York Times*, April 24, 2005): "Merck designed the trial, paid for the trial, ran the trial. . . . Merck came to me after the study was completed and said, 'We want your help to work on the paper.' The initial paper was written at Merck, and then it was sent to me for editing." Conflict-of-interest movement promoters seized on the comment as evidence for flagrant ghostwriting. But the *Annals* paper author, with whom I conversed by telephone, *had* actually participated in the clinical trial in question by enrolling patients and also had extensive interactions with the Merck clinical trial management team during the course of the trial. He believes that his contributions to the study were substantive and merited authorship.

28. M. Y. Peay and E. R. Peay, "The Role of Commercial Sources in the Adoption of a New Drug," *Soc Sci Med* 26(1988); R. F. Adair and L. R. Holmgren, "Do Drug Samples Influence Resident Prescribing Behavior?" *Am J Med* 118(2005); D. M. Hartung et al., "Effect of Drug Sample Removal on Prescribing in a Family Practice Clinic," *Ann Fam Med* 8(2010); J. M. Boltri, E. R. Gordon, and R. L. Vogel, "Effect of Antihypertensive Samples on Physician

Prescribing Patterns," *Fam Med* 34(2002); D. Brewer, "The Effect of Drug Sampling Solicits on Residents' Prescribing," *Fam Med* 30(1998); L. D. Chew et al., "A Physician Survey on Effect of Drug Sample Availability on Physicians' Behavior," *J Gen Int Med* 15(2000); R. G. Pinckney et al., "The Effect of Medication Samples on Self-Reported Prescribing Practices: A Statewide Cross-Sectional Survey," *J Gen Int Med* 26(2011).

29. D. Myers, "Conflict-of-Interest Policy Tightened and Clarified," *CU Medicine Today* 2012.

8. MISUNDERSTANDING INNOVATION

1. J. W. Scannell et al., "Diagnosing the Decline in Pharmaceutical R&D Efficiency," *Nat Rev Drug Discovery* 11(2012).

2. K. A. Getz et al., "Assessing the Impact of Protocol Design Changes on Clinical Trial Performance," *Am J Ther* 15(2008).

3. J. Arrowsmith, "Phase III and Submission Failures: 2007-2010," *Nat Rev Drug Disc* 10(2011); M. Hay et al., "Clinical Development Success Rates for Investigational Drugs," *Nat Biotechnol* 32(2014); I. Kola and J. Landis, "Can the Pharmaceutical Industry Reduce Attrition Rates?" *Nat Rev Drug Discov* 3(2004).

4. A. Cordiero and P. Loftus, "Warner Chilcott to Pay $3.1 Billion for P&G's Drug Business," *Wall Street Journal*, August 25, 2012.

5. J. D. Rockoff and A. Mattioli, "Build It or Buy It? Drug Bid Puts R&D in Focus," *Wall Street Journal*, June 11, 2014.

6. I. M. Cockburn and R. M. Henderson, "Scale and Scope in Drug Development: Unpacking the Advantages of Size in Pharmaceutical Resesarch," *J Health Econ* 20(2001).

7. J. Drews, "Drug Discovery: A Historical Perspective," *Science* 287(2000); DF Horrobin, "Innovation in the Pharmaceutical Industry," *J Roy Soc Med* 93(2000); "Realism in Drug Discovery—Could Cassandra Be Right?" *Nat Biotechnol* 19(2001); P Cuatrecasas, "Drug Discovery in Jeopardy," *J Clin Invest* 116(2006); B Munos, "Lessons from 60 Years of Pharmaceutical Innovation," *Nat Rev Drug Discovery* 8(2009).

8. Novartis, "Novartis Announces Portfolio Transformation, Focusing Company on Leading Businesses with Innovation Power and Global Scale: Pharmaceuticals, Eye Care and Generics," http://www.novartis.com/newsroom/media-releases/en/2014/1778515.shtml.

9. G. P. Pisano, *Science Business: The Promise, the Reality, and the Future of Biotech* (Harvard Business School Press, 2006).

10. R. S. Williams and S. Desmond-Hellman, "Making Translation Work," *Science* 332(2011); S. Olson and A. B. Claiborne, "Workshop Summary: Accel-

erating the Development of New Drugs and Diagnostics: Maximizing the Impact of the Cures, Acceleration Network, Forum on Drug Discovery, Development, and Translation," in *Board on Health Sciences Policy* (Washington, DC: Institute of Medicine, 2012); "National Dialogue for Healthcare Innovation," http://www. hlc.org/special-programs/national-dialogue-for-healthcare-innovation/.

11. M. Angell, *The Truth About the Drug Companies: How They Deceive Us and What to Do About It* (New York: Random House, 2004); J. Avorn, *Powerful Medicines: The Benefits, Risks and Costs of Prescription Drugs* (New York: Alfred A Knopf, 2004); D. W. Light and J. Lexchin, "Pharmaceutical R&D. What Do We Get for All That Money?" *BMJ* 345(2012).

12. M. Angell, "Big Pharma, Bad Medicine," *Boston Rev*, May/June (2010).

13. E. Chargaff, "Voices in the Labyrinth: Dialogues around the Study of Nature," *Perpect Biol Med* 18(1975).

14. M. Polanyi, *Personal Knowledge: Towards a Post-Critical Philosophy* (Chicago: University of Chicago Press, 1958).

15. O. H. Lowry et al., "Protein Measurement with the Folin Phenol Reagent," *J Biol Chem* 193(1951).

16. T. S. Kuhn, *The Structure of Scientific Revolutions*, 2nd ed. (Chicago: University of Chicago Press, 1970); RK Merton, "Priorities in Scientific Discovery," *Am Sociol Rev* 22(1957).

17. D. G. Contopoulos-Ioannidis, E. Ntzani, and J. P. Ioannidis, "Translation of Highly Promising Basic Science Research into Clinical Applications," *Am J Med* 114(2003).

18. A. Lam, "What Motivates Academic Scientists to Engage in Research Commercialization: 'Gold,' 'Ribbon,' or 'Puzzle'?" *Res Policy* 40(2011).

19. R. Kneller, "The Origins of New Drugs," *Nat Biotechnol* 23(2005); "The Importance of New Companies for Drug Discovery: Origins of a Decade of New Drugs," *Nature Rev Drug Discovery* 9(2010).

20. B. Zycher, J. A. DiMasi, and C. P. Milne, "Private Sector Contributions to Pharmaceutical Science: Thirty-Five Summary Case Histories," *Am J Ther* 17, no. 1 (2010); BN Sampat and FR Lichtenberg, "What Are the Respective Roles of the Public and Private Sectors in Pharmaceutical Innovation?" *Health Aff* 30(2011); AJ Stevens et al., "The Role of Public-Sector Research in the Discovery of Drugs and Vaccines," *N Engl J Med* 364(2011).

21. J. D. Watson and F. H. Crick, "Molecular Structure of Nucleic Acids: A Structure for Deoxyribose Nucleic Acid," *Nature* 171(1953).

22. J. H. Comroe and R. D. Dripps, "Scientific Basis for the Support of Biomedical Science," *Science* 192(1976); H. Y. Zoghbi, "The Basics of Translation," *Science* 239(2013); M. Kirschner, "A Perverted View of 'Impact,'" *Science* 340(2013); H. I. Miller, "Basic Research Is Often Best Appreciated in Retrospect," *Nat Biotechnol* 32(2014). As a lifelong academic researcher, I have

been and continue to be an ardent supporter of research for research's sake. Even when it doesn't generate many inventions, academic research continues to define characteristics of biology and disease processes that can contribute to innovation. For example, detailed descriptions of the properties of cancers help predict how patients respond to various therapies. Researchers employed by industry operate under the expectation that their efforts must advance their companies' interests, specifically by discovering product candidates and advancing them toward development. For this reason, they operate with the expectation that company research managers will often instruct them to stop working on projects and switch their attention to other ones.

Academic researchers, on the other hand, can persistently pursue research goals that interest them (provided they can obtain funding for the work). The story recounted in this chapter illustrates my own experience about how such persistent research did—completely and unpredictably—lead to possible invention and, with additional persistence, to possible innovation. Some academic investigators, however, have no interest in translating their research into practical outlets—and that is fine. What is most important is to assure that as many varieties of research take place as possible.

23. J. G. Thursby and M. C. Thursby, "Who Is Selling the Ivory Tower? Sources of Growth in University Licensing," *Management Sci* 48(2002); L. G. Zucker, M. R. Darby, and M. Torero, "Labor Mobility from Academe to Commerce," *J Labor Econ* 20(2002).

24. J. Friedman, "Popper, Weber, and Hayek: The Epistemology and Politics of Ignorance," *Crit Rev* 17(2005).

25. I. Ösholm, *Drug Discovery: A Pharmacist's Story* (Stockholm: Swedish Pharmaceutical Press, 1995).

26. D. E. Brown, "Medicine and Healthcare," in *Inventing Modern America: From the Microwave to the Mouse* (Cambridge, MA: MIT Press, 2009).

27. J. Flood, "A Legend at Heart: Thomas Fogarty Brings His Inventive Clout to El Camino Hospital," *Los Altos Town Crier*, http://www.losaltosonline.com/news/sections/news/215-news-briefs/26261-J24709.

28. M. Herper, "How a $440,000 Drug Is Turning Alexion into Biotech's New Innovation Powerhouse," *Forbes* 2012.

29. Alexion, "Alexion's Soliris Receives 2008 Prix Galien USA Award for Best Biotechnology Product," http://www.alxn.com/News/article.aspx?relid=336880.

30. J. H. Hartwig and T. P. Stossel, "Isolation and Properties of Actin, Myosin, and a New Actin-Binding Protein in Rabbit Alveolar Macrophages," *J Biol Chem* 250(1975); T. P. Stossel and J. H. Hartwig, "Interactions of Actin, Myosin and an Actin-Binding Protein of Rabbit Alveolar Macrophages. Macrophage Myosin Mg++ -Adenosine Triphosphatase Requires a Cofactor for Activation by

Actin," *J Biol Chem* 250(1975); T. P. Stossel and J. H. Hartwig, "Interactions of Actin, Myosin and an Actin-Binding Protein of Rabbit Pulmonary Macrophages. II. Role in Cytoplasmic Movement and Phagocytosis," *J Cell Biol* 68(1976). E. A. Brotschi, J. H. Hartwig, and T. P. Stossel, "The Gelation of Actin by Actin-Binding Protein," *J Biol Chem* 253(1978); J. H. Hartwig and T. P. Stossel, "Cytochalasin B and the Structure of Actin Gels.," *J Mol Biol* 134(1979).

31. H. L. Yin and T. P. Stossel, "Control of Cytoplasmic Actin Gel-Sol Transformation by Gelsolin, a Calcium-Dependent Regulatory Protein," *Nature* 281(1979); H. L. Yin and T. P. Stossel, "Purification and Structural Properties of Gelsolin, a Ca^{2+}-Activated Regulatory Protein of Macrophages," *J Biol Chem* 255(1980); H. L. Yin, K. S. Zaner, and T. P. Stossel, "Ca^{2+} Control of Actin Gelation," *J Biol Chem* 255(1980).

32. Entrez Pub Med, "Filamin," http://www.ncbi.nlm.nih.gov/pubmed?term= filamin; "Gelsolin," http://www.ncbi.nlm.nih.gov/pubmed?term=gelsolin.

33. https://www.researchgate.net/profile/Thomas_Stossel.

34. A. W. Husari et al., "Relationship between Intensive Care Complications and Costs and Initial 24h Events of Trauma Patients with Haemorrhage," *Emerg Med* 26(2009); S. V. Desai, T. J. Law, and D. M. Needham, "Long-Term Complications of Critical Care," *Crit Care Med* 39(2011).

35. W. M. Lee and R. M. Galbraith, "The Extracellular Actin-Scavenger System and Actin Toxicity," *N Engl J Med* 326(1992).

36. CA Vasconcellos et al., "Reduction in Viscosity of Cystic Fibrosis Sputum in Vitro by Gelsolin," *Science* 263(1994).

37. K. C. Mounzer et al., "Relationship of Admission Gelsolin Levels to Clinical Outcomes in Patients after Major Trauma," *Am J Respir Crit Care Med* 160(1999).

38. M. J. DiNubile et al., "Prognostic Implications of Declining Plasma Gelsolin Levels after Allogeneic Stem Cell Transplantation," *Blood* 100(2002); P-S. Lee et al., "Relationship of Plasma Gelsolin Levels to Outcomes in Critically Ill Surgical Patients," *Ann Surg* 243(2006); P-S. Lee et al., "Plasma Gelsolin, Circulating Actin, and Chronic Hemodialysis Mortality," *JASN* 20(2009).

39. P-S. Lee et al., "Plasma Gelsolin Is a Marker and Therapeutic Agent in Animal Sepsis," *Crit Care Med* 35(2007).

40. M. Angell, "Is Academic Medicine for Sale?" *N Engl J Med* 342(2000).

41. I. Cockburn and R. Henderson, "Public-Private Interaction in Pharmaceutical Research," *Proc Nat Acad Sci USA* 93(1996).

9. ECONOMIC ILLITERACY

1. H. Brody, *Hooked: Ethics, the Medical Profession, and the Pharmaceutical Industry* (Lanham, MD: Rowman & Littlefield, 2007).

2. B. J. Druker, "Perspectives on the Development of Imatinib and the Future of Cancer Research," *Nat Med* 15(2009).

3. M. Angell, *The Truth About the Drug Companies: How They Deceive Us and What to Do About It* (New York: Random House, 2004).

4. J. Avorn, *Powerful Medicines: The Benefits, Risks and Costs of Prescription Drugs* (New York: Alfred A Knopf, 2004).

5. N. Lydon, "Attacking Cancer at Its Foundation," *Nat Med* 15(2009).

6. H. Joensuu et al., "Effect of the Tyrosine Kinase Inhibitor Sti571 in a Patient with a Metastatic Gastrointestinal Stromal Tumor," *N Engl J Med* 344(2001).

7. G. D. Demetri et al., "Efficacy and Safety of Imatinib Mesylate in Advanced Gastrointestinal Stromal Tumor," *N Engl J Med* 347(2002).

8. C. R. Flowers and K. L. Melmon, "Clinical Investigators as Critical Determinants in Pharmaceutical Innovation," *Nat Med* 2(1997).

9. D. M. Cutler et al., "The Value of Antihypertensive Drugs: A Perspective on Medical Innovation. Why Don't Americans Do Better at Controlling Hypertension, If the Societal Return on Investment Is So High?" *Health Aff* 26(2007); D. M. Cutler, A. B. Rosen, and S. Vijan, "The Value of Medical Spending in the United States, 1960–2000," *N Engl J Med* 355(2006); F. R. Lichtenberg, "Are the Benefits of Newer Drugs Worth Their Cost? Evidence from the 1996 MEPS. The Newer the Drug in Use, the Less Spending on Nondrug Items," *Health Afff* 20(2001); "The Impact of New Drug Launches on Longevity: Evidence from Longitudinal, Disease-Level Data from 52 Countries, 1982–2001," *Int J Health Care Finance Econ* 5(2005); "The Effect of Using Newer Drugs on Admissions of Elderly Americans to Hospitals and Nursing Homes: State-Level Evidence from 1997 to 2003," *Phamacoeconomics* 24 Suppl 3(2006); K. M. Murphy and R. H. Topel, "Social Value and the Speed of Innovation," *Am Econ Rev* 92, no. 2 (2006); "The Value of Health and Longevity," *J Polit Econ* 114(2006); F. Lichtenberg, "Why Has Longevity Increased More in Some States than in Others? The Role of Medical Innovation and Other Factors," in *Medical Progress Report* (New York: Manhattan Institute for Policy Research, 2007); F. R. Lichtenberg, "The Impact of New Drugs on Us: Longevity and Medical Expenditure, 1990–2003: Evidence from Longitudinal, Disease-Level Data," *Am Econ Rev* 97(2007); Häussler et al., "The Impact of Pharmaceuticals on the Decline of Cardiovascular Mortality in Germany," *Pharmacoepidemiol Drug Safety* 16(2007); F. R. Lichtenberg, "Effects of New Drugs on Overall Health Spending: Frank Lichtenberg Responds," *Health Aff* 26(2007); Y. Zhang and S. B.

Soumerai, "Do Newer Prescription Drugs Pay for Themselves? A Reassessment of the Evidence. Reanalysis of an Important Study on Drug Pricing Suggests That the Health Cost-Reducing Effects of Newer Drugs Might Have Been Overstated," *Health Aff* 26(2007); F. R. Lichtenberg, "Alive and Working: How Access to New Drugs Has Slowed the Growth in America's Disability Rates" (Manhattan Institute for Policy Research, 2008); L. C. Paramore et al., "Value of Biologic Therapy: A Forecasting Model in Three Disease Areas," *Curr Med Res Opin* 26(2010); R. E. Santerre, "National and International Tests of the New Drug Cost Offset Theory," *South Econ J* 77(2011); F. Lichtenberg, "The Quality of Medical Care, Behavioral Risk Factors, and Longevity Growth," *Int J Health Care Finance Econ* 11(2011); D. Khayat, "Innovative Cancer Therapies: Putting Costs into Context," *Cancer* 118(2012); F Lichtenberg, "Contribution of Pharmaceutical Innovation to Longevity Growth in Germany and France, 2001-2007," *Pharmacoeconomics* 30(2012); "The Impact of Therapeutic Procedure Innovation on Hospital Patient Longevity: Evidence from Western Australia," *Soc Sci Med* 77(2013).

10. D. Baker and A. Fugh-Berman, "Do New Drugs Increase Life Expectancy? A Critique of a Manhattan Institute Paper," *J Gen Intern Med* 24(2009).

11. F. R. Lichtenberg, "Do New Drugs Save Lives?" *J Gen Intern Med* 24(2009).

12. J. Abramson, *Overdosed America* (New York: HarperCollins, 2004).

13. CMS, "National Health Expenditure Data" (Centers for Medicare and Medicaid Services, 2013). Recently, physicians specializing in treating patients with potentially crippling rheumatoid arthritis warmly welcomed the FDA's approval of a new drug, because even though effective medications have become available, patients respond idiosyncratically to them, and more options result in more favorable responses. Having so reacted, however, these physicians mimicked the lack of economic sophistication of their hematologist colleagues by complaining about the pricing of new products (K. Garber, "Pfizer's First-in-Class JAK Inhibitor Pricey for Rheumatoid Arthritis Market," *Nat Biotechnol* 31, no. 1 [2013]). Similar complaints invoking quantitatively unsupported references to "social justice" and societal "unsustainability" followed the FDA approval of a novel high-priced drug to treat the genetic disease cystic fibrosis. Among the complainants were physicians who were paid consultants of the company that developed the drug (B. P. O'Sullivan, D. M. Orenstein, and C. E. Milla, "Pricing for Orphan Drugs: Will the Market Bear What Society Cannot?" *JAMA* 310(2013)). The most recent objections to the pricing of lifesaving drugs concern stunningly effective medications for hepatitis C that ultimately reduce health care expenditures by eliminating hospitalizations and other costs previously incurred by this chronic disease (R. Steinbrook and R. F. Redberg, "The High Price of the New Hepatitis C Virus Drugs," *JAMA Internal Medicine* [2014]).

Unsurprisingly, health insurers are among the lead complainers (R Weisman, "Demand for Expensive Hepatitis C Drugs Strains Insurers," *The Boston Globe* 2014).

14. E. Rosenthal, "For Medical Tourists, Simple Math. US Estimate for a New Hip: Over $78,000. The Belgian Bill: $13,660," *New York Times*, August 4, 2013.

15. A. Pollack, "Doctors Denounce Cancer Drug Prices of $100,000 a Year," *New York Times*, April 26, 2013.

16. Experts in chronic myeloid leukemia, "The Price of Drugs for Chronic Myeloid Leukemia (CML); a Reflection of the Unsustainable Prices of Cancer Drugs: From the Perspective of a Large Group of CML Experts," *Blood* (2013).

17. B. Caplan, *The Myth of the Rational Voter: Why Democracies Choose Bad Policies* (Princeton, NJ: Princeton University Press, 2007).

18. T. C. De Campos and T. Pogge, "Pharmaceutical Firms and the Right to Health," *J Law Med Ethics* 40(2012).

19. L. von Mises, *Socialism: An Economic and Sociological Analysis (1922)*, trans. J. Kahane (Indianapolis: Liberty Fund, 1969); F. A. Hayek, "The Uses of Knowledge in Society," *Am Econ Rev* 35(1945).

20. C. S. Hemphill and B. N. Sampat, "Evergreening, Patent Challenges, and the Effective Market Life in Pharmaceuticals," *J Health Econ* 31(2012).

21. M. J. Higgins and S. J. H. Graha, "Balancing Innovation and Access: Patent Challenges Tip the Scales," *Science* 326(2009).

22. Doctors Without Borders, "Campaign for Access to Essential Medicines," (2007).

23. M. Kremer, "Pharmaceuticals and the Developing World," *J Econ Perspectives* 16(2002); P. A. Danzon and A. Towse, "Differential Pricing for Pharmaceuticals: Reconciling Access, R&D and Patents," *Int J Health Care Finance Econ* 3(2003).

24. J. A. DiMasi et al., "Cost of Innovation in the Pharmaceutical Industry," *J Health Econ* 10(1991); "Research and Development Costs for New Drugs by Therapeutic Category: A Study of the US Pharmaceutical Industry," *PharmacoEconomics* 7(1995); J. A. DiMasi, R. W. Hansen, and H. G. Grabowski, "The Price of Innovation: New Estimates of Drug Development Costs," *Health Econ* 22(2003); J. DiMasi and H. G. Grabowski, "The Cost of Biopharmaceutical R&D: Is Biotech Different?" *Managerial Decision Econ* 28(2007); J. A. Dimasi et al., "Trends in Risks Associated with New Drug Development: Success Rates for Investigational Drugs," *Clin Pharmacol Ther* 87(2010); Ed Silverman, "Developing a Drug Costs $2.6 Billion, but not Everyone Believes This," *The Wall Street Journal: Pharmalot*(2014), http://blogs.wsj.com/pharmalot/2014/11/18/developing-a-drug-costs-2-6-billion-but-not-everyone-believes-this/.

25. J. A. Vernon, J. H. Golec, and J. A. DiMasi, "Drug Development Costs When Financial Risk Is Measured Using the Fama-French Three-Factor Model," *Health Econ* (2009); J. W. Scannell et al., "Diagnosing the Decline in Pharmaceutical R&D Efficiency," *Nat Rev Drug Discovery* 11(2012); J-M. Fernandez, R. M. Stein, and A. W. Lo, "Commercializing Biomedical Research through Securitization Techniques," *Nat Biotechnol* 30(2012).

26. "Fortune 500 Index," (2013), http://money.cnn.com/magazines/fortune/fortune500/2013/full_list/index.html?iid=F500_sp_full.

27. C. P. Adams and V. V. Brantner, "Estimating the Cost of New Drug Development: Is It Really $802 Million?" *Health Aff* 25(2006).

28. H. Grabowski, J. Vernon, and J. A. DiMasi, "Returns on Research and Development for 1990s New Drug Introductions," *Pharmacoeconomics* 20 Suppl 3(2002).

29. J. A. DiMasi and C. Paquette, "The Economics of Follow-on Drug Research and Development," *Pharmacoeconomics* 22 Suppl 2(2004); J. A. DiMasi and L. B. Faden, "Competitiveness in Follow-on Drug R&D: A Race or Imitation?" *Nat Rev Drug Disc* 10(2011).

30. S. Gottlieb and J. Makower, "A Role for Entrepreneurs: An Observation on Lowering Healthcare Costs Via Technology Innovation," *Am J Prev Med* 44 Suppl 1(2013).

31. C. M. Christensen, J. H. Grossman, and J. Hwang, *The Innovator's Prescription: A Disruptive Solution for Health Care* (New York: McGraw-Hill, 2009).

32. Angell, *The Truth About the Drug Companies: How They Deceive Us and What to Do About It*; D. W. Light and R. N. Warburton, "Discussion: Setting the Record Straight in the Reply by Dimasi, Hansen and Grabowski," *J Health Econ* 24(2005); R. A. Epstein, "Response to Arnold S Relman's Review of Overdose: How Excessive Government Regulation Stifles Pharmaceutical Innovation," Manhattan Institute for Policy Research, http://www.medicalprogresstoday.com/spotlight/spotlight_indarchive.php?id=1726.

33. J. A. DiMasi, R. W. Hansen, and H. G. Grabowski, "Reply: Setting the Record Straight: Response to the Light and Warburton Rejoinder," *J Health Econ* 24(2005); "Reply: Extraordinary Claims Require Extraordinary Evidence," *J Health Econ* 24(2005).

34. D. W. Light, J. K. Andrus, and R. N. Warburton, "Estimated Research and Development Costs of Rotavirus Vaccine," *Vaccine* 27(2009).

35. Thomson Reuters Pharma, "Comprehensive Source of Global Pharmaceutical Competitor Inteligence" (2013).

36. T. Francis and J. Lublin, "CEO Pay Rising but Not for All," *Wall Street Journal*, March 26, 2014.

37. G. P. Pisano, *Science Business: The Promise, the Reality, and the Future of Biotech* (Harvard Business School Press, 2006).

38. R. E. Santerre, J. A. Vernon, and C. Giaccotto, "The Impact of Indirect Government Controls on US Drug Prices and R&D," *Cato J* Winter(2006).

39. A. S. Kesselheim and R. Rajkumar, "Who Owns Federally Funded Research? The Supreme Court and the Bayh-Dole Act," *N Engl J Med* 365(2011); J Avorn and AS Kesselheim, "The NIH Translational Research Center Might Trade Public Risk for Private Reward," *Nat Med* 17(2011).

40. L. Von Mises, *Human Action: A Treatise on Economics* (Irvington on Hudson: The Foundation for Economic Education, Inc, 1963); F Hayek, *The Fatal Conceit: The Errors of Socialism* (University of Chicago Press, 1988).

10. MISPLACED CRITICISM OF INCREMENTAL INNOVATION

1. M. Angell, "Big Pharma, Bad Medicine," *Boston Rev*, May/June (2010).

2. A. I. Wertheimer and T. M. Santella, "Pharmacoevolution: The Advantages of Incremental Innovation," in *IPN Working Papers on Intellectual Property, Innovation and Health* (London, UK: International Policy Network, 2005).

3. Contributing the discounting of important incremental innovation is an academic position that sometimes values "basic" over "applied" science or "science" over "technology" as mentioned in chapter 8. The immunologist and author, Lewis Thomas famously referred to iron lung respirators used to keep polio victims alive as examples of "halfway technology," inferior to definitive measures acquired through science such as the polio vaccine (L. Thomas, *Lives of a Cell* (New York: Viking Press, 1974). But in the absence of Utopian perfection, such interventions can and do have clear value. The iron lung was a stepping-stone to modern respiratory assist devices used in intensive care settings worldwide today (J. H. Maxwell, "The Iron Lung: Halfway Technology or Necessary Step," *Milbank Q* 64[1986]).

4. J. A. DiMasi and C. Paquette, "The Economics of Follow-on Drug Research and Development," *Pharmacoeconomics* 22 Suppl 2(2004); J. A. DiMasi and L. B. Faden, "Competitiveness in Follow-on Drug R&D: A Race or Imitation?" *Nat Rev Drug Disc* 10(2011).

5. L. J. Wastila, M. E. Ulcickas, and L. Lasagna, "The World Health Organization's Essential Drug List," *J Clin Res Drug Dev* 3(1989); J. Cohen, L. Cabanilla, and J. Sosnov, "Role of Follow-on Drugs and Indications on the Who Essential Drug List," *J Clin Pharmacy Therapeut* 31(2006).

6. Pharmaceutical Research and Manufacturers of America, "2013 Industry Profile."

7. T. Pincus and L. F. Callahan, "Clinical Use of Multiple Nonsteroidal Anti-Inflammatory Drug Preparations within Individual Rheumatology Private Practices," *J Rheumatol* 16(1989).

8. H Brody, *Hooked: Ethics, the Medical Profession, and the Pharmaceutical Industry* (Lanham, MD: Rowman & Littlefield, 2007).

9. E. Carreño et al., "Update on Twice-Daily Bromfenac Sodium Sequihydrate to Treat Postoperative Ocular Inflammation Following Cataract Extraction," *Clin Ophthalmol* 6(2012).

10. J. A. DiMasi, "Price Trends for Prescription: Pharmaceuticals 1995–1999," (Conference Report on Pharmaceutical Pricing Practices, Utilization and Costs, 2000).

11. DiMasi and Paquette, "The Economics of Follow-on Drug Research and Development; DiMasi and Faden, "Competitiveness in Follow-on Drug R&D: A Race or Imitation?"

12. M. King et al., "Medical School Gift Restriction Policies and Physician Prescribing of Newly Marketed Psychotropic Medications: Difference-in-Difference Analysis," *BMJ* 346(2013). This article misleadingly labels all medicine-industry interactions gifts, a rhetorical tactic discussed in chapter 13.

13. DJ Graham et al., "Incidence of Hospitalized Rhabdomyolysis Inpatients Treated with Lipid-Lowering Drugs," *JAMA* 292(2004).

14. H. Naci et al., "Dose-Comparative Effects of Different Statins on Serum Lipid Levels: A Network Meta-Analysis of 256,827 Individuals in 181 Randomized Controlled Trials," *Eur J Prev Cardiol* 20, no. 4 (2013).

15. C. P. Cannon et al., "Intensive versus Moderate Lipid Lowering with Statins after Acute Coronary Syndromes," *N Engl J Med* 350(2004).

16. R. SoRelle, "Baycol Withdrawn from Market," *Circulation* 104, no. 8 (2001).

17. P. Ridker et al., "Rosuvastatin to Prevent Vascular Events in Men and Women with Elevated C-Reactive Protein," *N Engl J Med* 359(2008).

18. R. F. Redberg and M. H. Katz, "Healthy Men Should Not Take Statins," *JAMA* 307(2012).

19. The following comment epitomizes the conflict-of-interest movement's denigration of wide prescribing of statins (D Healy, *Pharmaggedon* [Berkeley: University of California Press, 2012]): "For instance, a small number of people have a genetic disorder that leads to excessively high cholesterol levels and for them drugs like the statins can save lives. . . . The statins can also save lives of people who have had strokes or heart attacks and who also smoke or are overweight, but in this case hundreds of people have to be persuaded to take them for the rest of their lives in order for a handful of them to be saved." First, this critic is wrong in claiming that statins can lower blood cholesterol in the patients with the genetic disorder that causes very high cholesterol levels, leading to severe

vascular complications. The genetic defect, in fact, makes these patients *resistant* to statins (D. Steinberg, *The Cholesterol Wars: The Cholesterol Skeptics vs the Predonderance of Evidence* [Academic Press, 2007]). The critic then blames industry promotion for physicians, allegedly unnecessarily, prescribing statins for the vast majority of other individuals with high cholesterol. Would this critic also decry the facts that only a tiny fraction of motor vehicle operators—and especially impaired or incompetent ones—benefit markedly from the protective effects of mandated seat belts and air bags and that sometimes seat belts and air bags exacerbate rather than reduce injuries caused by motor vehicle accidents?

20. F. Sofi et al., "Accruing Evidence on Benefits of Adherence to the Mediterranean Diet on Health: An Updated Systemic Review and Meta-Analysis," *Am J Clin Nutr* 92(2010); S. W. Tracy, "Something New under the Sun? The Mediterranean Diet and Cardiovascular Health," *N Engl J Med* 368(2013).

21. P. M. Ridker et al., "Cardiovascular Benefits and Diabetes Risks of Statin Therapy in Primary Prevention: An Analysis from the Jupiter Trial," *Lancet* 380(2012); M. J. Blaha, K. Nasir, and R. S. Blumenthal, "Statin Therapy for Healthy Men Identified as 'Increased Risk'" *JAMA* 307(2012).

22. R. J. Simpson, Jr. et al., "Cardiovascular and Economic Outcomes after Initiation of Lipid-Lowering Therapy with Atorvastatin vs Simvastatin in an Employed Population," *Mayo Clin Proc* 84(2009).

23. D. C. Grabowski et al., "Large Social Value Resulting from Use of Statins Warrants Steps to Improve Adherence and Broaden Treatment," *Health Aff* 31(2012).

24. A. D. Sniderman et al., "The Necessity for Clinical Reasoning in the Era of Evidence-Based Medicine," *Mayo Clinic Proc* 88(2013).

25. Centers for Disease Control and Prevention, "An Estimated 1 in 10 US Adults Report Depression," http://www.cdc.gov/features/dsdepression/.

26. F. López-Muñoz and C. Alamo, "Monoaminergic Neurotransmission: The History of the Discovery of Antidepressants," *Curr Pharm Des* 15(2009).

27. A. Bass, *Side Effects: A Prosecutor, a Whistleblower, and a Bestselling Antidepressant on Trial* (Chapel Hill, NC: Algonquin Books of Chapel Hill, 2008).

28. M. J. Oldani, "Thick Prescriptions: Toward an Interpretation of Pharmaceutical Sales Practices," *Med Anthropology Q* 18, no. 3 (2004). *The Medical Letter* 40: 115–116, 1998. Cited in Oldani, "Thick Prescriptions".

29. D. J. Carlat, *Unhinged: The Trouble with Psychiatry—a Doctor's Revelations About a Profession in Crisis* (New York: Free Press, 2010).

30. A. J. Rush, "Star*D: What Have We Learned?" *Am J Pschiatry* 164(2007); A. J. Rush et al., "Acute and Longer-Term Outcomes in Depressed Outpatients Requiring One or Several Treatment Steps: A Star*D Report," *Am J Psychiatry* 163(2006).

31. S. M. Stahl, *Stahl's Essential Psychopharmacology*, 4th ed. (Cambridge, UK: Cambridge University Press, 2013).

32. US Food and Drug Administration, "Facts About Generic Drugs," http://www.fda.gov/drugs/resourcesforyou/consumers/buyingusingmedicinesafely / understandinggenericdrugs/ucm167991.htm.

33. GD Schiff et al., "Principles of Conservative Prescribing," *Arch Int Med* 171(2011).

34. Antihypertensive and Lipid-Lowering Treatment to Prevent Heart Attack Trial Collaborative Research Group, "Diuretic versus Alpha-Blocker as First-Step Antihypertensive Therapy: Final Results from the Antihypertensive and Lipid-Lowering Treatment to Prevent Heart Attack Trial (ALLHAT)," *Hypertension* 42(2003).

35. L. A. Hebert and CJ Hebert, "The Design of ALLHAT May Have Biased the Study's Outcome in Favor of the Diuretic Cohort," *Nat Clin Practice Nephrol* 3(2007).

36. A. Pollack, "The Evidence Gap: The Minimal Impact of a Big Hypertension Study," *New York Times*, November 27, 2008.

37. H. J. Demonaco, A. Ali, and E. von Hippel, "The Major Role of Clinicians in the Discovery of Off-Label Drug Therapies," *Pharmacotherapy* 26, no. 3 (2006).

38. L. Payer, *Disease Mongers: How Doctors, Drug Companies, and Insurers Are Making You Feel Sick* (New York: Wiley, 1994).

39. R. Moynihan, I. Heath, and D. Henry, "Selling Sickness: The Pharmaceutical Industry and Disease Mongering," *BMJ* 324(2002); L. M. Hunt, M. Kreiner, and H. Brody, "The Changing Face of Chronic Illness Management in Primary Care: A Qualitative Study of Underlying Influences and Unintended Outcomes," *Ann Fam Med* 10(2012).

40. S. Woloshin and L. M. Schwartz, "Giving Legs to Restless Legs: A Case Study of How the Media Helps Make People Sick," *PLoS Med* 3, no. 4 (2006).

41. P. J. Shaw and S. P. Duntley, "Neurologic Disorders: Towards a Mechanistic Understanding of Restless Legs Syndrome," *Curr Biol* 22(2012); S. Chokroverty, "Therapeutic Dilemma for Restless Legs Syndrome," *N Engl J Med* 370(2014).

42. H. G. Welch, L. M. Schwartz, and S. Woloshin, *Overdiagnosed: Making People Sick in the Pursuit of Health* (Boston, MA: Beacon Press, 2011).

11. RUSHING TO JUDGMENT WITH FALSE PRODUCT SAFETY ALARMS

1. M Hay et al., "Clinical Development Success Rates for Investigational Drugs," *Nat Biotechnol* 32(2014); I Kola and J Landis, "Can the Pharmaceutical Industry Reduce Attrition Rates?" *Nat Rev Drug Discov* 3(2004).

2. US Food and Drug Administration, "Reporting Adverse Events (Medical Devices)," http://www.fda.gov/MedicalDevices/DeviceRegulationandGuidance/PostmarketRequirements/ReportingAdverseEvents/default.htm.

3. "The Sentinel Initiative," http://www.fda.gov/downloads/Safety/FDAsSentinelInitiative/UCM233360.pdf.

4. K. E. Lasser et al., "Timing of New Black Box Warnings and Withdrawals for Prescription Medications," *JAMA* 287(2002).

5. T. J. Philipson et al., "Assessing the Safety and Efficacy of the FDA: The Case of the Prescription Drug Use Fee Acts," in *National Bureau of Economic Research* (2005); M. K. Olson, "Are Novel Drugs More Risky for Patients than Less Novel Drugs?" *J Health Econ* 23(2004).

6. D. Carpenter, E. J. Zucker, and J. Avorn, "Drug-Review Deadlines and Safety Problems," *N Engl J Med* 358(2008).

7. J. C. P. Weber, "Epidemiology of Adverse Reactions to Nonsteroidal Anti-Inflammatory Drugs," *Adv Inflamm Res* 6(1984); M. R. Southworth, M. E. Reichman, and E. F. Unger, "Dibigitran and Postmarketing Reports of Bleeding," *N Engl J Med* 368(2013).

8. R. J. Kelly et al., "Long-Term Treatment with Eculizumab in Paroxysmal Nocturnal Hemoglobinuria: Sustained Efficacy and Improved Survival," *Blood* 117(2011).

9. J. Avorn, "Dangerous Deception—Hiding the Evidence of Adverse Drug Effects," *N Engl J Med* 355(2006).

10. P. B. Fontanarosa, D. Rennie, and C. D. DeAngelis, "Postmarketing Surveillance—Lack of Vigilance, Lack of Trust," *JAMA* 292(2004).

11. R. S. Bresalier et al., "Cardiovascular Events Associated with Rofecoxib in a Colorectal Adenoma Chemoprevention Trial," *N Engl J Med* 352(2005).

12. C. Bombardier et al., "Comparison of Upper Gastrointestinal Toxicity of Rofecoxib and Naproxen in Patients with Rheumatoid Arthritis: Vigor Study Group," *N Engl J Med* 343(2000).

13. T. Nesi, *Poison Pills: The Untold Story of the Vioxx Drug Scandal* (Saint Martin's Press, 2008).

14. H. M. Krumholz et al., "What Have We Learnt from Vioxx?" *BMJ* 334(2007); BM Psaty and RA Kronmal, "Reporting Mortality Findings in Trials of Rofecoxib for Alzheimer Disease or Cognitive Impairment: A Case Study Based on Documents from Rofecoxib Litigation," *JAMA* 299(2008).

15. *Newsweek* similarly smeared Dr. Weinblatt's integrity and performance as chair of the Vioxx clinical trial data safety monitoring board in a 2014 article (S. Scutti, "The Sunshine Act Will Publicize Big Pharma's Undue Influence on Doctors," *Newsweek*, May 22, 2014).

16. US Senate Committee on Finance, *Testimony of Dr David Graham*, November 18, 2004; D. J. Graham et al., "Risk of Acute Myocardial Infarction and Sudden Cardiac Death in Patients Treated with Cyclo-Exygenase 2 Selective and Non-Selective Non-Steroidal Anti-Inflammatory Drugs: Nested Case-Control Study," *Lancet* 365(2005).

17. (G. D. Curfman, S. Morrissey, and J. M. Drazen, "Expression of Concern: Bombardier et al., 'Comparison of Upper Gastrointestinal Toxicity of Rofecoxib and Naproxen in Patients with Rheumatoid Arthritis,' N Engl J Med 2000;343:1520-8," *N Engl J Med* 353[2005]). The *Wall Street Journal* revealed that the "statement" was timed to deflect onto Merck media attention and possible legal action against the *NEJM* for its alleged complicity in promoting Vioxx use by publishing the VIGOR trial results (D Armstrong, "How the New England Journal Missed Warning Signs on Vioxx: Medical Weekly Waited Years to Report Flaws in Article That Praised Pain Drug. Merck Seen as 'Punching Bag,'" *Wall Street Journal*, May 15, 2006).

18. C. J. Hawkey, "Cox-2 Chronology," *Gut* 54(2005).

19. G. A. Fitzgerald, "Coxibs and Cardiovascular Disease," *N Engl J Med* 351(2004); U.S. Food and Drug Administration, "Advisory Committee Briefing Document: Cardiovascular Safety of Rosiglitazone" (2010).

20. M. A. Konstam et al., "Cardiovascular Thrombotic Events in Controlled Clinical Trials of Rofecoxib," *Circulation* 104(2001).

21. Psaty and Kronmal, "Reporting Mortality Findings in Trials of Rofecoxib for Alzheimer Disease or Cognitive Impairment: A Case Study Based on Documents from Rofecoxib Litigation; DY Graham, NP Newell, and FKL Chan, "Rofecoxib and Clinically Significant Upper and Lower Gastrointestinal Events Revisited Based on Documents from Recent Litigation," *Am J Med Sci* 342(2011); D Madigan et al., "Under-Reporting of Cardiovascular Events in the Rofecoxib Alzheimer Disease Studies," *Am Heart J* 164(2012).

22. For example, Elizabeth Sukkar, "Still Feeling the Vioxx Pain," *The Pharmaceutical Journal* 293(2014). These views were echoed by expert panels for both the FDA and Health Canadian, which voted to allow Vioxx to return to market shortly after its voluntary withdrawal (Meredith Wadman, "Vioxx May Go Back on Sale after Scraping Past FDA Panel," *Nature* 433, no. 7028 (2005); B. Sibbald, "Vioxx Should Be Allowed Back on the Market Advises Expert Panel," *Canadian Medical Association Journal* 175, no. 3 (2006)).

23. J. S. Martin, Jr., "Report of the Honorable John S. Martin, Jr. to the Special Committee of the Board of Directors of Merck & Co., Inc Concerning

the Conduct of Senior Management in the Development and Marketing of Vi-oxx" (Debevoise & Plimpton LLP, 2006).

24. Fontanarosa, Rennie, and DeAngelis, "Postmarketing Surveillance—Lack of Vigilance, Lack of Trust; B. Lo, "Conflicts of Interest: A Call for Professional Standards," *J Law Med Ethics* 40(2012).

25. A. W. Matthews and B. Martinez, "E-Mails Suggest Merck Knew Vi-oxx's Dangers at Early Stage," *Wall Street Journal*, November 1, 2004; A Beren-son, "Evidence in Vioxx Suits Shows Intervention by Merck Officials," *New York Times*, April 24, 2005.

26. Alan Silman, a member of the data safety monitoring board whom I consulted, gave the following response: "[N]one of us suggested stopping the trial, which was very close to its end anyway. I believe, and without recall of the exact details, that to have stopped the trial at that late point would have been unethical. We had no reason to believe that the severe event rate was sufficiently greater in either arm, that lives were being put at risk by continuing the random-ized treatment. We have to note that stopping a trial before it can reach its natural conclusion means that those who have participated have participated in vain."

27. H. Presley, "Vioxx and the Merck Team Effort," in *Case Studies in Ethics* (The Kenan Institute for Ethics at Duke University).

28. Hawkey, "Cox-2 Chronology; CD Salzberg and MR Weir, "Cox-2 Inhibi-tors and Cardiovascular Risk," *Subcell Biochem* 42(2007); S. D. Solomon et al., "Cardiovascular Risk of Celecoxib in 6 Randomized Placebo-Controlled Trials," *Circulation* 117(2008). A medical journal article that contained data revealing that nonselective NSAIDs also cause cardiovascular complications and an ac-companying editorial were notable for failing even to mention this fact; both texts focused only on the toxicity of Vioxx (Graham et al., "Risk of Acute Myocardial Infarction and Sudden Cardiac Death in Patients Treated with Cyclo-Exygenase 2 Selective and Non-Selective Non-Steroidal Anti-Inflammatory Drugs: Nested Case-Control Study").

29. M. Bäck, L. Yin, and E. Ingelsson, "Cyclooxygenase-2 Inhibitors and Cardiovascular Risk Ion a Nation-Wide Cohort Study after the Withdrawal of Rofecoxib," *Eur Heart J* 33(2012).

30. For example, D. M. McCarthy, "Comparative Toxicity of Nonsteroidal Anti-Inflammatory Drugs," *Am J Med* 107 Suppl 1(1999).

31. D. T. Mangano, I. C. Tudor, and C. Dietzel, "The Risk Associated with Aprotinin in Cardiac Surgery," *N Engl J Med* 354(2006); K. Karkouti et al., "A Propensity Score Case-Control Comparison of Aprotinin and Tranexamic Acid in High-Transfusion-Risk Cardiac Surgery," *Transfusion* 46(2006).

32. W. R. Hiatt, "Observational Studies of Drug Safety—Aprotinin and the Absence of Transparency," *N Engl J Med* 355(2006).

33. S. Schneeweiss et al., "Aprotinin During Coronary-Artery Bypass Grafting and Risk of Death," *N Engl J Med* 358(2008); A. D. Shaw et al., "The Effect of Aprotinin on Outcome after Coronary-Artery Bypass Grafting," *N Engl J Med* 358(2008); DA Fergusson et al., "A Comparison of Aprotinin and Lysine Analogues in High-Risk Cardiac Surgery," *N Engl J Med* 358(2008).

34. M. Franchini and P. M. Mannucci, "Adjunct Agents for Bleeding," *Curr Opin Hematol* 21, no. 6 (2014); Health Canada, "Health Canada Decision on Trasylol (Aprotinin)," http://www.hc-sc.gc.ca/ahc-asc/media/advisories-avis/_2011/2011_124-eng.php; European Medicines Agency, "European Medicines Agency Recommends Lifting Suspension of Aprotinin," http://www.ema.europa.eu/ema/pages/news_and_events/news/2012/02/news_detail_001447.jsp.

35. G. A. Chressanthis et al., "Can Access Limits on Sales Representatives to Physicians Affect Clinical Prescription Decisions? A Study of Recent Events with Diabetes and Lipid Drugs," *J Clin Hypertension* 14(2012).

36. W. R. Hiatt, S. Kaul, and R. J. Smith, "The Cardiovascular Safety of Diabetes Drugs—Insights from the Rosiglitazone Experience," *N Engl J Med* 369(2013); S. Tavernise and K. Thomas, "FDA Advisors' Vote Is a Minor Victory for a Troubled Diabetes Drug," *New York Times*, June 7, 2013; "FDA Requires Removal of Certain Restrictions on the Diabetes Drug Avandia," November 25, 2013, http://www.fda.gov/NewsEvents/Newsroom/PressAnnouncements/ucm376516.htm.

37. A. Besarab et al., "The Effects of Normal as Compared with Low Hematocrit Values in Patients with Cardiac Disease Who Are Receiving Hemodialysis and Epoetin," *N Engl J Med* 339(1998); AK Singh et al., "Correction of Anemia with Epoeten Alpha in Chronic Kidney Disease," *N Engl J Med* 355(2006); TB Drüeke et al., "Normalization of Hemoglobin Level in Patients with Chronic Kidney Disease and Anemia," *N Engl J Med* 355(2006).

38. C. L. Bennett et al., "Venous Thromboembolism and Mortality Associated with Recombinant Erythropoietin and Darbopoietin Administration for the Treatment of Cancer-Associated Anemia," *JAMA* 299(2008).

39. A. Phrommintikul et al., "Mortality and Target Haemoglobin Concentrations in Anaemic Patients with Chronic Kidney Disease Treated with Erythropoietin: A Meta-Analysis," *Lancet* 369(2007); J. Bohlius et al., "Recombinant Human Erythropoietins and Cancer Patients: Updated Meta-Analysis of 57 Studies Including 9353 Patients," *J Natl Cancer Inst* 98(2006); S. Elliot and A. Sinclair, "The Effect of Erythropoietin on Normal and Neoplastic Cells," *Biologics: Targets and Therapy* 6(2012).

40. M. A. Pfeffer et al., "A Trial of Darbepoietin Alfa in Type 2 Diabetes and Chronic Kidney Disease," *N Engl J Med* 361(2009).

41. P. Citron, "Ethics Considerations for Medical Device R&D," *Progr Cardiovasc Dis* 55(2012).

42. "Measuring Postmarket Performance and Other Select Topics: Workshop Report," in *The Public Health Effectiveness of the FDA 510(k) Clearance Process*, ed. T. Wizemann (The Institute of Medicine, 2011).

43. US Food and Drug Administration, "External Defibrillator Improvement Initiative," http://www.fda.gov/MedicalDevices/ProductsandMedicalProcedures/CardiovascularDevices/ExternalDefibrillators/ucm232302.htm.

44. The IOM report includes two studies on the recall rate for devices approved under the 510(k) system. The first found that 1.6% of devices were recalled in the first year, rising to 8.5% by the fifth year postapproval when all causes of recalls were considered. When only recalls of devices believed to pose a serious threat to consumer's health were considered, only 112, or 0.2% of all devices that had then been approved under the 510(k) system, were recalled over a five-year period ("Measuring Postmarket Performance and Other Select Topics: Workshop Report").

45. "Recalls Specific to Metal-on-Metal Hip Implants," http://www.fda.gov/MedicalDevices/ProductsandMedicalProcedures/ImplantsandProsthetics/MetalonMetalHipImplants/ucm241770.htm; DB Kramer, S Xu, and AS Kesselheim, "Regulation of Medical Devices in the United States and European Union," *N Engl J Med* 366(2012).

46. B. M. Ardaugh, S. E. Graves, and R. F. Redberg, "The 510(k) Ancestry of a Metal-on-Metal Hip Implant," *N Engl J Med* 368(2013).

12. DEMONIZING MARKETING IS FALSE ADVERTISING

1. L. Von Mises, *Human Action: A Treatise on Economics* (Irvington on Hudson: The Foundation for Economic Education, Inc, 1963).

2. D. Korn, "The Challenge of Public Expectations," *Boston Rev*, May/June (2010); JS Flier, "Dean's Corner: 2010 Recommendations: Dean's Perspective," (2010).

3. T. A. Brennan et al., "Health Industry Practices That Create Conflict of Interest: A Policy Proposal for Academic Medical Centers," *JAMA* 295(2006).

4. A. Wazana, "Physicians and the Pharmaceutical Industry: Is a Gift Ever Just a Gift?" *JAMA* 283(2000).

5. P. H. Rubin, "Pharmaceutical Marketing: Medical and Industry Biases," *J Pharmaceutical Finance, Econ & Policy* 13(2004); "An Uncertain Diagnosis," *Regulation*, Summer (2005); TS Huddle, "Drug Reps and the Academic Medical Center: A Case for Management Rather than Prohibition," *Persp Biol Med* 51(2008); TP Stossel, "Response to AMA's Council on Ethical and Judicial Affairs Draft Report on 'Ethical Guidance for Physicians and the Profession with

Respect to Industry Support for Professional Education in Medicine,'" *Medscape J Med* 10, no. 6 (2008).

6. R. Lesko, S. Scott, and T. P. Stossel, "Bias in High-Tier Medical Journals Concerning Physician-Academic Relations with Industry," *Nat Biotechnol* 30(2012).

7. F. Haayer, "Rational Prescribing and Sources of Information," *Soc Sci Med* 16(1982).

8. G. K. Spurling et al., "Information from Pharmaceutical Companies and the Quality, Quantity, and Cost of Physicians' Prescribing: A Systematic Review," *PLoS Med* 7, no. 10 (2010).

9. G. A. Chressanthis et al., "Can Access Limits on Sales Representatives to Physicians Affect Clinical Prescription Decisions? A Study of Recent Events with Diabetes and Lipid Drugs," *J Clin Hypertension* 14(2012).

10. C. D. May, "Selling Drugs by 'Educating ' Physicians," J Med Edu 36(1961).

11. No Free Lunch, http://www.nofreelunch.org/aboutus.htm.

12. Pharmaceutical Research and Manufacturers of America, "2011 Industry Profile."

13. L. Noah, "Medicine's Epistemology: Mapping the Haphazard Diffusion of Knowledge in the Biomedical Community," *Ariz L Rev* 44(2002); S. Saint et al., "Journal Reading Habits of Internists," *J Gen Intern Med* 15(2000).

14. Following approval of an implantable device, almost nobody is better equipped to train users than technicians employed by the device manufacturer's company. In some circumstances, ongoing monitoring of device implantation can extend well into a device's life cycle. Nevertheless, the conflict-of-interest movement recommends that physicians maintain an adversarial relationship with such experts. For example, at my institution, when in the operating room, device technicians must wear black scrub suits emblazoned with the sign "VENDOR." How this helps the physicians, attendants, and an anesthetized patient cope with the procedure is a mystery.

15. M. E. Porter, J. W. Lorsch, and N. Nohria, "Seven Surprises for New CEOs," *Harvard Bus Rev*, October 2004; R Fisman and T Sullivan, *The Org* (New York: Hachette Book Group, 2013).

16. M. A. Steinman, M. G. Shlipak, and S. McPhee, "Of Principles and Pens: Attitudes and Practices of Medicine Housestaff toward Pharmaceutical Industry Promotions," *Am J Med* 110(2001); Wazana, "Physicians and the Pharmaceutical Industry: Is a Gift Ever Just a Gift?; Kaiser Family Foundation, "National Survey of Physicians (2002)," (2003); A. S. Brett, W. Burr, and J. Moloo, "Are Gifts from Pharmaceutical Companies Ethically Problematic? A Survey of Physicians," *Arch Int Med* 163(2003); F. S. Sierles et al., "Medical Student's Exposure to and Attitudes About Drug Company Interactions. A National Survey," *JAMA*

294(2005); P. Manchanda and E. Honka, "The Effects and Role of Direct-to-Physician Marketing in the Pharmaceutical Industry: An Integrative Review," *Yale J Health Policy Law Ethics* 5(2005); S. Chimonas, T. A. Brennan, and D. J. Rothman, "Physicians and Drug Representatives: Exploring the Dynamics of the Relationship," *J Gen Intern Med* 22(2007); M. A. Fischer et al., "Prescribers and Pharmaceutical Representatives: Why Are We Still Meeting?" *J Gen Intern Med* 24(2009); D Korenstein, S Keyhani, and JS Ross, "Physician Attitudes toward Industry: A View across the Specialties," *Arch Surg* 145(2010); D. E. Grande et al., "Effect of Exposure to Small Pharmaceutical Promotional Items on Treatment Preferences," *Arch Int Med* 169(2009); K. E. Austad, J. Avorn, and A. S. Kesselheim, "Medical Students' Exposure to and Attitudes About the Pharmaceutical Industry: A Systematic Review," *PLoS Med* 8, no. 5 (2011); K. E. Austad et al., "Changing Interactions between Physician Trainees and the Pharmaceutical Industry: A National Survey," *J Gen Intern Med* 28(2013); J. S. Yeh and A. S. Kesselheim, "Same Song, Different Audience: Pharmaceutical Promotion Targeting Non-Physician Health Care Providers," *PLoS Med* 10(2013); Q. Grundy, L. Bero, and R. Malone, "Interactions between Non-Physician Clinicians and Industry: A Systematic Review," *PLoS Med* 10(2013).

17. P. Manchanda, Y. Xie, and N. Youn, "The Role of Targeted Communication and Contagion in Product Adoption," *Marketing Sci* 27(2008); C Van den Bulte and GL Lilien, "Medical Innovation Revisited: Social Contagion Versus Marketing Effort," *Am J Sociol* 106(2001); S Narayanan, P Manchanda, and PK Chintagunta, "Temporal Differences in the Role of Marketing Communication in New Product Categories," *J Marketing Res* 42(2005); Chressanthis et al., "Can Access Limits on Sales Representatives to Physicians Affect Clinical Prescription Decisions? A Study of Recent Events with Diabetes and Lipid Drugs."

18. A. T. Ching and M. Isihara, "Measuring the Informative and Persuasive Roles of Detailing on Prescribing Decisions," *Management Sci* 58(2012).

19. P. Azoulay, "Do Pharmaceutical Sales Respond to Scientific Evidence?" *J Econ Management Strategy* 11(2002); N. Mizik and R. Jacobson, "Are Physicians 'Easy Marks'? Quantifying the Effects of Detailing and Sampling on New Prescriptions," *Management Sci* 50(2004).

20. S. Narayanan and P. Machanda, "Heterogeneous Learning and the Targeting of Marketing Communication for New Products," *Marketing Sci* 28(2009).

21. S. Venkataraman and S. Stremersch, "The Debate on Influencing Doctors' Decisions: Are Drug Characteristics the Missing Link?" *Management Sci* 53(2007).

22. S. R. Majumdar, F. A. McAlister, and S. B. Soumerai, "Synergy between Publication and Promotion: Comparing Adoption of New Evidence in Canada and the United States," *Am J Med* 115(2003).

23. S. Stremersch and W. Van Dyke, "Marketing of the Life Sciences: A New Framework and Research Agenda for a Nascent Field," *J Marketing* 73(2009).

24. Pew Charitable Trust, "Prescription Project" (2009).

25. SS Andaleeb and RF Tallman, "Physician Attitudes toward Pharmaceutical Sales Representatives," *Health Care Manage Rev* 20(1995); JA Schneider et al., "Residents' Perception over Time of Pharmaceutical Industry Interactions and Gifts and the Effect of an Educational Intervention," *Acad Med* 81(2006).

26. J. A. Hopper, M. W. Speece, and J. Musial, "Effects of an Educational Intervention on Residents' Knowledge and Attitudes toward Interactions with Pharmaceutical Representatives," *J Gen Intern Med* 12(1997); B. B. McCormick et al., "Effect of Restricting Contact between Pharmaceutical Company Representatives and Internal Medicine Residents on Posttraining Attitudes and Behavior," *JAMA* 286(2001); S. Agrawal, I. Saluja, and J. Kaczorowski, "A Prospective before-and-after Trial of an Educational Intervention About Pharmaceutical Marketing," *Acad Med* 79(2004); J. A. Schneider et al., "Residents' Perception over Time of Pharmaceutical Industry Interactions and Gifts and the Effect of an Educational Intervention," *Acad Med* 81(2006); A. C. Kao et al., "Effect of Educational Interventions and Medical School Policies on Medical Students' Attitudes toward Pharmaceutical Marketing Practices: A Multi-Institutional Study," *Acad Med* 896(2011).

27. "Effect of Educational Interventions and Medical School Policies on Medical Students' Attitudes toward Pharmaceutical Marketing Practices: A Multi-Institutional Study."

28. American Medical Association, "Under Pressure? Making Sound Prescribing Decisions," www.soundprescribing.org.

29. K. Greenwood, C. H. Coleman, and K. M. Boozang, "Toward Evidence-Based Conflict of Interest Training for Physician-Investigators," *J Law Med Ethics* 40(2012).

30. J. Avorn and S. Soumerai, "Improving Drug-Therapy Decisions through Educational Outreach: A Randomized Trial of Academically Based 'Detailing,'" *N Engl J Med* 308(1983); J. Avorn, "Teaching Clinicians About Drugs—50 Years Later, Whose Job Is It?" *N Engl J Med* 364(2011); M. A. Fischer and J. Avorn, "Academic Detailing Can Play a Key Role in Assessing and Implementing Comparative Effectiveness Research Findings," *Health Aff* 31(2012).

31. "Academic detailing provides health care professionals with unbiased, noncommercial, evidence-based clinical information." "The Alosa Foundation, Inc. is a 501(c)(3) nonprofit organization which is not affiliated with any pharmaceutical company. Our clinical information is developed by research physicians and clinicians who have no personal financial relationships with any drug or device maker." Alosa Foundation, http://www.alosafoundation.org/. "Academic detailing is a method of outreach education that combines the interactive,

one-on-one communication approach of industry detailers with the evidence-based, noncommercial information of academia." National Resource Center for Academic Detailing. "About Academic Detailing," http://www.narcad.org/about/aboutad/.

32. M. A. O'Brien et al., "Educational Outreach Visits: Effects on Professional Practice and Health Care Outcomes," *Cochrane Database Syst Rev*, no. 4 (2007).

33. J. E. Dicken, "Drug Pricing: Research on Savings from Generic Drug Use" (Washington, DC: United States Government Accountability Office, 2012).

34. "Authorized Generic Drugs. Short-Term Effects and Long-Term Impact" (Federal Trade Commission, 2011); AJ Fein, "Pharmacy Profits from Authorized Generics," *Pembroke Consulting* (2012), http://www.drugchannels.net/2011/09/pharmacy-profits-from-authorized.html; "Pharmacy Profits over the Generic Life Cycle: Explaining the NARP-NADAC Data," http://www.drugchannels.net/2012/12/pharmacy-profits-over-generic-life.html.

35. CVS Caremark Corporation, "Form 10-Q. Quarterly Report Pursuant to Section 13 or 15(D) of the Securities Exchange Act of 1934. For the Quarterly Period Ended June 30, 2013," (2013); Walgreen Co, "Form 10-Q. Filed 06/28/13 for the Period Ending 05/31/13," (2013).

36. W. H. Shrank et al., "The Epidemiology of Prescriptions Abandoned at the Pharmacy," *Ann Int Med* 153(2010); W. H. Shrank et al., "The Use of Generic Drugs in Prevention of Chronic Disease Is Far More Cost-Effective than Thought, and May Save Money," *Health Aff* 30(2011).

37. CVS Caremark, "Advancing Medication Adherence" (2011).

38. R. J. Cooper et al., "The Quantity and Quality of Scientific Graphs in Pharmaceutical Advertisements," *J Gen Intern Med* 18(2003).

39. S. Woloshin et al., "Press Releases by Academic Medical Centers: Not So Academic?" *Ann Int Med* 150(2009).

40. P. Galewitz, "Hospitals Hire Reps to Sell Doctors on Patient Referrals," *USA Today*, December 13, 2011.

13. THE GIFT SMOKE SCREEN

1. M Mauss, *The Gift: The Form and Reason for Exchange in Archaic Societies*, trans. WD Halls (New York: W.W. Norton, 1990).

2. RM Emerson, "Social Exchange Theory," *Annu Rev Sociol* 2(1976); M Dufwenberg and G Kirchsteiger, "A Theory of Sequential Reciprocity," *Games and Econ Behav* 47(2004).

3. KE Austad et al., "Changing Interactions between Physician Trainees and the Pharmaceutical Industry: A National Survey," *J Gen Intern Med* 28(2013).

4.   MA Rodwin, "Reforming Pharmacuetical Industry-Physician Financial Relationships: Lessons from the United States, France, and Japan," *J Law Med Ethics* 39, no. 4 (2011).

5.   M-M Chren, S Landfield, and TH Murray, "Doctors, Drug Companies and Gifts," *JAMA* 362(1989); DA Katz, AL Kaplan, and J Merz, "All Gifts Large and Small: Toward an Understanding of Pharmaceutical Gift-Giving," *Am J Bioethics* 3(2003); H Brody, *Hooked: Ethics, the Medical Profession, and the Pharmaceutical Industry* (Lanham, MD: Rowman & Littlefield, 2007).

6.   EG Campbell, "Doctors and Drug Companies—Scrutinizing Influential Relationships," *N Engl J Med* 357(2007).

7.   L Kowalczyk, "For Physicians, Another Option on Education: Classes Won't Take Drug Firms' Money," *Boston Globe*, September 14, 2010.

8.   The biopharmaceutical industry spent approximately $31 billion on marketing in 2010, which is less than half of what they spent on research and development and approximately 1% of total U.S. national health expenditures that year (T Staton, "Does Pharma Spend More on Marketing Than R&D? A Numbers Check," *FiercePharma*(2013), http://www.fiercepharma.com/story/ does-pharma-spend-more-marketing-rd-numbers-check/2013-05-21; CMS, "National Health Expenditure Data" (Centers for Medicare and Medicaid Services, 2013)).

9.   Brody, *Hooked: Ethics, the Medical Profession, and the Pharmaceutical Industry.*

10.   A negative consequence of demonizing benefits is that the most successful entrepreneurial physicians and non-physician researchers in universities have discreetly kept their earnings from industry from consulting and other relationships—which in some cases have been and continue to be prodigious—under a bushel. As a result, the message that excellence and accomplishment in biomedical scholarship can not only result in promotions, recognition by influential peers, and awards but also in the financial rewards that accompany success in other endeavors has not aired. As described in Chapter 15, however, the "Sunshine" legislation enacted as part of health care reform will expose some of these winnings, but only those of licensed practitioners. The rewards to academics who are predominantly administrators or basic scientists will remain in the shadows.

11.   W Osler, "The Reserves of Life," *St Mary's Hosp Gaz* 13(1907).

12.   Wall Street Journal Health Blog, "Text of Obama's Speech to the AMA," (2008), http://blogs.wsj.com/health/2009/06/15/text-of-obamas-speech-before-the-ama/.

13.   D Wootton, *Bad Medicine: Doctors Doing Harm since Hippocrates* (New York: Oxford University Press, 2006).

14.   These products were actually not "patented." An expose series of articles titled "The Great American Fraud" published in the magazine *Colliers* beginning

in 1905 went a long way to putting the patent medical industry out of business and also contributed to passage of the 1906 Food and Drug Act described in Chapter 2 (Samuel Hopkins Adams, "The Great American Fraud," *Collier's Weekly*(1905)). A thriving modern equivalent of that industry offers health foods, supplements, and alternative medicine. Like its patent medicine forbears, these nutraceuticals and alternative medicine appeal to consumers whose needs mainstream medicine does not serve or who are fearful or suspicious of it and evade regulations. Chapter 14 discusses nutraceuticals further.

15. BM Bernheim, *Medicine at the Crossroads* (New York: William Morrow and Company, 1939).

16. *Goldfarb v. Virginia State Bar*, 421 U.S. 773(1975).

17. These developments were the subject of a published debate between *The New England Journal of Medicine* editor Arnold Relman and Princeton University health care economist, Uwe Reinhardt. Relman criticized Reinhardt for considering physicians no different than any other "purveyors of other goods and services." Reinhardt's responses featured clear historical facts, solid logic, and acerbic wit. A few of his laser sharp arguments follow (AS Relman and UE Reinhardt, "Debating For-Profit Health Care and the Ethics of Physicians," *Health Aff* 5(1986)): "The time is long past when as vast and technically complex a sector as the health care sector could be run by missionaries and candy stripers. It is a real industry now, whether we like it or not, and it must pay wages competitive with other industries.

"You . . . contrast the presumably venal 'business ethic' with your profession's presumably more lofty code of ethics. If you ever sat in on the board meetings of large corporations, you would be surprised to learn how often business people forgo easy profits for the sake of ethical standards. And you would be surprised to learn what they could get away with, if they were as venal as is implied in your use of the term 'business ethic.' I honestly believe that a corporation has as much concern over the decency with which it treats its customers as physicians have over their patients.

"But it so happens that I am more comfortable dealing with a well-trained, competitive, self-professed entrepreneur who drives a Lincoln than I am with a well-trained competitive, self-professed saint who insists on driving a Cadillac."

18. KJ Arrow, "Uncertainty and the Welfare Economics of Medical Care," *Am Econ Rev* 53(1963).

19. EG Campbell et al., "Physician Professionalism and Changes in Physician-Industry Relationships from 2004 to 2009," *Arch Int Med* 170, no. 20 (2010).

20. RH Tawney, *Religion and the Rise of Capitalism with a New Introduction by Adam B Seligman* (New Brunswick and London: Transaction Publishers, 2005 (1926)).

21. JP Orlowski and L Wateska, "The Effects of Pharmaceutical Firm Entice-ments on Physician Prescribing Patterns," *Chest* 102(1992); Katz, Kaplan, and Merz, "All Gifts Large and Small: Toward an Understanding of Pharmaceutical Gift-Giving; D Korenstein, S Keyhani, and JS Ross, "Physician Attitudes toward Industry: A View across the Specialties," *Arch Surg* 145(2010).

22. MJ Oldani, "Thick Prescriptions: Toward an Interpretation of Pharma-ceutical Sales Practices," *Med Anthropology Q* 18, no. 3 (2004).

23. RB Cialdini, *Influence: The Psychology of Persuasion* (New York: Harp-er, 2007).

24. TA Brennan et al., "Health Industry Practices That Create Conflict of Interest: A Policy Proposal for Academic Medical Centers," *JAMA* 295(2006).

25. AAMC, "Report of the AAMC Task Force on Industry Funding of Medi-cal Education to the AAMC Executive Council" (Washington DC: Association of American Medical Colleges, 2008).

26. S Sah and G Loewenstein, "Nothing to Declare: Mandatory and Volun-tary Disclosure Leads Advisors to Avoid Conflicts of Interest," *Psychol Sci* (2013).

27. DM Cain, G Loewenstein, and DA Moore, "When Sunlight Fails to Disinfect: Understanding the Perverse Effects of Disclosing Conflicts of Inter-est," *J Consumer Res* 37(2011).

28. D Chugh, MH Bazerman, and MR Banaji, "Bounded Ethicality as a Psychological Barrier to Recognizing Conflicts of Interest," in *Conflicts of Inter-est: Problems and Solutions from Law, Medicine and Organizational Settings*, ed. DA Moore, et al. (London: Cambridge University Press, 2005).

29. AAMC, "The Scientific Basis of Influence and Reciprocity: A Sympo-sium" (Washington, DC, 2007).

30. J Dana and G Loewenstein, "A Social Science Perspective on Gifts to Physicians from Industry," *JAMA* 290(2003), cited in AAMC, "The Scientific Basis of Influence and Reciprocity: A Symposium."

31. C Koch and C Schmidt, "Disclosing Conflicts of Interest—Do Experi-ence and Reputation Matter?" *Accounting Org Soc* 35(2010).

32. S Sah and G Loewenstein, "Effect of Reminders of Personal Sacrifice and Suggested Rationalizations on Residents' Self-Reported Willingness to Ac-cept Gifts," *JAMA* 304(2010); S Sah, "Conflicts of Interest and Your Physician: Psychological Processes That Cause Unexpected Changes in Behavior," *J Law Med Ethics* 40(2012).

33. N Bardsley, "Experimental Economics and the Artificiality of Altera-tion," *J Econ Methodol* 12(2005); M Voors et al., "Exploring Whether Behavior in Context-Free Experiments Is Predictive of Behavior in the Field: Evidence from Lab and Field Experiments in Rural Sierra Leone," *Econ Lett* 114(2012); U Gneezy and JA List, "Putting Behavioral Economics to Work: Testing for Gift

Exchange in Labor Markets Using Field Experiments," *Econometrica* 74(2006); SD Levitt and JA List, "What Do Laboratory Experiments Measuring Social Preferences Reveal About the Real World?" *J Econ Persp* 21(2007); "Viewpoint: On the Generalizability of Lab Behavior to the Field," *Can J Econ* 40(2007).

34. TS Huddle, "The Pitfalls of Deducing Ethics from Behavioral Economics: Why the Association of American Medical Colleges Is Wrong about Pharmaceutical Detailing," *Am J Bioethics* 10(2010); "Response to Open Peer Commentaries on 'The Pitfalls of Deducing Ethics from Economics: Why the Association of Medical Colleges Is Wrong about Pharmaceutical Detailing,'" *Am J Bioethics* 10(2010).

14. THE LAWYERS' BALL

1. D Wilson, "Glaxo Settles Cases with US for $3 Billion," *New York Times*, November 3, 2011; "Merck to Pay $950 Million over Vioxx," *New York Times*, November 23, 2011.

2. TJ Philipson and E Sun, "Is the Food and Drug Administration Safe and Effective?" *J Econ Perspect* 22(2008).

3. AS Kesselheim and J Avorn, "The Role of Litigation in Defining Drug Risks," *JAMA* 297(2007); CD DeAngelis and PB Fontanarosa, "Prescription Drugs, Products Liability, and Preemption of Tort Litigation," *JAMA* 300(2008); GD Curfman, S Morrissey, and JM Drazen, "Why Doctors Should Worry About Preemption," *N Engl J Med* 359(2008); LO Gostin, "The FDA, Preemption, and Public Safety," *Hastings Cent Rep* 41(2011).

4. PW Huber and KR Foster, *Judging Science: Scientific Knowledge and the Federal Courts* (Cambridge, MA: MIT Press, 1997).

5. *Riegel v Medtronic*, 552 U.S. 312(2007).

6. C Weaver and J Smith, "St. Jude Hit by Suits: Cases Could Challenge Liability Protection of Device Makers," *Wall Street Journal*, 2013.

7. DC Radley, SN Finckelstein, and RS Stafford, "Off-Label Prescribing among Office-Based Physicians," *Arch Int Med* 166(2006); AD Shaw et al., "The Effect of Aprotinin on Outcome after Coronary-Artery Bypass Grafting," *N Engl J Med* 358(2008); M Ratner and T Gura, "Off-Label or Off-Limits?" *Nat Biotechnol* 26(2008); CM Wittich, CM Burkle, and WL Lanier, "Ten Common Questions (and Their Answers) about Off-Label Drug Use," *Mayo Clin Proc* 87(2012). Eculizumab, the treatment discussed in the Preface that was given to my patient Grace for HUS, has not been approved for that indication—only for atypical HUS and for PNH (See Chapter 1).

8. Food and Drug Administration, "Good Reprint Practices for the Distribution of Medical Journal Articles and Medical or Scientific Reference Publications on Unapproved New Uses of Approved Drugs and Approved or Cleared Medical Devices" (2009), http://www.fda.gov/RegulatoryInformation/Guidances/ucm125126.htm.

9. HA Waxman, "A History of Adverse Drug Experiences: Congress Had Ample Evidence to Support Restrictions on the Promotion of Prescription Drugs," *Food & Drug L J* 58(2003).

10. *Franklin v Parke-Davis*, 147 F. Supp. 2d 39(2001); "Warner-Lambert to Pay $430 Million to Resolve Criminal & Civil Health Care Liability Relating to Off-Label Promotion" (2004).

11. MA Steinman et al., "Narrative Review: The Promotion of Gabapentin: An Analysis of Internal Industry Documents," *Ann Int Med* 145, no. 4 (2006); CS Landefeld and MA Steinman, "The Neurontin Legacy—Marketing through Misinformation and Manipulation," *N Engl J Med* 360(2009).

12. MA Rodwin, "Rooting out Institutional Corruption to Manage Inappropriate Off-Label Drug Use," *J Law Med Ethics* 41(2013).

13. S Sah, "Conflicts of Interest and Your Physician: Psychological Processes That Cause Unexpected Changes in Behavior," *J Law Med Ethics* 40(2012); AS Kesselheim, MM Mello, and DM Studdert, "Strategies and Practices in Off-Label Marketing of Pharmaceuticals: A Retrospective Analysis of Whistleblower Complaints," *PLoS Medicine* 8, no. 4 (2011).

14. K Outterson, "Punishing Health Care Fraud—Is the GSK Settlement Sufficient?" *N Engl J Med* 367(2012).

15. AS Kesselheim, DM Studdert, and MM Mello, "Whistle-Blowers' Experiences in Fraud Litigation against Pharmaceutical Companies," *N Engl J Med* 362(2010).

16. C Bray and J Whalen, "US Accuses Novartis of Kickbacks: Prosecutors Allege Drug Maker Gave Physicians Lavish Dinners, Fishing Trips to Prescribe Pills," *Wall Street Journal*, April 27, 2013.

17. T Eguale et al., "Drug, Patient, and Physician Characteristics Associated with Off-Label Prescribing in Primary Care," *Arch Int Med* 172(2012).

18. M Oates, "Facilitating Informed Medical Treatment through Production and Disclosure of Research into Off-Label Uses of Pharmaceuticals," *NY Univ LR* 80(2005); DM Fritch, "Speak No Evil, Hear No Evil, Harm the Patient— Why the FDA Needs to Seek More, Rather than Less, Speech from Drug Manufacturers on Off-Label Drug Treatments," *Mich St U J Med & L* 9(2005); RF Hall and RJ Berlin, "When You Have a Hammer Everything Looks Like a Nail: Misapplication of the False Claims Act to Off-Label Promotion," *Food and Drug Law* 61(2006); SL Johnson, "Polluting Medical Judgment? False Assumptions in the Pursuit of False Claims Regarding Off-Label Prescribing," *Minn J L Sci &*

Tech 9, no. 1 (2007); JH Krause, "Health Care Providers and the Public Fisc: Paradigms of Government Harm under the Civil False Claims Act," *Ga L Rev* 36(2007); C Young, "Will Everyone Get Their Best Medicine? Implications for Off-Label Use of Pharmaceuticals in an American Universal Healthcare Regime," *St Louis Univ J Health Law Policy* 2(2008); JE Osborn, "Can I Tell You the Truth? A Comparative Perspective on Regulating Off-Label Scientific and Medical Information," *Yale J Health Policy & Ethics* 10(2010); C Klasmeier and MH Redish, "Off-Label Prescription Advertising, the FDA and the First Amendment: A Study in the Values of Commercial Speech Protection," *Am J Law Med* 37(2011); G Conko, "Hidden Truth: The Perils and Protection of Off-Label Drug and Medical Device Promotion," *Health Matrix* 21(2011); G Masoudi and C Pruitt, "The Food and Drug Administration V. The First Amendment: A Survey of Recent FDA Enforcement," *Health Matrix* 21(2011); JH Beales, III, "Health Related Claims, the Market for Information, and the First Amendment," *Health Matrix* 21(2011); L Noah, "Truth or Consequences?: Commercial Free Speech vs. Public Health Promotion (at the FDA)," *Health Matrix* 21(2011).

19. *United States v GlaxoSmithKline*, No. 11-10398-RWZ 1-76(2011).

20. HA Silverglate, *Three Felonies a Day: How the Feds Target the Innocent* (New York, London: Encounter Books, 2009).

21. Ibid.

22. D Wilson, "Drug Makers' Feared Enemy Switches Sides, as Their Lawyer," *New York Times*, June 4, 2011.

23. "Who Else Is Paying Your Doctor? Soon, You Can Look It Up," *USA Today*, February 28 2012.

24. "AMA Database Licensing," http://www.ama-assn.org/ama/pub/about-ama/physician-data-resources/ama-database-licensing.page?.

25. *Sorrell v. IMS Health*, 10-779(2011).

26. *United States v. Caronia* (2010).

27. *Sorrell v. IMS Health.*

28. *United States v. Caronia.*

29. Radley, Finckelstein, and Stafford, "Off-Label Prescribing among Office-Based Physicians."

30. A sad aspect of this case was that Caronia's co-defendant, a physician named Gleason, committed suicide as a result of the prosecution (HA Silverglate, "A Doctor's Posthumous Vindication," *Wall Street Journal*, December 25, 2012).

31. GD Curfman, S Morrissey, and JM Drazen, "Prescriptions, Privacy, and the First Amendment," *N Engl J Med* 364, no. 21 (2011); MM Mello and NA Messing, "Restrictions on the Use of Prescribing Data for Drug Promotion," *N Engl J Med* 365(2011); A Kesselheim, MM Mello, and J Avorn, "FDA Regulation of Off-Label Promotion under Attack," *JAMA* 309(2013).

32. ReportLinker, "Nutraceutical Industry: Market Research Reports, Statistics and Analysis," http://www.reportlinker.com/ci02038/Nutraceutical.html.

33. US Food and Drug Administration, "GRAS Substances (SCOGS) Database," http://www.fda.gov/Food/IngredientsPackagingLabeling/GRAS/SCOGS/default.htm.

34. Dr. Paul Offit has nicely chronicled how the nutraceutical industry effectively exerted political pressure to avoid regulation and how celebrities' affinity for its nostrums have encouraged their widespread use, despite overwhelming evidence that most of them have no physiological benefits. Cases in which contaminated products and even uncontaminated ones have caused injury and to the extent that patients have resorted to ineffective nutraceuticals instead of accepting mainstream medical treatment for otherwise curable diseases point out that these products are far from completely harmless (PA Offit, *Do You Believe in Magic? The Sense and Nonsense of Alternative Medicine* (New York: Harper-Collins Publishers, 2013)). But then again, we do not ban certifiably damaging substances such as alcohol and tobacco.

15. THE PRICE WE PAY

1. DE Zinner et al., "Participation of Academic Scientists in Relationships with Industry," *Health Aff* 28(2009).

2. Association of University Technology Managers, "Surveys and Publication: AUTM Licensing Activity Surveys 1991-2011," http://www.autm.net/Surveys.htm.

3. Technology *licenses* rather than *patent applications* or *issued patents* are the proper metric for monitoring progress of innovation, because they require the partnership between the university and a commercial entity that is necessary for actual product development. Most patent applications do not issue, and most of those that do are abandoned rather than licensed.

4. JM Hockenberry et al., "Financial Payments by Orthopedic Device Makers to Orthopedic Surgeons," *Arch Int Med* 171(2011).

5. E Sagara to ProPublica, 2014, http://projects.propublica.org/graphics/d4d-slopegraph.

6. Massachusetts Department of Public Health, "Top 20 Manufacturers 2010-12," Pharmaceutical Code of Conduct: Data & Reports: Prepared Reports; "Top 50 Hospitals 2010-12," Pharmaceutical Code of Conduct: Data & Reports: Prepared Reports. http://www.mass.gov/eohhs/gov/departments/dph/programs/hcq/healthcare-quality/pharm-code-of-conduct/data/prepared-reports.html

7. A. S. Kesselheim et al., "Distributions of Industry Payments to Massachusetts Physicians," *N Engl J Med* 368(2013).

8. D. Korn, "The Challenge of Public Expectations," *Boston Rev*, May/June (2010); J. B. Martin, "The Pervasive Influence of Conflicts of Interest: A Personal Perspective," *Neurology* 74(2010).

9. National Institutes of Health, "History of Congressional Appropriations, Fiscal Years 2000-2012," http://officeofbudget.od.nih.gov/approp_hist.html.

10. "Accreditation Council for Continuing Medical Education: 2011 Annual Report Data," (2012). http://www.accme.org/news-publications/publications/annual-report-data

11. The *Wall Street Journal* article describing these corporate education expense reductions made no mention of informational consequences affecting physicians and patients. (P Loftus, "For Doctors, Fewer Perks, Free Lunches," *Wall Street Journal*, April 12, 2013).

12. M Angell and J Kassirer, "Editorials and Conflicts of Interest," *N Engl J Med* 335(1996).

13. For example, PM Ridker, "Incomplete Financial Disclosure for Study of Funding and Outcomes in Major Cardiovascular Trials," *JAMA* 295(2006).

14. K. Okike et al., "Accuracy of Conflict-of-Interest Disclosures Reported by Physicians," *N Engl J Med* 361(2009).

15. Hockenberry et al., "Financial Payments by Orthopedic Device Makers to Orthopedic Surgeons."

16. CMS, "Medicare, Medicaid, Childrens Health Insurance Programs; Transparency Reports and Reporting of Physician Ownership or Investment Interests. Final Rule," in *42 CFR Parts 402 & 403*, ed. Department of Health and Human Services. Center for Medicare and Medicaid Services (Federal Register, 2013).

17. Transparency Reports and Reporting of Physician Ownership or Investment Interests (Sunshine Legislation). 42 USC §1320a-7h(a).

18. O Ben-Shahar and CE Schneider, "The Failure of Mandated Disclosure" (University of Chicago Law School John M Olin Law & Economics Research Paper No. 516 and University of Michigan Law School Law & Economics, Empirical Legal Studies Center Paper No. 10-0082010); *More Than You Wanted to Know: The Failure of Mandated Disclosure* (Princeton University Press, 2014).

19. A chilling example is accessible in the 2006 film *The Lives of Others*. Set in 1980s East Germany, rampant and detailed state surveillance of citizens, ostensibly to protect and preserve socialism, was really a vehicle for taking political and personal advantage of others.

20. "Medicare, Medicaid, Childrens Health Insurance Programs; Transparency Reports and Reporting of Physician Ownership or Investment Interests. Draft Guidelines," in 42 CFR Parts 402 & 403, ed. Department of Health and Human Services. Centers for Medicare and Medicaid Services (Washington DC, 2011).

21. M Roseman et al., "Reporting of Conflicts of Interest in Meta-Analyses of Trials of Pharmacologic Treatments," *JAMA* 305(2011); M Roseman et al., "Reporting of Conflicts of Interest from Drug Trials in Cochrane Reviews: Cross Sectional Studies," *BMJ* 345(2012).

22. "ProPublica: About Us," http://www.propublica.org/about/.

23. M Arnold, "Dollars for Docs: Report Says Pharmas Pay Quacks to Hawk Drugs," *Medical Marketing and Media*, October 19, 2010.

24. ProPublica checked only disciplinary records for physicians from the 15 most populous states. According to the U.S. Census Bureau, the 15 most populous states have 66% of the U.S. population (United States Census Bureau, "Population Estimates: State Totals: Vintage 2013."). Correcting 250 for 66% sampling gives 379 physicians. Dividing 379 by 17,700 gives 2.1% of industry paid physicians with disciplinary records in the past 10 years according to their investigation.

25. National Practitioner Healthcare Integrity and Protection Databank, "NPDB Report Statistics for Physicians by State," (2001–2011).

26. "Medicare, Medicaid, Childrens Health Insurance Programs; Transparency Reports and Reporting of Physician Ownership or Investment Interests. Draft Guidelines."

27. The Knowledge Group CLE, "Sunshine Act: The Final Rule (Recording)," in *CPE Webcast Series* (2013).

28. A recent estimate of the number of pharmaceutical reps in the United States came to 80,000. Wikipedia, "Pharmaceutical Marketing," http://en.wikipedia.org/wiki/Pharmaceutical_marketing. They receive an average total annual compensation of $120,000. MedReps.com, "2012 Pharmaceutical Sales Salary Report," http://www.medreps.com/medical-sales-careers/2012-pharma-sales-rep-salary-report/. If these individuals each spend one hour a week keeping track of the value of educational materials, samples, meals, and other goods given to health care providers and reporting these sums to the company clerical personnel who deal with them, the cost of time comes to over $180 million per year, which doubles the CMS annual cost estimate.

29. JS Mill, "On Liberty," in *On Liberty and Other Writings*, ed. S Collini (Cambridge University Press, 1859).

16. WHAT IS TO BE DONE?

1. Rodney Dangerfields's standard comedic routine was to riff off the line "I don't get no respect."

2. In his remarks, the speaker piously pronounced that a company's product efficacy claims must be evidence based. This requirement must have been star-

tling news to Merck's director of research, a world-class chemist, who was in the audience.

3. BA Mansi et al., "Ten Recommendations for Closing the Credibility Gap in Reporting Industry-Sponsored Clinical Research: A Joint Journal and Pharmaceutical Industry Perspective," *Mayo Clinic Proc* 87, no. 5 (2012).

4. TP Stossel and LK Stell, "Commenting on Ten Recommendations for Closing the Credibility Gap in Reporting Industry-Sponsored Clinical Research," *Mayo Clin Proc* 87(2012).

5. J Collins and JI Porras, *Built to Last: Successful Habits of Visionary Companies* (New York: HarperCollins, 1994); L Timmerman, "12 Things the Pharma Industry Can Do to Rebuild Real Public Trust," http://www.xconomy.com/national/2013/12/09/12-things-pharma-industry-can-re-build-public-trust/.

6. J Avorn, "Keeping Science on Top in Drug Evaluation," *N Engl J Med* 357(2007).

7. http://www.mectizan.org/about

8. In fact, over the years, companies have occasionally made large financial investments in academic institutions to support research. These partnerships predictably evoked protests from anti-industry critics and from academics (who didn't directly benefit from them) that they were perverting the academic mission of "disinterested inquiry" (J. Washburn, *University, Inc.: The Corporate Corruption of Higher Education* (Basic Books, 2005)).

9. ZT Bloomgarden, "Summary of the ACRE Inaugural Meeting," *Endocrine Practice* 15(2009).

10. MA Weber et al., "Association of Clinical Researchers and Educators: A Statement on Relationships between Physicians and Industry," *Endocr Pract* 14(2012).

11. An example of such abuse was a Wall Street Journal article titled "Top Spine Surgeons Reap Royalties, Medicare Bounty" (J. Carreyrou and T. McGinty, "Top Spine Surgeons Reap Royalties, Medicare Bounty," *Wall Street Journal*, December 20, 2010). The narrative insinuated that certain surgeons overzealously perform spinal fusion operations and insert bone-stabilizing implants manufactured by the medical device corporation, Medtronic, because they receive large payments from that company. Using Medicare and Medicaid payment data, the reporters focused on the fact that 24% of spinal fusions performed at a Kentucky hospital were for degenerative disc disease in contrast to a national average of 17% and that surgeons at that particular hospital happened to be receiving Medtronic royalties. Although buried in the article is a comment by Medtronic stating that its relationships with surgeons advance device innovation, most readers are unaware that royalty payments (which is the only basis for such large payments from a company to surgeons) are rewards for contributions made

in the past that led to device innovation. If these payments are large, it takes device use by far more surgeons than those at a single Kentucky hospital to make them add up. In other words, the rewards are for contributions that have widely perceived value.

The article sported critical comments of a surgeon who specializes in denigrating the "ethics" of spine implant surgery. But this individual had no way to evaluate the specific appropriateness of the Kentucky surgeons' decisions based on aggregated payment information. Chapter 7 reviewed the importance of individual relationships and networks for innovation and its randomness. The fact that a cluster of surgeons based at one particular hospital has had specific and productive industry relationships is not unusual, surprising, or indicative of corruption. Moreover, the fact that these surgeons specialize in implant surgery arguably makes them more likely to receive referrals to perform it, partially explaining the modest increase in surgery frequency above the national average.

SELECT BIBLIOGRAPHY

A Working Group of the Advisory Committee to the Director, National Institutes of Health. "Report of the National Institutes of Health Blue Ribbon Panel on Conflict of Interest Policies." 2004.

AAMC. "Protecting Subjects, Preserving Trust, Promoting Progress—Policy and Guidelines for the Oversight of Individual Financial Interests in Human Subjects Research." 2001.

———. "Report of the AAMC Task Force on Industry Funding of Medical Education to the AAMC Executive Council." 34. Washington DC: Association of American Medical Colleges, 2008.

Abramson, J. *Overdosed America*. New York: HarperCollins, 2004.

"Accreditation Council for Continuing Medical Education. 2011 Annual Report Data." 2011.

Ackerley, N, J Eyraud, M Mazzotta, and Inc Eastern Research Group. "Measuring Conflict of Interest and Expertise on FDA Advisory Committees." 2007.

ADVAMED. "Code of Ethics on Interactions with Health Care Professionals." Advanced Medical Technology Association, 2008.

Angell, M. *The Truth About the Drug Companies: How They Deceive Us and What to Do About It.* New York: Random House, 2004.

Armstrong, D. "How the New England Journal Missed Warning Signs on Vioxx. Medical Weekly Waited Years to Report Flaws in Article That Praised Pain Drug. Merck Seen as 'Punching Bag.'" *Wall Street Journal*, May 15, 2006.

Arrowsmith, J. "Phase III and Submission Failures: 2007-2010." *Nat Rev Drug Disc* 10 (2011): 1.

Austad, KE, J Avorn, JM Franklin, MK Kowal, EG Campbell, and AS Kesselheim. "Changing Interactions between Physician Trainees and the Pharmaceutical Industry: A National Survey." *J Gen Intern Med* 28 (2013): 1064–71.

Austad, KE, J Avorn, and AS Kesselheim. "Medical Students' Exposure to and Attitudes About the Pharmaceutical Industry: A Systematic Review." *PLoS Med* 8, no. 5 (2011): 1–12.

"Avoid Financial Correctness." *Nature* 385 (1997): 469.

Avorn, J. *Powerful Medicines: The Benefits, Risks and Costs of Prescription Drugs.* New York: Alfred A. Knopf, 2004.

———. "Dangerous Deception—Hiding the Evidence of Adverse Drug Effects." *N Engl J Med* 355 (2006): 2169–71.

Avorn, J, and S Soumerai. "Improving Drug-Therapy Decisions through Educational Outreach: A Randomized Trial of Academically Based 'Detailing.'" *N Engl J Med* 308 (1983): 1457–63.

Azoulay, P. "Do Pharmaceutical Sales Respond to Scientific Evidence?" *J Econ Management Strategy* 11 (2002): 551–94.

Bäck, M, L Yin, and E Ingelsson. "Cyclooxygenase-2 Inhibitors and Cardiovascular Risk in a Nation-Wide Cohort Study after the Withdrawal of Rofecoxib." *Eur Heart J* 33 (2012): 1928–33.

Bauer, PT. *Reality and Rhetoric: Studies in the Economics of Development.* Cambridge, MA: Harvard University Press, 1984.

Begley, CG, and LM Ellis. "Raise Standards for Preclinical Cancer Research." *Nature* 483 (2012): 531–33.

Ben-Shahar, O, and CE Schneider. *More Than You Wanted to Know: The Failure of Mandated Disclosure.* Princeton University Press, 2014.

Blum, JA, K Freeman, RC Dart, and RJ Cooper. "Requirements and Definitions in Conflict of Interest Policies of Medical Journals." *JAMA* 302 (2009): 2230–34.

Boland, GL. "Federal Regulation of Prescription Drug Advertising and Labeling." *Boston Coll Law Rev* 12, no. 2 (1970): 202–66.

Bombardier, C, L Laine, A Reicin, D Shapiro, R Burgos-Vargas, B Davis, R Day, et al. "Comparison of Upper Gastrointestinal Toxicity of Rofecoxib and Naproxen in Patients with Rheumatoid Arthritis. Vigor Study Group." *N Engl J Med* 343 (2000): 1520–28.

Bosch, X, B Esfandiari, and L McHenry. "Challenging Medical Ghostwriting in US Courts." *PLoS Med* 9, no. 1 (2012): e1001163.

Bowden, ME, AB Crow, and T Sullivan. *Pharmaceutical Achievers: The Human Face of Pharmaceutical Research.* Philadelphia, PA: Chemical Heritage Press, 2003.

Brennan, TA, DJ Rothman, L Blank, D Blumenthal, S Chimonas, JJ Cohen, J Goldman, et al. "Health Industry Practices That Create Conflict of Interest. A Policy Proposal for Academic Medical Centers." *JAMA* 295 (2006): 429–33.

Brody, H. *Hooked: Ethics, the Medical Profession, and the Pharmaceutical Industry.* Lanham, MD: Rowman & Littlefield Publishers, 2007.

Cain, DM, G Loewenstein, and DA Moore. "When Sunlight Fails to Disinfect: Understanding the Perverse Effects of Disclosing Conflicts of Interest." *J Consumer Res* 37 (2011): 836–57.

Campbell, EG. "Doctors and Drug Companies—Scrutinizing Influential Relationships." *N Engl J Med* 357 (2007): 1796–97.

Carlat, DJ. "Dr Drug Rep." *New York Times Magazine,* November 25, 2007.

———. *Unhinged: The Trouble with Psychiatry—A Doctor's Revelations About a Profession in Crisis.* New York: Free Press, 2010.

Centers for Medicare and Medicaid Services. "Medicare, Medicaid, Childrens Health Insurance Programs; Transparency Reports and Reporting of Physician Ownership or Investment Interests. Final Rule." 42 CFR Parts 402 & 403. Federal Register, 2013.

Cervero, RM, and J He. "Final Report: The Relationship between Commercial Support and Bias in Continuing Medical Education Activities: A Review of the Literature." Accreditation Council on Continuing Medical Education, 2008.

Chargaff, E. "Voices in the Labyrinth: Dialogues around the Study of Nature." *Perpect Biol Med* 18 (1975): 313–30.

Ching, AT, and M Isihara. "Measuring the Informative and Persuasive Roles of Detailing on Prescribing Decisions." *Management Sci* 58 (2012): 1374–87.

Chressanthis, GA, P Khedkar, N Jain, P Poddar, and MG Seiders. "Can Access Limits on Sales Representatives to Physicians Affect Clinical Prescription Decisions? A Study of Recent Events with Diabetes and Lipid Drugs." *J Clin Hypertension* 14 (2012): 435–46.

Cialdini, RB. *Influence: The Psychology of Persuasion.* New York: Harper, 2007.

Cohen, J, L Cabanilla, and J Sosnov. "Role of Follow-on Drugs and Indications on the Who Essential Drug List." *J Clin Pharmacy Therapeut* 31 (2006): 585–92.

Contopoulos-Ioannidis, DG, E Ntzani, and JP Ioannidis. "Translation of Highly Promising Basic Science Research into Clinical Applications." *Am J Med* 114 (2003): 477–84.

Curfman, GD, S Morrissey, and JM Drazen. "Expression of Concern: Bombardier et al., 'Comparison of Upper Gastrointestinal Toxicity of Rofecoxib and Naproxen in Patients with Rheumatitis,'"*N Engl J Med* 353 (2005): 2813–14.

Curi, SD, and L Vernaglia. "Industry "'Gift Bans': Massachusetts and Beyond." 2010.

Cutler, DM, AB Rosen, and S Vijan. "The Value of Medical Spending in the United States, 1960–2000." *N Engl J Med* 355 (2006): 920–27.

Dana, J, and G Loewenstein. "A Social Science Perspective on Gifts to Physicians from Industry." *JAMA* 290 (2003): 252–55.

Danzon, PA, and A Towse. "Differential Pricing for Pharmaceuticals: Reconciling Access, R& D and Patents." *Int J Health Care Finance Econ* 3 (2003): 183–205.

DeAngelis, C. "The Influence of Money on Medical Science." *JAMA* 296 (2006): 996–98.

Del Parigi, A. "Industry Funded Clinical Trials: Bias and Quality." *Curr Med Res Opin* 28 (2012): 23–25.

Demonaco, HJ, A Ali, and E von Hippel. "The Major Role of Clinicians in the Discovery of Off-Label Drug Therapies." *Pharmacotherapy* 26, no. 3 (2006): 323–32.

DiMasi, JA, and LB Faden. "Competitiveness in Follow-on Drug R&D: A Race or Imitation?" *Nat Rev Drug Disc* 10 (2011): 1–5.

DiMasi, JA, RW Hansen, and HG Grabowski. "The Price of Innovation: New Estimates of Drug Development Costs." *Health Econ* 22 (2003): 151–85.

Ellison, JA, CH Hennekens, J Wang, GD Lundberg, and D Sulkes. "Low Rates of Reporting Commercial Bias by Physicians Following Online Continuing Medical Education Activities." *Am J Med* 122 (2009): 875–78.

Epstein, RA. *Overdose. How Excessive Government Regulation Stifles Pharmaceutical Innovation*. New Haven: Yale University Press, 2006.

FDA. "Good Reprint Practices for the Distribution of Medical Journal Articles and Medical or Scientific Reference Publications on Unapproved New Uses of Approved Drugs and Approved or Cleared Medical Devices." 1–6, 2009. http://www.fda.gov/ RegulatoryInformation/Guidances/ucm125126.htm.

———. "FDA Requires Removal of Certain Restrictions on the Diabetes Drug Avandia. November 25." http://www.fda.gov/NewsEvents/Newsroom/PressAnnouncements/ ucm376516.htm.

Fenton, JJ, SK Mirza, A Lahad, BD Stern, and RA Deyo. "Variation in Reported Safety of Lumbar Interbody Fusion: Influence of Industrial Sponsorship and Other Study Characteristics." *Spine* 32 (2007): 471–80.

Fontanarosa, PB, and CD De Angelis. "Conflicts of Interest and Independent Data Analysis in Industry-Funded Studies." *JAMA* 294 (2005): 2576–77.

Franklin v. Parke-Davis, 147 F. Supp. 2d 39 (2001).

Friedman, J. "Popper, Weber, and Hayek: The Epistemology and Politics of Ignorance." *Crit Rev* 17 (2005): 1–42.

Fritch, DM. "Speak No Evil, Hear No Evil, Harm the Patient—Why the FDA Needs to Seek More, Rather than Less, Speech from Drug Manufacturers on Off-Label Drug Treatments." *Mich St U J Med & L* 9 (2005): 315–68.

Fukuyama, F. *Trust: The Social Virtues and the Creation of Prosperity*. Simon & Schuster, 1995.

Godlee, F. "Withdraw Approval for Tamflu until NICE Has Full Data." *BMJ* 345 (2012): e8415.

Goldacre, B. *Bad Pharma. How Drug Companies Mislead Doctors and Harm Patients*. London, UK: Fourth Estate, 2012.

Goldberg, R. *Tabloid Medicine. How the Internet Is Being Used to Hijack Medical Science for Fear and Profit*. New York: Kaplan Publishing, 2010.

Grande, D, JA Shea, and K Armstrong. "Pharmaceutical Industry Gifts to Physicians: Patient Beliefs and Trust in Physicians and the Health Care System." *J Gen Int Med* 27 (2011): 274–79.

Greene, JA, and SH Podolsky. "Keeping Modern in Medicine: Pharmaceutical Promotion and Physician Education in Postwar America." *Bull Hist Med* 83 (2009): 331–77.

Hall, RF, and RJ Berlin. "When You Have a Hammer Everything Looks Like a Nail: Misapplication of the False Claims Act to Off-Label Promotion." *Food and Drug Law* 61 (2006): 653–77.

Hampson, LA, M Agrawal, S Joffe, CP Gross, J Vertrer, and EJ Emmanuel. "Patients' Views on Financial Conflicts of Interest in Cancer Research Trials." *N Engl J Med* 355 (2006): 2330–37.

"Harvard University Policy on Individual Financial Conflicts of Interest for Persons Holding Faculty and Teaching Appointments." 2012. http://vpr.harvard.edu/files/ovpr-test/files/harvard_university_fcoi_policy_4_0.pdf.

Hay, M, DW Thomas, JL Craighead, C Economides, and J Rosenthal. "Clinical Development Success Rates for Investigational Drugs." *Nat Biotechnol* 32 (2014): 40–51.

Hayek, FA. *The Fatal Conceit: The Errors of Socialism*. University of Chicago Press, 1988.

Healy, D. *Pharmaggedon*. University of California Press, 2012.

Hemphill, CS, and BN Sampat. "Evergreening, Patent Challenges, and the Effective Market Life in Pharmaceuticals." *J Health Econ* 31 (2012): 327–29.

Higgins, MJ, and SJH Graha. "Balancing Innovation and Access: Patent Challenges Tip the Scales." *Science* 326 (2009): 370–71.

Hilts, PJ. *Protecting America's Health: The FDA, Business, and One Hundred Years of Regulation*. New York: Alfred A. Knopf, 2003.

Hirsch, LJ. "Conflicts of Interest, Authorship, and Disclosures in Industry-Related Scientific Publications: The Tort Bar and Editorial Oversight of Medical Journals." *Mayo Clin Proc* 84 (2009): 811–21.

Huddle, TS. "Drug Reps and the Academic Medical Center: A Case for Management Rather than Prohibition." *Persp Biol Med* 51 (2008): 251–60.

———. "The Pitfalls of Deducing Ethics from Behavioral Economics: Why the Association of American Medical Colleges Is Wrong About Pharmaceutical Detailing." *Am J Bioethics* 10 (2010): 1–8.

Ioannidis, JP. "Why Most Published Research Findings Are False." *PLoS Med* 2 (2005): e124.

———. "How Many Contemporary Medical Practices Are Worse than Doing Nothing or Doing Less?" *Mayo Clin Proc* 88 (2013): 779–81.

Jacobs, J. *Systems of Survival*. New York: Vintage, 1992.

Johnson, S, J Krause, R Saver, and RF Wilson. "Estate of Gelsinger v. Trustees of University of Pennsylvania." In *Health Law and Bioethics: Cases in Context*, 229–61: Aspen Publishers, 2009.

Jones, DK, AN Barkum, Y Luk, R Enns, P Sinclair, M Martel, I Gralnek, et al. "Conflict of Interest Ethics: Silencing Expertise in the Development of International Clinical Practice Guidelines." *Ann Int Med* 156 (2012): 809–16.

Jones, J. "Record 64% Rate Honesty, Ethics of Members of Congress Low. Ratings of Nurses, Pharmacists, and Medical Doctors Most Positive." *Gallop Politics* (2011). http://www.gallup.com/poll/151460/record-rate-honesty-ethics-members-congress-low.aspx.

Katz, DA, AL Kaplan, and J Merz. "All Gifts Large and Small: Toward an Understanding of Pharmaceutical Gift-Giving." *Am J Bioeth* 3 (2003): 40–46.

Katz, E, and PF Lazarsfeld. *Personal Influence: The Part Played by People in the Flow of Mass Communication*. Glencoe, IL: The Free Press, 1955.

Kenney, M. *Biotechnology: The University-Industrial Complex*. New Haven: Yale University Press, 1986.

Kesselheim, AS, CT Robertson, JA Myers, SL Rose, V Gillet, KM Ross, RJ Glynn, S Joffe, and J Avorn. "A Randomized Study of How Physicians Interpret Research Funding Disclosures." *N Engl J Med* 367 (2012): 1119–27.

Kesselheim, AS, CT Robertson, K Siri, P Batra, and JM Franklin. "Distributions of Industry Payments to Massachusetts Physicians." *N Engl J Med* 368 (2013): 2049–52.

Khan, NA, JI Lombeida, M Singh, HJ Spencer, and KD Torralba. "Association of Industry Funding with the Outcome and Quality of Randomized Controlled Trials of Drug Therapy for Rheumatoid Arthritis." *Arthritis Rheum* 64 (2012): 2059–67.

Khayat, D. "Innovative Cancer Therapies: Putting Costs into Context." *Cancer* 118 (2012): 2367–71.

Kneller, R. "The Importance of New Companies for Drug Discovery: Origins of a Decade of New Drugs." *Nature Rev Drug Discovery* 9 (2010): 867–82.

———. "The Origins of New Drugs." *Nat Biotechnol* 23 (2005): 529–30.

Koch, C, and C Schmidt. "Disclosing Conflicts of Interest—Do Experience and Reputation Matter?" *Accounting Org Soc* 35 (2010): 95–107.

Korenstein, D, S Keyhani, and JS Ross. "Physician Attitudes toward Industry: A View across the Specialties." *Arch Surg* 145 (2010): 570–77.

Kuhn, TS. *The Structure of Scientific Revolutions* (2nd ed.). Chicago: University of Chicago Press, 1970.

Kuran, T, and CR Sunstein. "Availability Cascades and Risk Regulation." *Stanford Law Rev* 51, no. 4 (1999): 683–768.

Laine, C, E Guallar, C Mulrow, DB Taichman, JE Cornell, D Cotton, ME Griswold, et al. "Closing in on the Truth About Recombinant Human Bone Morphogenetic Protein-2: Evidence Synthesis, Data Sharing, Peer Review, and Reproducible Research." *Ann Int Med* 158 (2013): 916–18.

Lam, A. "What Motivates Academic Scientists to Engage in Research Commercialization: 'Gold,' 'Ribbon,' or 'Puzzle?'" *Res Policy* 40 (2011): 1354–68.

LaMattina, JL. *Devalued and Distrusted: Can the Pharmaceutical Industry Restore Its Broken Image?* New York: Wiley, 2013.

———. *Drug Truths: Dispelling the Myths About Pharma R&D*. Hoboken, NJ: Wiley, 2009.

Lasser, KE, PD Allen, SJ Woolhandler, DU Himmelstein, SM Wolfe, and DH Bor. "Timing of New Black Box Warnings and Withdrawals for Prescription Medications." *JAMA* 287 (2002): 2215–20.

Leenan v. Canadian Broadcasting System et al., 54 O.R. (3d) 612 (2001).

Lesko, R, S Scott, and TP Stossel. "Bias in High-Tier Medical Journals Concerning Physician-Academic Relations with Industry." *Nat Biotechnol* 30 (2012): 320–22.

Levitt, SD, and JA List. "Viewpoint: On the Generalizability of Lab Behavior to the Field." *Can J Econ* 40 (2007): 347–70.

———. "What Do Laboratory Experiments Measuring Social Preferences Reveal About the Real World?" *J Econ Persp* 21 (2007): 153–74.

Lexchin, J. *The Real Pushers: A Critical Analysis of the Canadian Drug Industry*. Vancouver: New Star Books, 1984.

Lexchin, J, LA Bero, B Djulbegovic, and O Clark. "Pharmaceutical Industry Sponsorship and Research Outcome and Quality: Systematic Review." *BMJ* 326 (2003): 1127–30.

Lichtenberg, FR. "Are the Benefits of Newer Drugs Worth Their Cost? Evidence from the 1996 MEPS. The Newer the Drug in Use, the Less Spending on Nondrug Items." *Health Aff* 20 (2001): 241–51.

———. "Do New Drugs Save Lives?" *J Gen Intern Med* 24 (2009): 1356.

———. "The Impact of New Drug Launches on Longevity: Evidence from Longitudinal, Disease-Level Data from 52 Countries, 1982–2001." *Int J Health Care Finance Econ* 5 (2005): 47–73.

———. "The Impact of New Drugs on US Longevity and Medical Expenditure, 1990–2003: Evidence from Longitudinal, Disease-Level Data." *Am Econ Rev* 97 (2007): 438–44.

Light, DW, and J Lexchin. "Pharmaceutical R&D: What Do We Get for All That Money?" *BMJ* 345 (2012): 22–25.

Lo, B, and M Field. "Conflict of Interest in Medical Research, Education, and Practice." 360: Institute of Medicine, 2009.

Lurie, P, CM Almeida, N Stine, AR Stine, and SM Wolfe. "Financial Conflict of Interest Disclosure and Voting Patterns at Food and Drug Administration Drug Advisory Committee Meetings." *JAMA* 295 (2006): 1921–28.

Mansi, BA, J Clark, FS David, TM Gesell, S Glasser, J Gonzalez, DG Haller, et al. "Ten Recommendations for Closing the Credibility Gap in Reporting Industry-Sponsored Clinical Research: A Joint Journal and Pharmaceutical Industry Perspective." *Mayo Clinic Proc* 87, no. 5 (2012): 424–29.

Mill, JS. "On Liberty." In *On Liberty and Other Writings*, edited by S Collini, 289 pp: Cambridge University Press, 1859.

———. *Utilitarianism*. Oxford University Press, 1998.

Movsesian, M. "Intramural Conflicts of Interest Warrant Scrutiny, Too." *Nat Med* 17, no. 5 (2011): 534.

Moyhihan, R. "Key Opinion Leaders. Independent Experts or Drug Representatives in Disguise." *BMJ* 336 (2008): 1402–03.

Moynihan, R, I Heath, and D Henry. "Selling Sickness: The Pharmaceutical Industry and Disease Mongering." *BMJ* 324 (2002): 888–91.

Munos, B. "Lessons from 60 Years of Pharmaceutical Innovation." *Nat Rev Drug Discovery* 8 (2009): 959–68.

Murphy, KM, and RH Topel. "The Value of Health and Longevity." *J Polit Econ* 114 (2006): 871–904.

Nesi, T. *Poison Pills: The Untold Story of the Vioxx Drug Scandal*. Thomas Dunne Books—Saint Martin's Press, 2008.

NIH. "Responsibility of Applicants for Promoting Objectivity in Research for which PHS Funding is Sought." (2011). 42 CFR Part 50, Subpart F.

Noah, L. "Medicine's Epistemology: Mapping the Haphazard Diffusion of Knowledge in the Biomedical Community." *Ariz L Rev* 44 (2002): 374–466.

No Free Lunch. http://www.nofreelunch.org/aboutus.htm.

O'Brien, M. A., S. Rogers, G. Jamtvedt, A. D. Oxman, J. Odgaard-Jensen, D. T. Kristoffersen, L. Forsetlund, et al. "Educational Outreach Visits: Effects on Professional Practice and Health Care Outcomes." [In Engish]. *Cochrane Database Syst Rev*, no. 4 (2007): CD000409.

O'Sullivan, BP, DM Orenstein, and CE Milla. "Pricing for Orphan Drugs: Will the Market Bear What Society Cannot?" *JAMA* 310 (2013): 1343–44.

Olson, MK. *The Logic of Collective Action*. Boston: Harvard University Press, 1971.

———. "Are Novel Drugs More Risky for Patients than Less Novel Drugs?" *J Health Econ* 23 (2004): 1135–58.

Osborn, JE. "Can I Tell You the Truth?: A Comparative Perspective on Regulating Off-Label Scientific and Medical Information." *Yale J Health Policy & Ethics* 10 (2010): 299–356.

Payer, L. *Disease Mongers: How Doctors, Drug Companies, and Insurers Are Making You Feel Sick*. New York: Wiley, 1994.

Pew Charitable Trust. "Prescription Project." 2009. http://www.pewtrusts.org/our_work_detail. aspx?id=206.

Pharmaceutical Research and Manufacturers of America (PhRMA). "Code on Interactions with Healthcare Professionals," 2008.

Philipson, TJ, ER Berndt, AHB Gottschalk, and MW Strobeck. "Assessing the Safety and Efficacy of the FDA: The Case of the Prescription Drug Use Fee Acts." In *National Bureau of Economic Research*, 1–41, 2005.

Presley, H. "Vioxx and the Merck Team Effort." In *Case Studies in Ethics*. The Kenan Institute for Ethics at Duke University.

Prinz, F, T Schlange, and K Asadullah. "Believe It or Not: How Much Can We Rely on Published Data on Potential Drug Targets?" *Nat Rev Drug Dev* (2011).

Radley, DC, SN Finckelstein, and RS Stafford. "Off-Label Prescribing among Office-Based Physicians." *Arch Int Med* 166 (2006): 1021–26.

Ratner, M, and T Gura. "Off-Label or Off-Limits?" *Nat Biotechnol* 26 (2008): 867–75.

Rennie, DC. "Thyroid Storm." *JAMA* 277 (1997): 1238–44.

"Report 1 of the Council on Ethical and Judicial Affairs (CEJA Report 1a-08). Industry Support of Professional Education in Medicine (Reference Committee on Amendments to Constitution and Bylaws)." American Medical Association, 2008.

Research!America. "America Speaks: Poll Data Summary, Volume 5." 2004. http://www. researchamerica.org/uploads/AmericaSpeaksV5.pdf.

———. "America Speaks: Poll Data Summary, Volume 11." 2010. http://www. researchamerica.org/uploads/AmericaSpeaksV11.pdf.

Ridker, PM, and J Torres. "Reported Outcomes in Major Cardiovascular Clinical Trials Funded by for-Profit and Not-for-Profit Organizations: 2000–2005." *JAMA* 295 (2006): 2270–74.

Rosenthal, E. "For Medical Tourists, Simple Math: US Estimate for a New Hip: Over $78,000. The Belgian Bill: $13,660." *New York Times*, August 4, 2013.

Ross, JS, KP Hill, DS Egilman, and HM Krumholz. "Guest Authorship and Ghostwriting in Publications Related to Rofecoxib: A Case Study of Industry Documents from Rofecoxib Litigation." *JAMA* 299 (2008): 1800–12.

Rothman, KJ. "Conflict of Interest: The New McCarthyism in Science." *JAMA* 269 (1993): 2782–84.

Rothman, KJ, and S Evans. "Extra Scrutiny for Industry Funded Trials: JAMA's Demand for an Additional Hurdle Is Unfair—and Absurd." *BMJ* 331 (2005): 1350–51.

Rubin, PH. "Pharmaceutical Marketing: Medical and Industry Biases." *J Pharmaceutical Finance, Econ & Policy* 13 (2004): 65–79.

———. "An Uncertain Diagnosis." *Regulation*, Summer (2005): 34–39.

Sagara, E. "Doctor Payments on the Decline." In *ProPublica*, 2014. https://projects.propublica.org/graphics/d4d-slopegraph.

Sah, S. "Conflicts of Interest and Your Physician: Psychological Processes That Cause Unexpected Changes in Behavior." *J Law Med Ethics* 40 (2012): 482–87.

Sah, S, and G Loewenstein. "Nothing to Declare: Mandatory and Voluntary Disclosure Leads Advisors to Avoid Conflicts of Interest." *Psychol Sci* (2013).

Sampat, BN. "Patenting and US Academic Research in the 20th Century: The World before and after Bayh-Dole." *Res Policy* 35 (2006): 772–89.

Sampat, BN, and FR Lichtenberg. "What Are the Respective Roles of the Public and Private Sectors in Pharmaceutical Innovation?" *Health Aff* 30 (2011): 332–39.

Santerre, RE. "National and International Tests of the New Drug Cost Offset Theory." *South Econ J* 77 (2011): 1033–43.

Santerre, RE, JA Vernon, and C Giaccotto. "The Impact of Indirect Government Controls on US Drug Prices and R&D." *Cato J* Winter (2006): 143–58.

Scannell, JW, A Blanckley, H Boldon, and B Warrington. "Diagnosing the Decline in Pharmaceutical R&D Efficiency." *Nat Rev Drug Discovery* 11 (2012): 191–200.

Shuchman, M. *The Drug Trial: Nancy Olivieri and the Science Scandal That Rocked the Hospital for Sick Children.* Canada: Random House, 2005.

Sibbald, B. "Vioxx Should Be Allowed Back on the Market Advises Expert Panel." *CMAJ: Canadian Medical Association Journal* 175, no. 3 (2006): 234–35.

Sierles, FS, AC Brodkey, LM Cleary, FA McCurdy, M Mintz, J Frank, DJ Lynn, et al. "Medical Student's Exposure to and Attitudes About Drug Company Interactions: A National Survey." *JAMA* 294 (2005): 1034–42.

Silverglate, HA. *Three Felonies a Day: How the Feds Target the Innocent.* New York: Encounter Books, 2009.

———. "A Doctor's Posthumous Vindication." *Wall Street Journal*, December 25, 2012.

Simpson, RJ, Jr, J Signorovitch, H Birnbaum, J Ivanova, C Connolly, Y Kidolezi, and A Kuznik. "Cardiovascular and Economic Outcomes after Initiation of Lipid-Lowering Therapy with Atorvastatin vs Simvastatin in an Employed Population." *Mayo Clin Proc* 84 (2009): 1065–72.

Smith, JS. *Patenting the Sun: Polio and the Salk Vaccine: The Dramatic Story Behind of the Greatest Achievements of Modern Science.* New York: Morrow, 1990.

Sorrell v. Ims Health, 10-779 (2011).

"Special Issue: Symposium: Institutional Corruption and the Pharmaceutical Industry." *J Law Med Ethics* 41 (2013): 544–746.

Spurling, GK, PR Mansfield, BD Montgomery, J Lexchin, J Doust, N Othman, and AI Vitry. "Information from Pharmaceutical Companies and the Quality, Quantity, and Cost of Physicians' Prescribing: A Systematic Review." *PLoS Med* 7, no. 10 (2010): e1000352.

Stark, A. *Conflict of Interest in American Public Life.* Cambridge, MA: Harvard University Press, 2000.

Riegel v. Medtronic. 552 U.S. 312 (2007).

Steinberg, D. *The Cholesterol Wars: The Cholesterol Skeptics vs the Predonderance of Evidence.* Academic Press (Elsevier), 2007.

Steinbrook, R. "Conflicts of Interest at the NIH: Resolving the Problem." *N Engl J Med* 351 (2004): 955–57.

Steinbrook, R, and B Lo. "Medical Journals and Conflicts of Interest." *J Law Med Ethics* 40 (2012): 488–99.

Steinman, MA, LA Bero, M-M Chren, and CS Landefeld. "Narrative Review: The Promotion of Gabapentin: An Analysis of Internal Industry Documents." *Ann Int Med* 145, no. 4 (2006): 284–93.

Stelfox, HT, G Chua, K O'Rourke, and AS Detsky. "Conflict of Interest in the Debate over Calcium-Channel Antagonists." *N Engl J Med* 338 (1998): 101–06.

Stell, LK. "Drug Reps Off Campus! Promoting Professional Purity by Suppressing Commercial Speech." *J Law Med Ethics* 37 (2009): 431–43.

Stevens, AJ, JJ Jensen, K Wyller, P Kilgore, S Chatterjee, and ML Rohrbaugh. "The Role of Public-Sector Research in the Discovery of Drugs and Vaccines." *N Engl J Med* 364 (2011): 535–41.

Stossel, TP. "Free the Scientists! Conflict-of-Interest Rules Purport to Cure a Problem That Doesn't Exist—and Are Stifling Medical Progress." *Forbes*, February 14, 2005, 40.

———. "Mere Magazines." *Wall Street Journal*, December 29, 2005.

———. "Regulating Academic-Industry Research Relationships—Solving Problems or Stifling Progress." *N Engl J Med* 353 (2005): 1060–65.

Stossel, TP, and LK Stell. "Commenting on Ten Recommendations for Closing the Credibility Gap in Reporting Industry-Sponsored Clinical Research." *Mayo Clin Proc* 87 (2012): 925–26.

Stroebe, W, T Postmes, and R Spears. "Scientific Misconduct and the Myth of Self-Correction in Science." *Persp Psychol Sci* 7 (2011): 670–88.

Sulmasy, DP. "What's So Special About Medicine?" *Theoret Med* 14 (1993): 27–42.

Sunstein, CR. "Deliberative Trouble? Why Groups Go to Extremes." *Yale Law J* 110 (2000): 71–119.

Swann, JP. *Academic Scientists and the Pharmaceutical Industry*. Baltimore: The Johns Hopkins University Press, 1988.

Thompson, D. "Understanding Financial Conflicts of Interest." *N Engl J Med* 329 (1993): 573–76.

Thompson, J, P Baird, and J Downie. *The Olivieri Report. The Complete Text of the Report of the Independent Inquiry Commissioned by the Canadian Association of University Teachers*. Toronto: James Lorimer and Company Ltd, 2001.

Timmerman, L. "12 Things the Pharma Industry Can Do to Rebuild Real Public Trust." http://www.xconomy.com/national/2013/12/09/12-things-pharma-industry-can-rebuild-public-trust/.

Tobell, D. *Pills, Power and Policy: The Struggle for Drug Reform in Cold War America and Its Consequences*. Berkeley: University of California Berkeley Press, 2012.

Transparency Reports and Reporting of Physician Ownership or Investment Interests (Sunshine Legislation). 42 Usc §1320a-7h(a). 42 USC §1320a-7h(a).

Tregaskis, S. "A New Diet for Docs. No Free Lunches. No Swag. And Patients Have Everything to Gain." *Pitt Med*, no. Spring (2008): 17–21.

United States Department of Justice. "Warner-Lambert to Pay $430 Million to Resolve Criminal & Civil Health Care Liability Relating to Off-Label Promotion." 2004. http://www.justice.gov/archive/opa/pr/2004/May/04_civ_322.htm.

United States v. Caronia (2010).

Van den Bulte, C, and GL Lilien. "Medical Innovation Revisited: Social Contagion versus Marketing Effort." *Am J Sociol* 106 (2001): 1409–35.

Von Mises, L. *Human Action: A Treatise on Economics*. Irvington on Hudson: The Foundation for Economic Education, Inc, 1963.

———. *Socialism: An Economic and Sociological Analysis (1922)*. Translated by J Kahane. Indianapolis: Liberty Fund, 1969.

Voors, M, T Turley, A Kontoleon, E Bulte, and JA List. "Exploring Whether Behavior in Context-Free Experiments Is Predictive of Behavior in the Field: Evidence from Lab and Field Experiments in Rural Sierra Leone." *Econ Lett* 114 (2012): 308–11.

Wadman, M. "Vioxx May Go Back on Sale after Scraping Past FDA Panel." *Nature* 433, no. 7028 (02/24 print 2005): 790–90.

Wager, E, R Mhaskar, S Warburton, and B Djulbegovic. "*JAMA* Published Fewer Industry-Funded Studies after Introducing a Requirement for Independent Statistical Analysis." *PLoS One* 5, no. 10 (2010): e135691.

Waxman, HA. "A History of Adverse Drug Experiences: Congress Had Ample Evidence to Support Restrictions on the Promotion of Prescription Drugs." *Food & Drug L J* 58 (2003): 299–312.

Wazana, A. "Physicians and the Pharmaceutical Industry: Is a Gift Ever Just a Gift?" *JAMA* 283 (2000): 373–80.

Welch, HG, LM Schwartz, and S Woloshin. *Overdiagnosed: Making People Sick in the Pursuit of Health*. Boston, MA: Beacon Press, 2011.

Wertheimer, AI, and TM Santella. "Pharmacoevolution: The Advantages of Incremental Innovation." In *IPN Working Papers on Intellectual Property, Innovation and Health*. London, UK: International Policy Network, 2005.

Wittich, CM, CM Burkle, and WL Lanier. "Ten Common Questions (and Their Answers) About Off-Label Drug Use." *Mayo Clin Proc* 87 (2012): 982–90.

Woloshin, S, LM Schwartz, SL Casella, AT Kennedy, and RJ Larson. "Press Releases by Academic Medical Centers: Not So Academic?" *Ann Int Med* 150 (2009): 613–18.

Woolley, KL, RA Lew, S Stretton, JA Ely, NJ Bramich, JR Keys, JA Monk, and MJ Woolley. "Lack of Involvement of Medical Writers and the Pharmaceutical Industry in Publications Retracted for Misconduct: A Systematic, Controlled, Retrospective Study." *Curr Med Res Opin* 27 (2011): 1175–82.

Woosley, RL. "One Hundred Years of Drug Regulation: Where Do We Go from Here?" *Annu Rev Pharmacol Toxicol* 53 (2013): 255–73.

Wyeth v. Levine, 555 U.S. 555 (2008).

Young, NS, JPA Ioannidis, and O Al-Ubaydli. "Why Current Publication Practices May Distort Science: The Market for Exchange of Scientific Information: The Winner's Curse, Artificial Scarcity, and Uncertainty in Biomedical Publication." *PLoS Medicine* 5 (October 2008): e201–e19.

Zinner, DE, B Bjankovic, B Clarridge, D Blumenthal, and EG Campbell. "Participation of Academic Scientists in Relationships with Industry." *Health Aff* 28 (2009): 1814–25.

Zinner, DE, CM DesRoches, SJ Bristol, B Clarridge, and EG Campbell. "Tightening Conflict-of-Interest Policies: The Impact of 2005 Ethics Rules at the NIH." *Acad Med* 85 (2010): 1685–91.

Zycher, B, JA DiMasi, and CP Milne. "Private Sector Contributions to Pharmaceutical Science: Thirty-Five Summary Case Histories." *Am J Ther* 17, no. 1 (2010): 101–20.

INDEX